P9-DOE-444

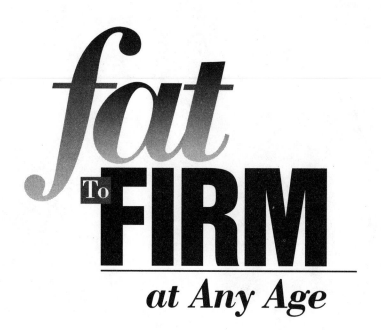

fat To FIRM

at Any Age

fat To FIRM

By Alisa Bauman,
Sarí Harrar,
and the editors of
PREVENTION
Health Books
for Women™

at Any Age

How You Can Have a Slimmer, Well-Toned Body at Age 30, 40, and Beyond

RODALE

Notice

This book is intended as a reference volume only, not as a medical manual. The information given here is designed to help you make informed decisions about your health and weight-loss needs. It is not intended as a substitute for any treatment or dietary advice that may have been prescribed by your doctor. If you suspect that you have a medical problem, we urge you to seek competent medical help. If you have not participated in an exercise program regularly or recently, we encourage you to work with your physician to determine the activity level that is best for you.

© 1998 by Rodale Inc.
Illustrations © 1998 by Chris Duke

All rights reserved. No part of this publication may be reproduced or transmitted in any form or by any means, electronic or mechanical, including photocopying, recording, or any other information storage and retrieval system, without the written permission of the publisher.

Prevention Health Books for Women and Fat-to-Firm Program are trademarks of Rodale Inc.

Printed in the United States of America
on acid-free ∞, recycled paper ♻

Library of Congress Cataloging-in-Publication Data

Bauman, Alisa.
    Fat to firm at any age : how you can have a slimmer, well-toned body at age 30, 40, and beyond / by Alisa Bauman, Sarí Harrar, and the editors of Prevention Health Books for Women.
        p.   cm.
    Includes index.
    ISBN 0–87596–412–5 hardcover
    1. Weight loss.   2. Women—Health and hygiene.   3. Middle-aged women—Health and hygiene.   4. Overweight women.   I. Harrar, Sarí. II. Prevention Magazine Health Books.   III. Title.
    RM222.2.B387   1997
    613.7'045—DC21   97–22062

    ISBN 1–57954–128–3 paperback

Distributed to the book trade by St. Martin's Press

		8	10	9	7					hardcover
2	4	6	8	10	9	7	5	3		paperback

Visit us on the Web at www.rodalebooks.com,
or call us toll-free at (800) 848-4735.

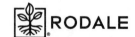

WE **INSPIRE** AND **ENABLE** PEOPLE TO IMPROVE
THEIR LIVES AND THE WORLD AROUND THEM

FAT TO FIRM AT ANY AGE
EDITORIAL STAFF

MANAGING EDITOR: **SHARON FAELTEN**

WRITERS: **ALISA BAUMAN**
SARÍ HARRAR

RECIPE CONTRIBUTOR: **DAVID JOACHIM**

ASSISTANT RESEARCH MANAGER: **ANITA C. SMALL**

LEAD RESEARCHER: **SUSAN E. BURDICK**

EDITORIAL RESEARCHERS: **LORI DAVIS**
CAROL J. GILMORE
SARAH WOLFGANG HEFFNER
JENNIFER L. KAAS
NICOLE A. KELLY
TERRY SUTTON KRAVITZ
STACI ANN SANDER
CAROL SPICIARICH MAHONEY
TERESA A. YEYKAL
SHEA ZUKOWSKI

COPY EDITOR: **KAREN NEELY**

ASSOCIATE ART DIRECTOR: **DARLENE SCHNECK**

COVER DESIGNER: **LYNN N. GANO**

INTERIOR DESIGNERS: **TANJA L. LIPINSKI**
ELIZABETH YOUNGBLOOD

TECHNICAL ARTIST: **ANDREW MACBRIDE**
DONNA G. ROSSI

MANUFACTURING COORDINATOR: **MELINDA B. RIZZO**

OFFICE MANAGER: **ROBERTA MULLINER**

OFFICE STAFF: **JULIE KEHS**
SUZANNE LYNCH
BERNADETTE SAUERWINE
MARY LOU STEPHEN

RODALE
HEALTH AND FITNESS BOOKS

VICE PRESIDENT AND EDITORIAL DIRECTOR: **DEBORA T. YOST**

EXECUTIVE EDITOR: **NEIL WERTHEIMER**

DESIGN AND PRODUCTION DIRECTOR: **MICHAEL WARD**

RESEARCH MANAGER: **ANN GOSSY YERMISH**

COPY MANAGER: **LISA D. ANDRUSCAVAGE**

BOOK MANUFACTURING DIRECTOR: **HELEN CLOGSTON**

Board of Advisors for Rodale Women's Health Books

DIANE L. ADAMS, M.D.
Associate clinical professor and coordinator of the cultural diversity and women's health program at the University of Maryland Eastern Shore in Princess Anne, Maryland

ROSEMARY AGOSTINI, M.D.
Clinical associate professor of orthopedics at the University of Washington and staff physician at the Virginia Mason Sports Medicine Center, both in Seattle

BARBARA D. BARTLIK, M.D.
Clinical assistant professor in the department of psychiatry at Cornell University Medical College in New York City

MARY RUTH BUCHNESS, M.D.
Chief of dermatology at St. Vincent's Hospital and Medical Center in New York City and associate professor of dermatology and medicine at New York Medical College in Valhalla

TRUDY L. BUSH, PH.D.
Professor of epidemiology and preventive medicine at the University of Maryland School of Medicine at Baltimore and principal investigator for the Heart and Estrogen/Progestin Replacement Study (HERS) and for the Postmenopausal Estrogen/Progestin Intervention (PEPI) Safety Follow-Up Study at the Johns Hopkins Women's Research Core in Lutherville, Maryland

DIANA L. DELL, M.D.
Assistant professor of obstetrics and gynecology at the Duke University Medical Center in Durham, North Carolina, past president of the American Medical Women's Association (AMWA), and co-director of their breast and cervical cancer physician training project

LEAH J. DICKSTEIN, M.D.
Professor and associate chairperson for academic affairs in the department of psychiatry and behavioral sciences and associate dean for faculty and student advocacy at the University of Louisville School of Medicine in Kentucky and past president of the American Medical Women's Association (AMWA)

JEAN L. FOURCROY, M.D., PH.D.
Past president of the American Medical Women's Association (AMWA) and past president of the National Council of Women's Health, Inc., in New York City

CLARITA E. HERRERA, M.D.
Clinical instructor in primary care at the New York Medical College in Valhalla and associate attending physician at Lenox Hill Hospital in New York City

DEBRA RUTH JUDELSON, M.D.
Senior partner with the Cardiovascular Medical Group of Southern California in Beverly Hills, fellow of the American College of Cardiology, and past president of the American Medical Women's Association (AMWA)

JOANN E. MANSON, M.D.
Associate professor of medicine at Harvard Medical School and co-director of women's health at Brigham and Women's Hospital in Boston

MARY LAKE POLAN, M.D., PH.D.
Professor and chairperson of the department of gynecology and obstetrics at Stanford University School of Medicine

ELIZABETH LEE VLIET, M.D.
Clinical associate professor in the department of family and community medicine at the University of Arizona College of Medicine and founder and medical director of HER Place: Health Enhancement and Renewal for Women, Inc., both in Tucson

LILA AMDURSKA WALLIS, M.D.
Clinical professor of medicine at Cornell University Medical College in New York City, past president of the American Medical Women's Association (AMWA), founding president of the National Council on Women's Health, director of continuing education programs for physicians, and Master and Laureate of the American College of Physicians

CARLA WOLPER, R.D.
Nutritionist and clinical coordinator at the Obesity Research Center at St. Luke's/Roosevelt Hospital Center in New York City

Contents

PART 1: Discover Your True Weight-Loss Needs

Chapter 1

It's Not Your Fault

In a push-button world, gaining weight is almost automatic.
Fortunately, losing it can be just as easy.

Chapter 2

Nourishing Your Heart and Soul

Ninety-five percent of overweight problems have an *emotional* cause,
say scientists. But you can "feed" your feelings without food.

Chapter 3

The Best Benefit

Looking good isn't the only reason women go from fat to firm. Here's
how to lose a little weight—and gain a lot of health.

PART 2: Eating Food and Loving It

Chapter 7

Here are more than 100 easy, effective strategies for declaring victory
over high-fat foods.

Chapter 8

Hidden calories and hefty portions can sabotage your weight-loss
efforts—even if you eat low-fat foods. It's time to clear up the
confusion and start losing weight.

PART 3: The Exercise Equation

Chapter 15
The Unexpected Benefits of Getting Fit 205

From an easier menopause to harder bones, there are plenty of reasons besides losing weight for a woman to start exercising.

Chapter 16
Muscle vs. Fat 219

Muscle burns lots of calories; fat burns few. So how do you get more muscle? Read on.

Chapter 17
Walking: A Giant Step toward Slimness 233

Easy, convenient, low-cost, and injury-free, walking is the one exercise that women can stick with.

Chapter 18
More Fat-to-Firm Aerobic Options 249

When it comes to aerobic exercise, "easy does it" is the key to weight loss, firming, and better health. Here's how to pick the best easy exercise for you.

Chapter 19
Strength Training: Boost Your Metabolism in an Hour a Week 263

Here's the best way to firm your body, lose weight faster, slow aging, and look great in clothes.

Chapter 20
Taming Your Trouble Spots 288

You probably can't look like a supermodel, say the experts, but you can look like the best possible version of yourself.

Chapter 26

Don't wait until you reach your "ideal" weight. Self-esteem can start today.

PART 5: The Fat-to-Firm Recipe Collection

Chapter 27

You can still eat the foods you love—now they're not only tasty but also slimming. Cook on.

Chapter 28

A few dollops of fatty salad dressing can derail weight loss. Try these low-fat (and high-yum) versions—they're a salad-lover's best friend.

Chapter 29

There's nothing "mini" about the taste, nutrition, and stomach-satisfying gusto of these low-fat treats.

For the best interactive guide to weight loss, fitness, nutrition, and living a more fulfilling life, visit our Web site at http://www.healthyideas.com.

Acknowledgments

The authors convey their thanks to the many physicians, nutritionists, and other health professionals consulted for this book. In particular, we thank the following for their contributions in shaping key elements of the Fat-to-Firm Program.

ANDREA L. DUNN, PH.D.
Exercise psychologist and associate director of the division of epidemiology and clinical applications at the Cooper Institute for Aerobics Research in Dallas

DIANE GRABOWSKI-NEPA, R.D.
Nutritionist with the Pritikin Longevity Center in Santa Monica, California

JONI JOHNSTON, PSY.D.
Clinical psychologist in private practice in Del Mar, California

CATHY KAPICA, R.D., PH.D.
Associate professor of nutrition and clinical dietetics at Finch University of Health Sciences/Chicago Medical School in North Chicago

MICHAEL POLLOCK, PH.D.
Exercise physiologist and professor of medicine and exercise science at the University of Florida in Gainesville

JAMES C. ROSEN, PH.D.
Psychologist and professor of psychology at the University of Vermont in Burlington

CARLA WOLPER, R.D.
Nutritionist and clinical coordinator at the Obesity Research Center at St. Luke's/Roosevelt Hospital Center in New York City

Introduction

Halt Female Flab Forever

If you've squashed your hips into control-top pantyhose, held your breath to zip up your jeans, or struggled into last year's bathing suit, you've experienced firsthand the sobering truth about female body flab: Left alone, it expands by stunning leaps and bounds. In fact, researchers from the University of Maryland at Baltimore have discovered that unless a woman takes action, her body fat increases by 26 percent with each decade of age while a man's increases by a more modest 17 percent. It hardly seems fair.

No wonder one in three American women is overweight. Or that two out of three of us feel flabby and long to firm up. Or that we are so desperate to slim down that we spend more than $4,000,000,000 a year on weight-loss programs, fat substitutes, and diet drugs. That's right—$4 billion. So why does our flab keep on growing? Obesity experts say that we are overlooking the real forces conspiring to make us overweight, forces you can control with the Fat-to-Firm Program.

■ **Our fast-lane lifestyles.** Three out of four of us are so busy that we can't find the time for regular physical activity—even though we would like to exercise. And the modern conveniences meant to help us save time and effort—such as remote-control televisions, department-store escalators, and drive-through bank machines—are actually adding inches to our hips and waists because they keep us sedentary. Researchers from the United Kingdom estimate that we burn 800 fewer calories a day now, compared to 1970, thanks to labor-saving devices.

■ **Fat-free food.** Overindulging in fat-free foods—from cookies to mayonnaise, ice cream to popcorn, soup to lunchmeat—may be the reason that American women are eating more calories than ever, says nutrition expert John Allred, Ph.D., a biochemist and professor of nutrition in the department of food science and technology at Ohio State University in Columbus and author of *Taking the Fear Out of Eating.* Ironically, fat-free foods aren't helping us reduce fat much either—our fat consumption has fallen by a mere 6 calories a day, about the amount in one large droplet of corn oil.

■ **Dieting.** Yes, dieting can leave you flabby. Low-calorie eating plans encourage your body to burn fewer calories and hoard the body fat that you're trying to lose, notes G. Ken Goodrick, Ph.D., assistant professor of medicine at Baylor College of Medicine and associate director of the Behavioral Medicine Research Center, both in Houston. And special weight-loss programs don't give you the skills you need for a lifetime of healthy, satisfying eating. As a result, more than nine out of 10 dieters on organized weight-loss programs regain lost pounds within five years.

■ **Eating out.** We spend about 44 cents of every food dollar eating away from home these days, nearly twice as much as we did 40 years ago, according to the National Restaurant Association. With super-size portions and gobs of hidden fat, restaurant meals and take-out food have become a way of life guaranteed to pad hips and thicken waistlines especially for women, 41% of whom eat out on an average day.

■ **Clothing size inflation.** As American woman gain girth, fashion designers are giving us more space—with roomy, oversize clothing and elastic waistbands that accommodate spreading tummies. Such amenities could fool you into thinking you have lost weight, or are staying the same size, when you're really gaining girth.

A Plan All Your Own

Fortunately, you can defeat the forces of flab. In this book you'll discover simple, powerful new weight-loss techniques drawn from the experiences of real women who have shed anywhere from 10 to 250 pounds (and then stayed slim). Endorsed by weight-loss experts, these new techniques don't require you to follow a special diet or a rigid exercise regimen. It's simply a custom-fit program tailored to your likes, your lifestyle, and your budget.

What's so special about customizing? When a woman adapts a healthy eating plan and physical activity program to fit her needs, she can stick to it for years—even when life is stressful and the going gets tough, according to research from the University of Pittsburgh Medical Center. In contrast, a one-size-fits-all diet that ignores your unique needs is a set-up for disappointment—because it doesn't flex to accommodate you.

When you mold the Fat-to-Firm healthy eating plan and gentle physical fitness program to suit yourself, you'll stop gaining body fat. You'll enjoy permanent weight loss. You'll feel more energetic and improve your health. And you'll never go hungry or find yourself stuck in an exercise routine that's unpleasant or uncomfortable. You'll see that there's room for treats like chocolate, pizza, and even filet mignon if you like—and room for exploring to find the fitness style that is exactly right for you.

That's the promise of the Fat-to-Firm Program. In every chapter you'll discover exactly how to identify your unique needs and then customize the program to meet them. Throughout, you'll find the newest scientific research on weight loss translated into a practical program that you can use at home. You'll read the best advice from hundreds of experts—including nutritionists, weight-loss researchers, exercise physiologists, psychologists, professional chefs, and fashion designers. And you'll meet women who have already made the journey from fat to firm—not movie stars with personal trainers, but real people who work, raise families, run households, and care for spouses and parents.

In part 1 you'll find out how to set a healthy, realistic weight goal geared to your body type, your health needs, and your habits. You'll find new motivation, in the latest scientific evidence on the health benefits offered by weight loss. And you'll discover sympathetic, expert advice on dealing with emotional eating—an obstacle to weight loss for many women.

In part 2 you'll find mouthwatering details of the Fat-to-Firm eating plan. You'll never go hungry because it makes room for three meals and three snacks a day. This plan includes all the foods women need—from treats like cookies and pasta to super-nutritious edibles vital for strong bones and disease prevention to high-energy foods that fuel our busy lives. It shows you how to dine out, without gaining an ounce, and how to overcome weight-loss obstacles like stress-induced eating and cooking for a family that doesn't like low-fat food.

In part 3 you'll discover a gentle, timesaving fitness program guaranteed to boost fat burning 24 hours a day. You can use it in your living room, on your lunch hour, or while you are climbing the stairs to your office or bedroom. You'll find out why strong muscles are a woman's best friend—and how in just 20 minutes a day you can firm up your curves and rev up your metabolism. The Fat-to-Firm exercise program gives you a wide variety of calorie-burning exercise options to choose among. And you'll see why taking the stairs or parking at the far end of the supermarket parking lot could, over time, help you win the battle against flab.

In part 4 you'll find practical tips on dressing to flatter your special body type and on boosting self-esteem so that you can lead the life you have always wanted—right now. We firmly believe there's no reason to put your life on hold until you have lost weight.

In part 5 you'll find the Fat-to-Firm recipe collection. These recipes are designed to help women spring their own fat traps—with low-fat, high-flavor versions of your favorite salad dressings; traditional family main dishes and side dishes, like meat loaf and onion rings; and delicious desserts, like chocolate chip cheesecake and peanut butter cookies.

The Fat-to-Firm Program could also help you avoid diet drugs. You may be wondering whether new, highly publicized weight-loss medications like Redux are right for you. The truth is, while diet medications may help severely overweight women shed pounds and reduce serious health risks like heart disease, diabetes, or high blood pressure, experts on the National Task Force on the Prevention and Treatment of Obesity warn against widespread, long-term use of these pills. For women whose weight is not an immediate health risk, lifestyle changes advocated by the Fat-to-Firm Program are your best bet.

Real Women, Real Success

Throughout this book you'll meet real women who have successfully lost weight with this no-diet, custom-fit approach. Their stories are inspiring and will give you new ideas for overcoming weight-loss obstacles. Among them are the following.

■ **Annie Schneider, a 34-year-old marketing manager for a Chicago cable-television network,** who makes a point to include pizza and chocolate in her healthy-eating plan. "It's easy to adapt to a healthy lifestyle when you don't deny yourself your favorite foods," she says. "I indulge when I have a taste for pizza. I have a few slices and get rid of the rest of the pie." Annie's lost 40 pounds.

■ **Doris Anglin, an insurance specialist from Houston,** who found that eating three meals a day plus snacks is a weight-loss essential. "If I skip meals, I overeat like crazy," says Doris, who keeps an emergency snack kit in her car to escape fat traps like vending-machine items and fast-food burgers. She's lost 258 pounds.

■ **Joyce Stoner, an administrative assistant from New Carrolton, Maryland,** who added a gentle weight-training routine to her fitness program and turned over-40 flab into firm buttocks and a trim tummy. "And I just love my arms," she says. "Now, I wear sleeveless tops without hesitation." Joyce discovered that sometimes, firming up—rather than losing weight—is all you need.

■ **Meg Larsen, 46, a San Francisco lawyer and mother of two,** who turned to an old-fashioned Crock-Pot–type slow-cooker and healthy take-out food to satisfy her hungry family without blowing her own low-fat eating plan. "Time is at an absolute premium in my life," says Meg. "I've found ways to eat healthy, keep my sons and husband happy, and not gain weight." She's lost 32 pounds.

■ **Mary Smith, 33, an administrative assistant from Champaign, Illinois,** who totes her own "alternative treats" so that she can enjoy office parties without succumbing to cookies, cakes, and doughnuts. "This way, I feel like I'm part of the social side of eating without gaining weight," Mary says. She's lost 160 pounds.

■ **Sue Dole, a representative of a private foundation in St. Joseph, Illinois,** who lost weight despite a job that requires her to eat out at least three nights a week. She uncovers delicious, low-fat choices often hidden on restaurant menus by asking the waiter lots of smart questions. "I get what I want now," says Sue, 49. "And I really enjoy my meals." She's lost 32 pounds.

■ **Donna Gettings, 42, an administrative assistant from Williamsburg, Virginia,** who snapped monthly photographs of herself to create a personal weight-loss picture show that boosts her motivation. "Now I look at them and think, 'Daggone! I can't believe I was ever like that,'" she says. Donna has lost 111 pounds.

▪ **Crystal Thompson, an accounting supervisor from Fort Washington, Maryland,** who practiced two simple exercises that eliminated the need for a surgery to raise her sagging bosom. "Now, my husband looks at me and says I don't need to have the breast lift done—and I agree," says 37-year-old Crystal.

We hope you'll be as inspired and motivated by these success stories as we were. Enjoy the book—and in a few months, share your own Fat-to-Firm success story by writing to us at

Prevention Health Books
Attn.: Sharon Faelten
33 East Minor Street
Emmaus, PA 18098-0099

Sarí Harrar and Alisa Bauman
Prevention Health Books

Part 1

Discover Your True Weight-Loss Needs

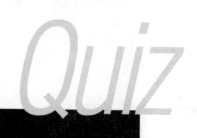

Are You at Risk for Emotional Eating?

Do you eat when you're blue, angry, lonely, or stressed? Uncovering the triggers that lead to emotional eating could help decipher your eating patterns and resolve the problem of unwanted pounds.

Find out if—and how much—your feelings rule your food choices with this quiz developed for the Fat-to-Firm Program by Joni Johnston, Psy.D., a clinical psychologist in Del Mar, California, and author of *Appearance Obsession: Learning to Love the Way You Look.* You'll also find advice on unraveling your emotional connections to food. Read the following statements, then rate your own eating habits by using this scoring system:

1 = Never
2 = Rarely
3 = Sometimes
4 = Often
5 = Always
You can tally your score below.

____ **1.** I eat to control stress.

____ **2.** Eating is one of the big pleasures in my life.

____ **3.** I eat well past the point of physical fullness at least two times a week.

____ **4.** When I'm lonely, food comforts me.

____ **5.** I find myself eating to put off things that I don't really want to do.

____ **6.** When my life seems out of control, I have a hard time controlling what I eat.

____ **7.** Sometimes I eat just for fun.

____ **8.** Eating, or trying not to eat, is on my mind a lot.

____ **9.** I eat a lot more when I'm alone than when I'm with others.

_____ **10.** Eating soothes me when I feel blue or anxious.

_____ **11.** When I was a child, food was a "home remedy" in our house, a source of comfort and love.

_____ **12.** Food helps me numb painful feelings and makes me feel better.

_____ **13.** When I'm angry, I find myself stuffing the anger down with food.

_____ **14.** Sometimes I just can't stop eating.

_____ **15.** In a difficult situation I might retreat and turn to food rather than deal with a problem directly.

_____ **Total Score**

Scoring: Add up your points for all answers to determine your total score, then read on for the results.

If you scored 15 to 35 points, you have a peaceful relationship with food and are unlikely to routinely respond to difficult emotional situations by eating. Reinforce your healthy attitude by giving yourself weekly self-nurturing treats like a candlelit bubble bath or a massage and by building a strong support system with friends and family. Use relaxation and physical activity to help handle stress. Learning positive coping techniques when life is good keeps the munchies away when times are tough.

If you scored 36 to 59 points, you eat for emotional reasons some of the time. Your eating is sending the message that certain feelings and events in your life need attention. Learn to identify these triggers by keeping a journal of your eating and your feelings. Then, develop new ways to relieve stress, fight boredom, or get comfort.

If you scored 60 to 75 points, food has become a major coping strategy—one you probably find less than effective. You have taken the first step toward change by taking this quiz. Now, develop a support network or friends and family you can trust to guide and support you in dealing with feelings and food more effectively.

Chapter 1

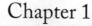

It's Not Your Fault

In a push-button world, gaining weight is almost automatic. Fortunately, losing it can be just as easy.

Click! Remote control in hand, Mindy Kane channel-surfs the 50 stations on her color TV—without leaving the comfort of her living-room couch.

R-R-Ring! There's the telephone. "I'll let the answering machine take a message," says Mindy. "I get so many annoying sales calls in the evening these days."

Whoosh! That's the dishwasher. Thanks to this "electronic servant," Mindy no longer has to soap, scrub, or rinse her kitchenware. She's free to sit, snack, and view CNN, her favorite TV network, until bedtime.

Ah, the good life. Small wonder that until two years ago, Mindy was 50 pounds overweight. Despite trying "every fad diet in the book," she wore a size 20 dress, never let the world glimpse her in a bathing suit, and shied away from social events that involved sports, like office softball games.

"I never got any physical activity," admits this 38-year-old project support manager at a Houston engineering company. "At home, I have all the modern conveniences. At work, I stare at a computer screen all day long. I take the elevator to my office. And when I get there, I don't even have to raise a finger to flip on a light switch. The lights come on automatically."

More Conveniences Equal More Pounds

If you're hauling around unwanted pounds as Mindy was, if you feel as if someone held your body over a copy machine and punched the enlarge button, stop blaming yourself. Modern life is fattening.

"Our civilization has worked hard to achieve a high standard of living," says obesity expert Richard L. Atkinson, M.D., professor of medicine and nutritional sciences at the University of Wisconsin in Madison and past president of the American Society for Clinical Nutrition. "We enjoy a rich diet. We have labor-saving devices. But we also work long hours and have no time for physical activity. The inevitable consequence is overweight."

When scientists from the National Center for Health Statistics of the Centers for Disease Control and Prevention in Hyattsville, Maryland, weighed a representative sample of Americans, they were startled to discover just how fattening our remote-control lifestyle can be: One in three women was overweight, up from one in four in 1960.

The researchers estimate that from the mid-1970s to the 1990s, the average woman gained 8 pounds. Many gained far more. What's more, the pounds-on trend seems to be hitting women earlier than ever. While the number of overweight women in their forties has increased somewhat, the proportion of overweight women in their thirties went from one in five to one in three. For those in their twenties, overweight doubled from one in 10 to one in five.

All told, 32 million of us tip the scales significantly above our ideal body weights.

Blame Bacon-Cheese Tacos and Three-TV Households

Experts are quick to blame our sedentary ways for this collective corpulence, calling the phenomenon an "epidemic of inactivity."

"We don't move anymore," says Sue Cummings, R.D., assistant professor at the Institute of Health Professions and a clinical dietitian who specializes in weight loss at Massachusetts General Hospital,

Battling the Nine-to-Five Bulge

At first glance, opera divas and female executives, file clerks and women doctors seem to have little in common on the job. Except this: Working could be hazardous to their waistlines.

"The majority of working women in United States hold down sedentary jobs these days," says Abby King, Ph.D., assistant professor of medicine and health research and policy at Stanford University School of Medicine. "At work, we mostly move our fingers at keyboards and move our mouths, talking. We don't move our bodies."

Small wonder, then, that one-third of American women are overweight. Even the 100,000 women in the construction trades probably get less exercise than they used to. "The jobs are so mechanized, that there's little continuous activity," Dr. King adds.

Thanks to mechanization, many of the little activities that once burned workaday calories have been supplanted by computers, elevators, fax machines, copiers, and answering machines.

"People used to climb stairs more often," notes Ralph Paffenbarger, M.D., Dr.P.H., professor emeritus of epidemiology at Stanford University School of Medicine who has studied physical activity on the job. "They typed on typewriters and had to press the keys down. If you needed a file, you hopped up and went to the filing cabinet. If you had to make a copy of something, you pulled out the carbon paper and started typing. There's been a big shift away from physical activity in our working lives."

The antidote? Create more physical activity at work. "You can make small changes that will help prevent obesity and lower your risk for diseases related to obesity such as heart disease and diabetes," Dr. King notes. "And there's a bonus: These activities also help fight stress."

Her top suggestions: Take the stairs instead of the elevator. Deliver messages in person, not by phone or electronic mail. Take a walking break or even schedule a meeting as a walk.

"If you can work in three 10-minute sessions of exercise a day, it goes a long way toward helping prevent overweight and improving health," she says. "Aim for moderate intensity—the pace of a brisk walk."

Try organizing lunchtime walking teams and have a friendly competition—see which teams can walk for the most time in a month, adds Dr. King.

both in Boston. "You can even press a button to roll down the car window."

In fact, a combination of too many modern conveniences, too little leisure time, too much stress, and too much food best explains our expanding waistlines. Consider these "firm-to-fat" trends.

- American women now eat 200 to 300 more calories a day than they did 15 years ago.

- Three out of four of us would like to exercise, but we say that we just can't find the time.

- More than one out of two women reduce dinner-hour stress by buying ready-to-eat or take-out food some of the time.

- At least clean-up is easy—58 percent of us have dishwashers.

- Women dine out an average of three times a month, choosing pizza as their most popular restaurant food, followed by hamburgers.

- We spend more than $103 billion a year on fast food.

- While burger and taco stands have added lower-fat fare, they're also "super-sizing" everything, from fries to soft drinks, and cramming bacon and cheese into pizza, burgers, and even tacos. That means more calories, more fat.

- We watch more than 30 hours of television a week.

- Seven in 10 American households have at least two television sets, while nearly four in 10 have three or more TVs.

- Four out of five of our homes have at least two telephones, but there's no need to answer—six in 10 also have answering machines.

- Bored with TV? Tired of conversing with friends and family? You can always browse in cyberspace or play a video game—more than three in 10 households now have personal computers.

The bottom line?

"It's especially tough to be active these days," notes clinical psychologist Abby King, Ph.D., assistant professor of medicine and health research and policy at the Stanford University School of Medicine. "When the greater percentage of the choices before us are sedentary, and only a few are active, it's easier to go with the TV or the computer, or to let a machine do work for us. Walking outside, riding a bike, and raking the lawn just don't look like as much fun."

Fat Pharm: Pills That Pack on Pounds

More than 100 prescription medications may cause some women to gain unwanted pounds. This unsettling side effect impacts less than 2 percent of people who take those drugs. But if you're among them, here's what the experts have to say about how to handle the worst offenders.

Check your mood meds. Antidepressants and other psychiatric drugs can be the most notorious weight-gain instigators, often simply because the medication makes you feel so much better that you socialize more, according to Madelyn H. Fernstrom, Ph.D., associate professor of psychiatry at the University of Pittsburgh School of Medicine.

Possible culprits include amitriptyline, bupropion, phenelzine sulfate, paroxetine (when used on a long-term basis), clomipramine, and alprazolam.

If you think a psychiatric drug is behind your weight gain, think about your recent eating habits: Have they changed drastically as your mood lifted? If appetite has increased, use low-fat eating strategies to control calories. Add exercise to burn more calories, too. If these tactics don't help, says Dr. Fernstrom, ask your doctor about switching to a different drug.

Watch out for antihistamines. The same medicines that dry out your nose may pack on the pounds, says Charles Lacy, Pharm.D., drug-information specialist at Cedars-Sinai Medical Center in Los Angeles and author of the *Drug Information Handbook*. They may act on the brain's appetite-control center or just make you feel thirsty—and in need of more liquids.

Culprits include newer, nonsedating antihistamines such as astemizole and loratadine.

If exercising and watching your diet don't help, ask your doctor about switching prescriptions, suggests Dr. Lacy. One cau-

Dead-End Diets

So, in an effort to head off creeping weight gain, we diet. Liquid meals. Public weigh-ins. Prepackaged "diet cuisine." Super-low-calorie regimens. While we desperately want these weight-loss systems to

tion: The older antihistamines, such aschlorpheniramine, may be a better bet but are more likely to cause drowsiness. Or consider a timing change, he suggests. If allergies are worst in the morning, perhaps you can make it through the afternoon and evening without the drugs.

Scrutinize blood-pressure-control drugs. Blood-pressure-lowering drugs can cause water-weight gain, often seen as swelling of the ankles or other parts of the body.

Culprits include guanadrel, methyldopa, and guanethidine, Dr. Lacy says. Betaxolol and pindolol can cause weight gain not related to water retention. He suggests that you ask your doctor about a diuretic to flush excess water from your body. For weight gain that's not related to water retention, try a lower-fat diet and more exercise. If the weight doesn't budge, ask about a different drug.

Ask: Is it a steroid? Corticosteroids used to treat asthma, arthritis, and allergies may increase appetite, cause water retention, or, again, improve well-being so that you simply feel like eating more, says Arthur Jacknowitz, Pharm.D., chairperson of the department of clinical pharmacy at West Virginia University Health Sciences Center School of Pharmacy in Morgantown.

Culprits include prednisone and inhaled asthma drugs beclomethasone dipropionate and flunisolide. Medications used to treat endometriosis such as leuprolide acetate, nafarelin acetate, and danazol may all help you put on a few pounds.

If you take these drugs, Dr. Jacknowitz suggests that you pay close attention to how much you're eating. Consider using a food diary. If watching your food intake and getting a little extra exercise doesn't reverse a weight-gain trend, he recommends that you talk with your doctor about alternatives.

work—so much so that Americans spend about $33 billion a year in the quest for leaner physiques—the truth is, they don't.

In fact, our weight-loss efforts leave us fatter. At least two-thirds of all dieters in organized programs regain all their lost flab within one year. Some become even heavier than before their diets began.

Blame the "Chubby" Gene

One memorable summer vacation, Nicolle Johnson, of North Wales, Pennsylvania, and her sister-in-law, Lisa Anderson, of Edmonds, Washington, threw dietary caution to the winds, enjoying buttery pastries, robust luncheon cheeses, dinners drenched in cream sauce and, often, Belgian chocolate for dessert.

After two lip-smacking weeks, Lisa was as willowy as ever. But poor Nicolle was 5 pounds pudgier. Why? In part, experts say, it's a tale of two gene pools.

"It's not fair, but some people are born with the genetic tendency to gain weight, and others are predisposed to be lean," says obesity expert Richard L. Atkinson, M.D., professor of medicine and nutritional sciences at the University of Wisconsin in Madison and past president of the American Society for Clinical Nutrition.

As researchers unlock more of the mysteries of human genetics, the link between heredity and the shape we're in grows stronger. Our bodies, for example, seem to defend a "set point"—a certain weight or fat level—by regulating appetite, activity levels, and metabolism, says Dr. Atkinson.

One messenger sending signals to the brain's body-weight thermostat may be leptin, a protein programmed by the so-called obesity gene and released by fat cells. In laboratory experiments, a defective ob gene never sent the signal that enough fat was on board.

"Ninety-five percent of the people who lose weight regain it all within five years," says Cummings. And despite the bounty of low-fat, fat-free, and diet foods crowding supermarket shelves, the long-term prospects aren't any better.

Nutrition researchers suspect that those new low-fat and nonfat foods may actually make us fatter in the first place, says John Allred, Ph.D., a biochemist and professor of nutrition in the department of food science and technology at Ohio State University in Columbus and author of *Taking the Fear Out of Eating*. Overindulging in "guilt-free" goodies, he says, may account for the extra calories American women are now consuming.

"People tend to think that they can eat a lot of these low-fat items, but the truth is that sweet foods and snack foods still have a lot of calo-

But don't be too quick to blame the obesity gene yet for pudgy thighs. A combination of 24 different genes may have an impact on how much you weigh—and even where you pack the pounds. And lifestyle factors, such as food choices and physical activity levels, seem to play an even bigger role.

"Genetics is responsible for maybe 20 to 50 percent of the weight differences in our society, while factors such as how much you eat and how often you exercise are responsible for 50 to 80 percent," Dr. Atkinson notes. "I personally believe those factors are what's critical. Genetics simply determines what happens if you overeat or don't exercise."

That's good news if you, like Nicolle, seem genetically predisposed to chubbiness. "You have some control," Dr. Atkinson says. "If you look at your family—particularly parents, grandparents, aunts, and uncles—and see overweight people, you are likely to have the same tendency. But you also have a great deal of control over whether or not it happens."

The Fat-to-Firm Program can help you find a form of physical activity that you can perform at least three days a week for at least 30 minutes. And it will show you how to convert slowly to a healthy, low-fat diet. And it will help you determine a weight-loss goal that's realistic for you, genetically.

ries," he says. "There's no magic in low-fat foods. If you take in more calories than you burn—whether the calories are from a fat-free fig bar or a slab of chocolate cake—then you'll be fatter."

The New "Thin" Thinking

Happily, the Fat-to-Firm Program described in this book offers a new promise for success. The cornerstone? It's a program you create for yourself. "If a person has power over her food choices and exercise program, then that person will be successful in any weight-loss attempt," says Anne Dubner, R.D., nutrition consultant in Houston and a spokesperson for the

American Dietetic Association. "The key is, you have to play a part in all the decisions."

The foundation, proved in studies of women who have successfully lost weight and kept it off, isn't a diet at all. The Fat-to-Firm Program is based on a new way of thinking. "It's all about redefining success," says Cummings. "You have to think about your own life and your own body and what's right for you."

Following the Fat-to-Firm Program requires creative problem-solving. You can melt down modern-day barriers that keep you from achieving a healthy weight by devising a program that flexes with the demands of your unique life, says Susan Kayman, R.D., Dr.P.H., program coordinator of regional health education for the Kaiser-Permanente Medical Group in Oakland, California. Every step of the way, you'll find useful and innovative strategies for customizing your program.

"A woman may have to learn some coping skills to handle what's going on in her life. It's the first and most powerful step," says Dr. Kayman, who studied women who succeeded in maintaining their goal weight. "Without these skills, you may eat to feel good rather than thinking about and resolving the real issue bothering you. Or you end up watching TV instead of exercising."

Of course, the Fat-to-Firm Program includes a healthy eating program, but one tailored to your own needs and desires. One that leaves you feeling satisfied, includes your favorite foods, and focuses on nutritious, low-fat meals. One that helps you deal with the weak moments when you're most vulnerable to overeating.

It also includes a fitness plan—the kind you enjoy and have the time to do. And if you must set pound-shedding goals, it calls for small, smart, reasonable steps—such as losing weight in increments of no more than 5 to 10 pounds at a time.

So whether you're among the three out of five Americans hoping to lose weight for health reasons or the one in five Americans who simply hope to look better, the Fat-to-Firm Program can be your ally for an entire lifetime.

"If you eat healthy food, find time for fitness, and work on problem solving, you can stabilize at a lower weight and improve your health risks a lot," says G. Ken Goodrick, Ph.D., assistant professor of medicine at Baylor College of Medicine and associate director of the Behavioral Medicine Research Center, both in Houston. "You'll lower your risk of cardiovascular disease, diabetes, high blood pressure, and some forms of cancer. And, you'll have more energy."

Resist the Remote Control

When it comes to fitness, the Fat-to-Firm Program maximizes healthy weight loss by taking advantage of your body's three-way calorie-burning system. "Every day, 60 percent of the calories you use up are burned by your lean muscles during everyday activities," says Cummings. "Another 30 percent are burned by intense physical activity, and 10 percent are burned during digestion."

Start with something aerobic. To follow the Fat-to-Firm Program, you can choose an aerobic fitness activity, such as walking, biking, swimming, or aerobic dance (in a gym, or at home with a video), whatever you can engage in three times a week. "Aerobic exercise mobilizes fat," says Cummings. "See if you have 30 minutes anywhere in your day for physical activity."

Add strength training. Call it body sculpting, weight lifting, or resistance training, strength training is the secret weapon of the Fat-to-Firm Program. With simple weights, you can build more muscle. Doing so will not only burn more calories during exercise, but it will also rev up the rate at which your body burns calories to sustain itself all day, says Cummings.

In one study at Tufts University in Boston, 19 women who participated for one year in a program of strength-training exercises such as leg lifts, sit-ups, and knee extensions increased muscle power by 35 to 76 percent. And when muscle replaced fat, they increased the calorie-burning speed of their metabolisms and burned an extra 442 calories a week. Physiques took on a trimmer look, too. One woman went down two dress sizes.

Get up and around. Leave your chair at work or your sofa at home, too, suggests Dr. King. After all, for every flight of stairs you climb, you burn 8 to 10 calories. "The more activity, the better—for your health, your weight, and your stress levels," she notes.

See Food in a New Light

Skipping meals and going without food are not part of the Fat-to-Firm Program. When 99 normal-weight women revealed their weight-maintenance secrets to researchers at Winthrop University in Rock Hill, South Carolina, the value of regular eating was obvious: These women ate three meals a day—and most added at least one snack. They even indulged in occasional fried foods, desserts, sweet sodas, or rich sauces. So "they actually ate a few more calories than women who skipped meals," says researcher Patricia Giblin Wolman, R.D., Ed.D., professor of human nutrition and chairperson of the department of human nutrition at Winthrop University. "But," she adds, "they seemed to burn it off."

Why? "Frequent eating works with your metabolism, which speeds up a little each time you eat," says Dr. Wolman. "Also, if you eat regular meals, you'll be less likely to feel ravenously hungry and overeat at one meal." So the Fat-to-Firm Program calls for regular meals—and then some.

What's on the plates of successful weight maintainers? It's not "diet" food. In Dr. Kayman's study, women who kept weight off didn't think of their food choices as temporary weight-loss plans.

"It wasn't something special or temporary," Dr. Kayman says. "While relapsers—people who regained weight they lost—tried special diet foods and formulas, maintainers adjusted to a meal plan they could follow all the time." The basic elements follow.

Bring on the fiber. The best plan turns out to be a high-fiber, low-fat eating plan that you can enjoy for a lifetime, says Dr. Goodrick. So, the Fat-to-Firm Program calls for choosing more fruits, vegetables, and whole grains.

Give fat the slip. At the same time, the Fat-to-Firm Program shies away from full-fat dairy products, fat-marbled meats, oils, and fried foods.

Dr. Goodrick advocates slowly reducing the amount of fat in your diet to 30 percent or less of total calories—down from the 37 percent that most women eat. "Your weight slowly falls to a level you can maintain," he says. "It's a no-diet approach."

Remember: Customize the Program

Do you adore brownies? Hate getting up in the morning? Love dining out? Or loathe the idea of toting lunch to the office?

If so, you should keep eating brownies, enjoying restaurant dinners, and buying lunch. Oh, and think twice about signing up for that early-morning walking club.

"No food and no personal preference should be off-limits in a healthy weight-loss plan," says Dubner. "If you think your favorite food is a bad food, then sneaking just a little could lead to a binge. If you know it's fine to enjoy it, a serving can be satisfying."

As for exercise, "if you don't like a particular form of exercise or if the timing doesn't work for you, you'll have trouble sticking with it," says Dr. Kayman.

When 1,000 women and men revealed their weight-control secrets to obesity researchers of the National Weight-Loss Registry at the University of Pittsburgh Medical Center, the value of a personalized plan became clear, says Mary Lou Klem, Ph.D., a clinical psychologist and medical center senior fellow.

"We knew so little about maintainers—that is, people who lose weight successfully—that we asked people to write to us," says Dr. Klem. "We wanted to hear from people who had lost at least 30 pounds and kept it off for at least one year. One of our early findings is that these people tailored eating plans and exercise programs to their own specific situations.

In California Dr. Kayman saw the same pattern when she studied women who were considered weight maintainers and relapsers. One maintainer, who loved ice cream, would cut a half-gallon of ice cream into small cubes, then freeze the cubes individually. She ate one cube a day—reveling in the taste without consuming too many calories, or gaining any weight.

Lessons from a Master: Mindy's Story

Mindy Kane is living proof that this custom-tailored approach works. Today, she's 50 pounds lighter, a trim size 8. Yet she still eats in restaurants, grabs convenience-food dinners on busy nights, and watches television.

"I had to change my priorities and reorganize my schedule a little," says Mindy. "But I never gave up my favorite foods or my favorite activities. I'm sure that's why I've kept the weight off."

Socializing with friends at a restaurant, she's likely to choose a low-fat entrée such as pasta with marinara sauce instead of fried chicken. "But I still make room for treats," she said. "On a recent Saturday night, I had a chocolate–peanut butter pie that was incredibly good. Like many women, I find that if I don't eat what I like once in a while, the danger is that I'll end up bingeing."

When pressed for time, Mindy now grabs a quick dinner at the supermarket salad bar. "It's just as fast as ordering a burger, fries, and milk shake at a drive-through but less fattening," she notes.

Mindy succeeded, in part, because she made healthy eating a priority—"plenty of fruits and vegetables, not so much of the meat and fried foods I grew up with." So did a body-sculpting routine that features regular walking and a gentle workout with weights. "I reorganized my workday to fit in exercise," she says. "Sometimes, I work straight through lunch so that I can leave at five o'clock to get to the gym."

Mindy has also outwitted modern life, fitting in plenty of small "bonus" activities, also part of the Fat-to-Firm Program.

"I climb the stairs at work instead of riding the elevator," she says. "A lot of times, I park in a faraway parking spot and walk to the office door." And while she still loves CNN, she often watches while walking on a treadmill at the local gym.

The paybacks go beyond being svelte. "I have more energy," Mindy says. "And when I walk after work, I arrive home with a clear head. The stress of the day is behind me. I sleep really well."

Leap the Mental Barriers

Mindy's story also proves another point: Your mind is your number one weight-loss tool. That's what Dr. Kayman discovered when she compared two groups of women: 30 women who shed pounds and kept them off and 44 others who lost weight and then regained it.

"Maintainers made decisions to lose weight and then solved problems that stood in the way, like stress and time constraints," she says. "They persisted until new ways of eating and exercising were established. If the first thing they tried didn't work for them, they didn't give up."

But when life threw the relapsers a curve ball, they responded by overeating and skipping exercise sessions.

"Both groups of women faced the same kinds of stressful problems, from cars breaking down to arguments with a spouse and from money trouble to job problems," Dr. Kayman says. "The difference was how they dealt with it. Women who put their well-being first got over the problem barriers. They found ways to keep eating healthy food and to keep on exercising. But the relapsers didn't. They would say, 'Oh, I was on vacation. I couldn't eat my special food.' or 'Oh, I was upset with my children and couldn't exercise.'"

Maintainers, in contrast, found ways to overcome obstacles encountered, like a time crunch. "One working mother did aerobics two nights a week, when her husband could be home with the kids," Dr. Kayman says.

To overcome your own weight-loss barriers, first identify the real problem, Dr. Kayman suggests. If you overeat at night, the real problem may be that you're overworked and come home feeling stressed-out. "Then you ask yourself, 'Why am I working so hard? How can I change this?'" she says. "You may try talking to your boss, socializing more with co-workers, or delegating more work. The point is that you find solutions that work for you, and you keep experimenting until you find the one that's right for you."

Redefine Success

At Baylor University's Behavioral Medicine Research Center, Dr. Goodrick and other weight-loss experts have identified other themes among women who have stepped off the diet roller coaster and stayed off: These women focused on health rather than appearance, built new levels of self-esteem, and set realistic weight goals.

"The theory we go by is that being happy, having a constructive and meaningful life, and enjoying good relationships are the ultimate goals, and they're things you can have whether or not you're thin," Dr. Goodrick says. "We want to reverse the thinking that says, 'I can't be happy until I lose weight.'"

"Success is not a low number on the bathroom scale," says Cummings. "It's about better health and a more fulfilling life. You can significantly improve your health by losing just 10 or 15 pounds. I work with one woman whose weight went from 188 to 170, and she feels great about herself. She's exercising every day, eating well, and even got out of a lousy job because she worked on self-esteem. Work to reach your natural weight not some fictitious ideal."

Welcome to the Fat-to-Firm Program

So let's take a summary look at all the benefits and features of the Fat-to-Firm Program.

■ More weight-loss triumphs. With a lower-fat eating plan and a gentle fitness routine, you can achieve realistic weight-loss goals with tangible health benefits, says Ralph W. Cygan, M.D., clinical professor of medicine and director of the weight-management program at the University of California, Irvine, College of Medicine.

■ Better weight maintenance. People who focus on health, rather than pounds on the bathroom scale, are more successful at maintaining a lower body weight, according to a researcher at the Brigham and Women's Hospital in Boston.

■ More food. "Severe weight-loss programs are hard on your body and difficult to stick with," says Kathy McManus, R.D., manager of clinical nutrition at Brigham and Women's Hospital. "A lower-fat eating plan is healthier, and it teaches you how to eat for the rest of your life."

■ More culinary adventures. A healthy eating plan also brings new dining pleasures—chilled strawberry-cantaloupe soup, anyone? "As you add new fruits and vegetables and grains to your diet, your palate expands, and it's likely you'll find many new foods you're going to like," says Susanna Cunningham-Rundles, Ph.D., associate professor of immunology at Cornell University Medical Center in New York City.

■ Better fat-burning. By combining three kinds of physical activity— aerobic workouts, strength training, and "unplanned exercise" (such as taking the stairs instead of the "Up" escalator at the mall)—you'll boost your metabolism and burn more calories all day long, says Wayne Westcott, Ph.D., strength consultant in Quincy, Massachusetts, for the national YMCA.

■ More toning. The Fat-to-Firm Program tones you two ways by burning bulges of excess fat and shaping underlying muscles, says Dr. Westcott. The results? A flatter stomach. Sleeker hips. Firmer upper arms and thighs.

■ Better self-esteem. "You'll feel better about yourself," says McManus. "It's amazing the sense of control and sheer pleasure that women start to feel when they're doing something for themselves. As wives, mothers, daughters, and workers, so many women do things for other people. They can feel so obligated. It's a wonderful new experience to begin doing something just for yourself, especially if you've been feeling bad about yourself because you're overweight."

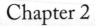

Chapter 2

Nourishing Your Heart and Soul

Ninety-five percent of overweight problems have an *emotional* cause, say scientists. But you can "feed" your feelings without food.

Like many women who struggle with their weight, Wendy Jarvis traces overeating to an emotional link. In Wendy's case, she says she found herself home alone with "the crazies."

"My husband was at work, my four children were at school," says Wendy, 52, of Devore, California. "Suddenly, I would start feeling insecure and out of control. Then my eating would get out of control, too."

Hershey bars. Milky Ways. Whatever she'd bought for the kids' lunch boxes or for her husband. "It was always chocolate," she says. "Not cake or pies or anything else. I would eat in the kitchen, the living room, the bedroom—all over the house. The more I tried to stop, the more I would eat. That's why I call it the crazies."

Ellie Klenske overate in response to worries about the family business. "There are times in any business when the cash flow is tight," she says. "But when things got stressful, I found myself staring into the refrigerator. And eating."

Frozen vanilla yogurt with nuts, potato chips, or cookies—"always fat-free, of course, but in such copious quantities that it was a lot of calories," says Ellie, also 52, of Redlands, California. "That's why I call food my drug of choice. It's my companion, but it's not necessarily my friend."

Feeding a Deep-Down Hunger

Food is comfort. From chicken soup when you're sick to a big bowl of mint–chocolate chip ice cream when you're blue to a peanut butter cookie Mom offered after you fell off your first two-wheeled bike, the soothing powers of food are a natural part of most every childhood, culture, or stage of life.

These days, the emotional impact of food has also become its prime selling point. "We hear about fun-size candy bars, about how making cookies will "bake someone happy," and about how chocolate is love," says Susan Moore, R.D., program manager and senior nutritionist of the obesity-management program at George Washington University in Washington, D.C. Small wonder we consume an average of more than 10 pounds of chocolate a year. Or that between ages 30 and 60, women eat significantly more chocolate than men do.

Yet if eating becomes your emotional lifeline—a way that you can soothe, cover up, or numb your feelings—then you may find yourself trapped in a vicious cycle of overeating, guilt feelings, and weight gain.

"Everyone does some emotional eating," says Donna Ciliska, R.N., Ph.D., associate professor of health sciences at McMaster University in Hamilton, Ontario, and author of *Beyond Dieting*. "But when a woman overeats for emotional reasons, it becomes a problem."

Emotional eating contributes to overweight and to the medical conditions that come with unhealthy amounts of body fat, says Dr. Ciliska. If comfort foods like ice cream, chips, chocolate, and pie take the place of healthy edibles in a woman's diet, she is also missing out on vital nutrients that provide optimal energy, prevent disease, and maintain strong bones, she adds. At the same time, it may also indicate that important inner needs are being ignored.

When is emotional eating a problem? When food becomes a distraction, a substitute for love, or even an "anesthesia." When overeating becomes a way to block out anger or depression or to soothe feelings of stress, loneliness, or boredom. These are all signs that your emotions may be a factor in your eating patterns, says Dianne Lindewall, Ph.D., supervising behavioral psychologist of the obesity-management program at George Washington University.

Emotional eating seems to "resonate more for women than men," says Dr. Lindewall. Identifying and dealing with the emotional component to weight loss is often a necessary part of the solution. And so making peace with the feelings that underlie eating problems is often the most important step a woman can take toward reaching or maintaining a healthy weight.

No Comfort in Carrots

Why is it that when that inner voice growls, "Things aren't right—I've gotta eat something!" we're likely to reach for apple pie but not an apple, for carrot cake but not a carrot, for a chocolate milk shake but not a glass of milk?

The answer is simple: Fat- and sugar-laden treats taste good and feel good in our mouths, providing instant pleasure that elevates a bad mood—if only for a few fleeting moments, notes Dr. Lindewall. "On that level," she says, "it's hard for a carrot to compete with a bowl of ice cream."

But our choices of comfort foods are also windows on the past. "One thing we always ask women is, 'What was eating like in your house when you were growing up?' " says nutritionist Barbara Dickinson, R.D., director of nutrition in the Weight Management Center at the Center for Health Promotion and co-leader of the Women and Food support group, both at Loma Linda University in California.

"We tend to go for the same kinds of foods and to eat them in the same way—we may overeat because in our families, feeling extra-full meant satisfaction," Dickinson says.

Foods like ice cream, cake, and candy are rich in carbohydrates that may also elevate levels of a feel-good brain chemical called serotonin, temporarily boosting a woman's sense of well-being, says Dr. Lindewall.

This carbohydrate connection may be especially strong for a woman during the second half of her menstrual cycle, after ovulation. At that time, progesterone levels rise, causing a drop in blood sugar and increased food cravings, according to Elizabeth Lee Vliet, M.D., author of *Screaming to Be Heard: Hormonal Connections Women Suspect...And Doctors Ignore.*

Breaking the Trance: Your Mood-Food Journal

Resisting the siren call of Ben and Jerry, Sara Lee, Famous Amos, the Keebler elf, the Pillsbury doughboy, and all the rest requires self-exploration—not sheer willpower.

"The best solution is to cope with the situation that's driving you to eat," says Dr. Lindewall. "And the first step in coping is becoming aware of what's bothering you. Yet instead of putting energy into dealing with the emotional issues, we often avoid them to the point that women tell me they find themselves staring into the refrigerator as if in a trance. They don't know how they got there."

To break the trance, you need to take steps to meet your emotional needs directly instead of through food. Begin with two simple tools: a pencil and paper, says Dr. Ciliska.

Jot your thoughts in a pocket-size notebook, in your day planner, or on a 3- by 5-inch card. Whatever system you use, the format should be as convenient as possible. That way, you can easily turn to your mood-food journal as soon as you find yourself on the threshold of an emotional eating episode, says Dr. Lindewall.

Use your journal when you feel driven to eat: when you have that sudden, inexplicable urge for a doughnut after a rough morning meeting with the boss, for instance, or when you find yourself reaching into that box of cookies during the lonely hours after dinner. On a blank page or card, answer these questions.

- Am I physically hungry?
- What do I want to eat?
- What am I eating, and how much?
- What am I feeling?
- What am I saying to myself?
- Who is with me?
- What's been going on in the past hours or the past day?

Even if you don't stop eating at first, simply developing the ability to pause before you eat and to identify your true needs—emotional or physical hunger—is a victory, Dr. Ciliska says. "Once you identify the emotions, the long-term goal is finding new ways to cope." Coping could mean anything from trying a new eating plan to learning to ask your spouse for emotional support.

Dig for Clues

After keeping a mood-food journal for a week or more, review your notes and search for your emotional-eating triggers.

Perhaps you're bored at night and eat for excitement. Maybe you eat after angry arguments with your spouse instead of saying what you feel. Maybe you find yourself in the bathroom gobbling Twinkies when your oh-so-critical mother comes to visit. Perhaps you're lonely.

Look for patterns. Your trigger may be a particular feeling or a certain time of day or a high-risk situation, suggests Dr. Lindewall.

Defusing Your Trigger Times

Once you've uncovered your own unique triggers, you can take steps to defuse inappropriate eating episodes and meet your emotional needs directly, Dr. Ciliska says. Customize your approach by choosing from among coping strategies that focus on your personal emotional-eating issues. Experiment until you find the best ways to feed underlying needs as well as the best ways to limit overeating. Every woman's solutions will be slightly different.

Soothe yourself. As soon as you notice agitated, upset feelings, quickly comfort yourself with a brief, relaxing time-out, suggests Dr. Lindewall. Try a short walk or 5 minutes of deep-breathing exercises, she says.

Think it through. Ask yourself, "What do I need right now?" Try writing your feelings down or calling a friend and talking about what's happening, suggests Dr. Ciliska. Even talking into a tape recorder can help. This step is vital. When you take a moment to sort out what you really need, you reinforce your self-worth and, at the same time, prepare for effective problem-solving.

Take action. If you can resolve the issue immediately, do so. You may have to cancel one of two conflicting appointments or make plans to get takeout for dinner on a busy night or clear the air with your spouse, kids, boss, or a co-worker, Dr. Lindewall says.

If the issue cannot be resolved immediately, write the solution down and get on with your day. Writing helps clear your head. On the other hand, if you just think about the solution, chances are you'll have trouble getting it out of your mind, she says.

Stress Busters

Thought you'd heard all the arguments against dieting? Here's one more reason to stop: Skimping on meals raises your risk for a stress-induced feeding frenzy.

"If you aren't eating as much as your body requires, several pressures kick in. Food smells more enticing. It tastes better. Just looking at it makes you want to eat," says Richard Straub, Ph.D., professor of psychology and chairperson of the behavioral sciences department at the University of Michigan in Dearborn. "You can resist these pressures under normal circumstances, but when you throw stress into the mix, you can lose all restraint." In our society, women are even more vulnerable to stress-prone eating than men because women diet more, he says. In a study at the University of Michigan, Dr. Straub compared the eating habits of women and men watching two movies—a stressful film about industrial accidents and a ho-hum travelogue. While unstressed men ate more than anyone, stressed women outpaced unstressed women and chose more sweet, creamy foods.

"I don't think it's really a gender issue," he says. "The stressed-out women ate more because, in general, women are dieters. They restrain their appetites and lose control under stress."

How can you stress-proof your eating habits? First, don't diet, says Dr. Straub. He recommends following a healthy, low-fat eating plan like the Fat-to-Firm Program to reduce your vulnerability to stress. Here are more stress-busting strategies for high-anxiety days.

Schedule stress-reducing breaks. Especially on pressure-filled days, clear room in your schedule for a walk or a talk with a friend, Dr. Straub suggests. "Exercise is especially effective. But talking with someone is also a helpful way to blow off steam."

Try a morning meal. Stress levels rise when your body's low on fuel, says Susan Moore, R.D., program manager and senior nutri-

Satisfying Your Emotional Needs—Without Food

As you gain insight into emotional issues that trigger overeating, the Fat-to-Firm Program offers many satisfying strategies to help you nurture yourself and find support. To customize these strategies to your particular needs, experiment to find what works best for you.

tionist of the obesity-management program at George Washington University in Washington, D.C. "Experiment with a combination of foods until you find out what gives you long-lasting energy. Some women need more than a bagel and juice—a little protein and fat, like a dab of peanut butter, gives you staying power."

Add a snack. Small pick-me-ups at midmorning and midafternoon can keep at bay the low energy that leads to anxiety and stress, says nutritionist Barbara Dickinson, R.D., director of nutrition in the Weight Management Center at the Center for Health Promotion and co-leader of the Women and Food support group, both at Loma Linda University in California.

Drink lots of water. Fit in eight 8-ounce glasses of water a day—and drink before you get thirsty, Dickinson suggests. Dehydration can cause headaches and fatigue, so that you think you need a snack when all you really need is cool, clear water, she says.

Go easy on sugar. After eating sugary foods, some women may experience reactive hypoglycemia—blood sugar levels rise, then fall dramatically, causing weakness and fatigue, notes Paul J. Rosch, M.D., clinical professor of medicine and psychiatry at New York Medical College and president of the American Institute of Stress, both in New York City.

Think twice about that cocktail. Drinking alcohol is a dangerous substitute for dealing with stressful situations, notes Dickinson.

And if you only drink occasionally, there's still reason to be wary. In one study of the effects of alcohol and stress on 60 women and men, researchers at the Addiction Research Foundation in Ontario, Canada, found that feelings of intoxication were muted under stress. That may lead to increased alcohol use, the researchers note. And the more you drink, the more excess calories you consume in the form of alcohol.

Talk about it. Gain new support and learn new coping techniques by sharing your experience with others, suggests Dr. Ciliska. Check with local hospitals or churches to find out about support groups in your area. "In a group, we really find out that we're not alone. It helps with problem solving and getting in touch with emotions," she says. "Behavior change is easier, too."

Problem Solved

Make Peace with Emotional Eating

Your emotional life is unique—and your emotions change from day to day, hour to hour, even minute to minute. So it makes sense that dealing with emotional eating would require a whole set of unique, tailored-made solutions. That's what experts like Susan Moore, R.D., program manager and senior nutritionist of the obesity-management program at George Washington University in Washington, D.C., suggest. "Trust yourself to find the best solutions," she says. "And realize that over time, you may need new solutions. Constantly adapting is the secret to the mystery of coping with emotional eating."

Ellie Klenske, 52, of Redlands, California, discovered that secret. "When an eating urge hits, I take a walk," says Ellie. "Walking helps me get into focus. And in order to treat myself well, I give myself some sort of nonfood reward when I've handled something really well. I might get a pedicure or buy a new blouse—even just a T-shirt. I also try to get a lot of fun into my life. I go for short hikes in the mountains. I also go fishing, basically ocean bottom fishing and lake fishing for trout, with my daughter-in-law."

Why it works: Ellie has combined many coping techniques to meet many needs. Diversity gives her the flexibility to meet new situations and respond to different feelings successfully, says Moore.

Exercise is an excellent way to relieve anxiety and boost self-esteem. "It also buys you some time before you eat, time for thinking about what the real issue is and how you can solve it," says Diane Lindewall, Ph.D., supervising behavioral psychologist of the obesity-management program at George Washington University.

Finding nonfood rewards gives you a well-deserved celebration—without landing you right back in the eat-guilt-eat cycle, says Donna Ciliska, R.N., Ph.D., associate professor of health sciences at McMaster University in Hamilton, Ontario, and author of *Beyond Dieting*.

Finding time for fun fills our human need for play that serious, responsibility-burdened adults often forget about, says Sue Irish, a psychotherapist who helps lead the Women and Food support group at the Weight Management Center at Loma Linda University in California.

"So often, eating is the only time we let ourselves relax and have a good time," she says. "We forget we need time for recreation."

Self-nurture. Take care of yourself, suggests Dr. Ciliska. You may need more rest, more creative and intellectual stimulation, or the opportunity to express your feelings and have them heard.

You may need new sources of comfort, nurture, and love—from setting aside time for a relaxing bath or listening to your favorite music to developing new friendships or asking old friends for hugs and attention.

Encourage yourself. Listen to how your self-talk is going throughout the day, suggests Dickinson. Is your inner voice critical or self-defeating or full of commands? Counter negative messages with truthful, positive responses. For example, turn a comment like "I can't talk with my new co-workers; they won't like me" into "I'd like to get to know them better; I'll begin with some questions about our office during coffee break."

Speak your mind. If you stuff down anger, then learning to ask assertively for what you need can help, Dr. Ciliska says. This may require taking an assertiveness training class, she says.

"I don't know any women, myself included, who haven't benefited from some assertiveness training," notes Dr. Lindewall. "Many times, changing a situation involves dealing effectively with other people. Learning to speak up for yourself without being timid or intimidating is a very important skill."

Make time for simply doing nothing. Stressed? Are mealtimes and snack times the only times you allow yourself to relax? If so, you may be eating just to get a breather from a nonstop routine, notes Sue Irish, a psychotherapist and co-leader of the Women and Food support group, sponsored by the Weight Management Center at Loma Linda University.

"A lot of women feel tremendous guilt if they stop working for even a minute," she says. "You work hard all day, eat lunch at your desk, and then spend the evening doing laundry, taking care of the kids, and cleaning the house. You may have a snack or spend a long time over dinner because for most of us it's the only time we give ourselves permission to stop working. Next time, try simply sitting and doing nothing." That could mean listening to music, reading, watching a movie, or simply not doing anything at all, she says.

Put some excitement in your life. Bored? Instead of perking up a dull day with chocolate-covered cherries, seek new job challenges, revive a long-lost hobby, or find a new one, suggests Dr. Ciliska.

"I've known people to ask their supervisors for more diverse job responsibilities," she says. "If you feel bored at home, think about past activities you've enjoyed—like a sport or a handicraft." Or, peruse the community calendar of your local newspaper for new activities—from volunteer opportunities to quilting circles, tennis classes to wildflower-identification walks.

Coping with Comfort Food

Understanding the hot-button issues that push you beyond the comfort zone can take time, says Dr. Lindewall. While you work out better ways to nourish emotional needs, you can also take steps to make your relationship with your favorite comfort foods healthier—and less likely to pack on added pounds or lead to guilty feelings, she says.

Here are some alternative strategies.

Redesign your food environment. Common sense says, don't stock up on the high-fat, high-calorie foods that you're mostly likely to grab when the going gets tough. "If you're upset and the only thing available is air-popped popcorn, then eating a lot of that has far fewer calories than, say, premium ice cream or a bag of cookies," Dr. Lindewall says.

Introduce new "convenience" foods. With high-fat fare out of the way, bring in precut vegetables and fruits, suggests Chris Rosenbloom, R.D., Ph.D., associate professor in the department of nutrition and dietetics at Georgia State University in Atlanta. "If you open the refrigerator and find a bowl of sliced peaches, chances are you'll try them," she says.

Eat every 4 hours. Skimping on breakfast and lunch can leave you hungry, irritable, and vulnerable to emotional eating, says Dickinson. The antidote? Eat the right foods, at the right time.

Most people find that a substantial breakfast totaling about 400 calories is helpful, says Moore.

Include a protein food (such as low-fat or skim milk, yogurt, or cottage cheese), grains (like whole-wheat toast, oatmeal, or a high-fiber cereal), and fruits, says Dickinson.

"Plan on eating lunch 4 hours later and dinner 4 hours after that," says Dickinson. "Waiting any longer makes most women really hungry. Include foods from at least three of these foods groups: proteins, grains, fruits, and vegetables. It's also good to have a small amount of a healthy fat from avocado, peanut butter, nuts, canola oil, or olive oil. These fats—composed largely of mono and polyunsaturated fats—help lower blood cholesterol and help make you feel satisfied."

If your stomach growls at midmorning or midafternoon, honor your hunger with a snack such as fruit, low-fat yogurt, or whole-wheat crackers and low-fat cheese, she suggests.

Do something with your hands. For some women, unwinding with food can be easily replaced by gardening, a craft, or even computer games—"anything that involves fine motor movement of fingers and hands," says Irish. Somehow, small, repeated movements help us chill out after a long day.

"Visualize a spring getting coiled really tight," says Irish. "Everybody gets their internal spring wound up tight all day. Sometimes, we eat at the end of the day just to unwind that spring—and it's really the repetitive motion of eating, not the food, that helps us unwind. I play solitaire on my computer, for example. Other people flip through magazines."

Stop, look, and listen. Take a 5- to 10-minute time-out before that first bite and think about what's going on. "Sometimes, you just need a few minutes to pull yourself together," says Moore. "You might get a cup of coffee or call a friend. You may be able to identify what's bothering you and decide to put it on the back burner till tomorrow, when you have the time or energy to deal with it directly."

Figure out what you want. If you've paused and still want to nosh, think of ways to minimize the binge. Before you reach for three candy bars or a big slice of cake, be clear about the food experience you're seeking, suggests Moore. "Find out what you really want," she says. "Will a cup of coffee do? Or do you really need a candy bar? Are you looking for a specific taste or do you want to fill yourself up? If it's a special taste, then maybe a small candy bar is all you need. If it's volume you're after, maybe fruit or popcorn is a smart choice."

Bargain down the size. Once you've decided what you want, ask yourself how much you really need, says Moore. Will one candy bar do instead of two or three? Will half a piece of cake satisfy you? "By keeping the size down—maybe to just a taste—you control overeating," she says.

Interrupt before the next bite. If you find yourself on automatic pilot, mindlessly reaching into the cookie bag, stop for a moment. "Ask yourself if this is really what you want to be doing and if there is anything else that you'd rather be doing instead," suggests Dickinson. "Often, emotional eating is done quickly. You don't even realize what's going on until the food is all gone. This gives you a chance to pause and be aware."

Balance the calories. Think about how much your indulgence will cost in terms of calories, then plan accordingly. You can compensate for the extra calories that come with an episode of emotional eating by eating less at another meal or two or by getting more physical activity, says Moore.

For example, compensating for a 250-calorie chocolate bar would mean skipping bread and butter at dinner and walking an extra mile.

"If you think about balancing the calories ahead of time, you might decide that the candy bar just isn't worth it," explains Moore. "That's when fruits, and vegetables like little baby carrots, start looking really good."

Or, you might decide that the candy bar is worth it. "And that's okay," Moore says. "The point is, you're not a bad person for eating this way. You simply have to adjust to avoid gaining weight."

Defuse high-risk times. Your mother's coming for a visit? Almost time for the annual family holiday gathering—and all the tense moments that come with it? "If you can predict high-risk situations and get ready for them, you can balance out the added calories in some way," Dr. Lindewall says. "You can always eat a little less before and afterward."

Challenge all-or-nothing thinking. If you do find yourself crunching instead of coping, don't despair. "That doesn't make you a bad person or mean that you've ruined everything," says Dickinson. "Even if you still experience some overeating, remember that you're making a change. It takes time. Don't lose sight of that."

When Overeating Gets Totally Out of Control

Kathi Geisler couldn't stop eating. She devoured bags of potato chips, then bought replacements so that her husband and daughters wouldn't discover her secret. She munched cookies in the bathroom, running the faucet to muffle the sound. After two years of bingeing episodes, she gained 100 pounds.

"I would go into what I call a food fog," says Kathi, 43, a public relations executive from Chelmsford, Massachusetts. "Time stops. You don't care about anything else. You get lost in this limbo world inhabited by just you and food. You don't know why, but you're compelled to keep eating."

Kathi later discovered that she had binge-eating disorder, a specific type of eating behavior that doctors have just recognized within the past few years. While it's hard to say just how common the problem is, binge-eating disorder affects one in three overweight women who seek help from university weight-loss clinics and nearly one in five who sign up for commercial weight-loss programs. "The binge eaters who come to us for treatment are often women over 35 who seek solace by eating large quantities of food and who feel out of control during a binge," says Marlene Schwartz, Ph.D., co-director of the Center for Eating and Weight Disorders at Yale University.

During a binge a woman often chooses foods that she regards as forbidden or dangerous or fattening—from to chips to slice after slice of toast slathered with peanut butter. She may feel as if she's in a trance, the state Kathi describes as a food fog.

Unlike women with bulimia, another behavioral problem, binge eaters do not purge afterward, Dr. Schwartz says. And unlike women who overeat once in a while, binge eaters are caught in a cycle that repeats itself several times a week.

"This isn't the same as eating too much at Thanksgiving dinner," Dr. Schwartz says. "Women with this condition have usually binged at least twice a week for at least six months. Food has become a way to cope, but then it ends up making them feel worse about themselves."

Bingeing or Simply Overeating?

Researchers are still debating the best ways to tell if a woman has binge-eating disorder. But, they say, you may have binge-eating disorder, and not a simple overeating problem, if you frequently eat abnormally large amounts of food, feel unable to control what or how much you eat, and you also have at least two of these experiences or feelings during a binge.

- Eat more rapidly than usual
- Eat until uncomfortably full
- Eat alone or in secret
- Feel depressed, guilty, or ashamed afterward

Another way to check is by asking yourself these four questions. If you answer yes to two or more, you may have binge-eating disorder, says Denise Wilfley, Ph.D., director of the Center for Weight Control and Eating Disorders at San Diego State University and the University of California, San Diego.

1. Are there times during the day when you could not have stopped eating, even if you wanted to?
2. Do you ever find yourself eating unusually large amounts of food in a short period of time?
3. Do you ever feel extremely guilty or depressed afterward?
4. Do you ever feel even more determined to diet or to eat healthier after the overeating episode?

Biggest, Baddest Bingeing Triggers

What prompts a binge? Loneliness, anger, sadness, frustration, and stress are often the triggers, Dr. Schwartz notes. Dieting, or severely restricting certain foods, can also lead to a binge episode.

"A woman who takes care of everything else in her life—her children, her spouse, her job, and her home—may not take the time to take care of herself. She may not feel entitled to put her own needs on the front burner," Dr. Schwartz says.

She may feel uncomfortable about conflict and find it easier to sweep her feelings under the rug, rather than sharing them with the people she's close to, Dr. Schwartz says. Or, she may simply be so busy that she has no time to sit down and sort out uncomfortable emotions.

And so she eats. She may hide the evidence, as Kathi did, or even stay home from social engagements, work, or school in order to eat.

"Bingeing temporarily soothes bad feelings by numbing you out," says Dr. Wilfley. "But afterward, a binge eater feels worse and tries to punish herself. She may resolve not to eat at all the next day, or to severely restrict certain foods."

But inevitably, she does eat again—for either emotional reasons, or simply out of hunger, or in response to the lure of forbidden food. "It's a natural reaction to eat when hungry," Dr. Wilfley says. "But just by eating, a woman who binge-eats may feel that she has blown her diet. She feels bad. So she eats more. And so the cycle of bingeing begins again. In this way, dieting and restricting foods can actually lead to more binge eating."

Breaking Free

Kathi overcame binge-eating disorder and has returned to her pre-binge weight by discovering and honoring her deepest emotional needs.

She kept a journal to track her feelings and makes it a priority to talk with friends and family members when there's a problem or she just needs to unwind. She goes for walks to tame stress—overriding one of her strongest binge-eating triggers. Kathi also found a therapist who helped her deal with a sexual assault from her teenage years, a deeply painful experience she had brushed aside for decades.

"That was a major experience I needed to understand, but I also had to stop turning to food for comfort in lots of situations," she says. "I still use food for comfort sometimes. But now, I don't criticize myself about it. And a small indulgence doesn't lead to a cycle of bingeing."

If you have, or suspect you have, binge-eating disorder, Dr. Wilfley says that you can overcome it by discovering and meeting your own emotional needs and by developing the habit of eating regular meals and snacks.

"A woman can try self-help techniques," Dr. Schwartz says. "Then, if she finds that she's not able to make changes on her own, finding a therapist or a support group is an excellent idea."

The Fat-to-Firm Program offers these ways to begin helping yourself overcome this disorder.

Write it all down. Keep a mood-food journal, as you would for simple emotional overeating. Use it to monitor all the foods you eat. Note when and how much you eat and how you were feeling at the time, suggests Dr. Wilfley. You may find that you skip meals, then binge out of hunger, or that certain situations trigger emotions that lead to bingeing.

Stick with regular meals and snacks. That means eating breakfast, lunch, and dinner as well as snacks in between to ward off hunger, Dr. Wilfley says. Follow this schedule even if it means having a meal soon after a binge, she says.

"After a binge, work even harder to get back into a regular schedule, rather than depriving yourself," she says. "You might have a small dinner if you binged beforehand, but the idea is to slowly become accustomed to regular eating and get out of the cycle of getting most of your calories from binges and little energy or nutrition from regular meals."

Worried about weight gain? In reality, your weight will probably stay the same or even drop as normal eating patterns replace high-calorie binges.

Put your needs first. The same steps toward self-esteem that help women overcome emotional eating are vitally important for women with binge-eating disorder as well, says Dr. Wilfley. So remember to take time to nurture yourself, challenge critical self-talk, and ask for what you need from others in an assertive way.

Problem-solve. Once you've identified your personal trigger emotions and situations for binge eating, try to spot them before a binge begins. Then, consider and evaluate solutions other than food. You may feel lonely, for example, and could call a friend, watch TV, or go for a walk. After considering the alternatives, act on your best solution.

Reach out. Many women find that a therapist or support group is invaluable in making the journey beyond binge eating, Dr. Wilfley says. "Just remember that this condition is just gaining recognition. Be sure to ask any therapist or group leader you're considering about their experience in treating binge-eating disorder."

To find a support group for eating disorders, contact your local hospital. The staff may also be able to refer you to qualified therapists. Or, for a list of university-based eating-disorder treatment centers, contact the Weight-Control Information Network, run by the National Institutes of Health, at 1 WIN Way, Bethesda, MD 20892-3665.

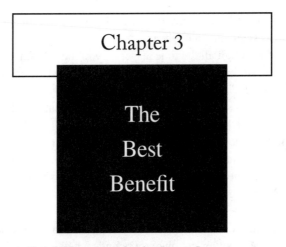

Chapter 3

The Best Benefit

**Looking good isn't the only reason
women go from fat to firm. Here's how to
lose a little weight—and gain a lot of health.**

Diane Sallemi was an expert on high blood pressure—her own. At home she ate heaping plates of buttery rigatoni with meaty red sauce; on the road, fast food was her cuisine of choice. And about the only "vigorous exercise" she got was brushing her teeth. By the time she was in her early forties, her blood pressure was in the danger zone and getting more threatening almost every day.

"I was gaining weight and getting scared," says this 46-year-old mother and bookstore clerk from Fountain Valley, California. "Despite taking two different medications every day, my blood pressure was still going up. Nothing was working."

Having high blood pressure meant that Diane's heart was working harder than normal, which put her at high risk for a heart attack or stroke.

"My father and his 10 brothers and sisters all had heart attacks," she says. "So I knew it could happen to me. When I was up to 245 pounds, I realized I had to do something. It was time to lose some weight."

(continued on page 38) ▶

Kicking the Habit:
When Extra Pounds Can Wait

When Ondie Neifert gave up her pack-a-day cigarette habit, she gained a dress size—and a big health bonus.

"I used to cough all the time, especially in the morning. Now that's stopped. And when I play softball, I don't have to work so hard to catch my breath," says Ondie, 40, a computer analyst from Easton, Pennsylvania, who smoked for 20 years. "It feels great—and I know I've lowered my risk for some big health problems."

A smoker since age 19, Ondie got serious about quitting after her doctor warned her about a precancerous sore in her mouth. "She was always after me to quit, telling me how women who smoke have a bigger chance of getting breast cancer and lung cancer, too," she recalls.

But like many women smokers, Ondie was afraid she would gain weight. "My mother put on extra pounds when she quit," she says. "It was one of my biggest worries."

To conquer it, she went shopping.

"I decided it would be okay to gain a few pounds. So I went out and bought some nice suits for work in a size 8, instead of my usual size 6," she says. "I also bought some casual clothes. I wanted to feel good about how I looked, instead of trying to squash into too-tight clothes."

Her strategy paid off. With the help of a nicotine patch, Ondie no longer craves cigarettes. Now, she's planning a new, healthy strategy for losing the 8 pounds she had put on.

"Those 8 pounds were worth it," she says. "The best thing in the world now is that my cigarette addiction is gone. I can fly across the country in an airplane and not go crazy waiting to smoke when it's over. The craving is gone."

Worth the Weight

Ondie's not alone. At the Cleveland Clinic Foundation's smoking-cessation program in Cleveland, director Garland DeNelsky, Ph.D., says that many women smokers who are reasonably satisfied with their weight worry that they're "going to gain a bundle of pounds" if they bid *adieu* to cigarettes.

"And for most women that fear just doesn't come true," he says. "After one year, the average weight gain is about 5 pounds."

And despite the health risks associated with weight gain, maintaining a low weight by smoking does not protect a woman's health. The opposite is true. "For any woman who smokes, there is no bigger health benefit than quitting," he says. "One statistic I've heard is that quitting a pack-a-day habit is as good for your heart as it would be for an extremely overweight person to lose 85 pounds. That's dramatic."

So are the rest of the facts about smoking's impact on women's health. About 140,000 women die each year from smoking-related diseases, including heart disease, lung cancer, chronic lung disease, and cancers of the pancreas, mouth, esophagus, urinary tract, and cervix. Women who smoke have a higher risk of breast cancer, reach menopause earlier, and experience more infertility than nonsmokers.

Our children don't escape the ill effects either. Smoking during pregnancy is associated with stillbirth, low birth weight, respiratory problems for babies, and even sudden infant death syndrome.

Quitting reduces or eliminates these risks. Studies show that after snuffing out the cigarettes, a woman's risk of heart disease drops by half within one year. The risk of lung cancer falls by up to half within 10 years. Quitters also experience fewer colds and less bronchitis, lower cancer risk, and better fertility.

"In addition, your breath is fresher. Your clothes stop smelling like stale smoke. The premature aging of the face—which can etch deep wrinkles around your eyes and mouth, thanks to reduced blood circulation—stops, and your skin looks better." Dr. DeNelsky says.

Be a Slimmer Quitter

You don't have to gain weight when you stop smoking. "Reach for smart substitutes, instead of something high in calories, when you want a cigarette," Dr. DeNelsky suggests. "Try sugarless gum or low-calorie soft drinks." Add some easy physical activity, such as walking, to your day. "Exercise boosts your metabolism in a healthy way, replacing the unhealthy boost it got from cigarettes."

But don't worry about a small weight gain in the midst of a smoking-cessation program, Dr. DeNelsky adds. "Quitting is your first priority. You can always work on weight loss later. Getting rid of the smoking habit is a gateway to better health."

And she did. She prepared low-fat versions of her beloved pasta and other favorite foods. She started an easy-does-it fitness routine. Slowly but very surely, the pounds began to disappear (55 at last count)—and so did her high blood pressure. After only nine months it was normal, and she no longer needed medication.

"I like the way I look," she says. "My husband even bought me some new clothes; he was so proud of me. But even more, I love the way I feel. I love being healthy."

The Drug-Free Way to Better Health

Feeling healthier—that's the number one reason to embrace the low-fat eating plan and the enjoyable, personalized exercise routine that you'll discover in the Fat-to-Firm Program, according to Ralph W. Cygan, M.D., clinical professor of medicine and director of the weight-management program at the University of California, Irvine, College of Medicine.

"The fact of the matter is, through better eating, moderate exercise, and small amounts of weight loss, you can often improve health problems like high blood pressure, diabetes, and high cholesterol," Dr. Cygan says. "You may not even need medication anymore. And if you have a family history of these medical problems, you can lower your risk for getting them in the first place."

And by preventing or reversing those three health problems—high blood pressure, high cholesterol, and diabetes—you also decrease your risk of dying from heart disease or stroke. Scientific studies reveal that "small amounts of weight loss" can bring a great deal of other health benefits, too. A reduction in your risk of breast and colon cancers. Less back pain and fewer aches in your knees and other joints. Less risk of a painful gallstone attack. More energy. Possibly, better sleep. Even more self-esteem.

"Losing small amounts of weight, if you sustain that weight loss, can yield significant health benefits," explains James M. Rippe, M.D., associate professor of medicine at Tufts University School of Medicine in Boston, director of the Center for Clinical and Lifestyle Research in Shrewsbury, Massachusetts, and author of *Fit Over Forty.* "Yet, few women truly understand how increased weight is harming their health—or how weight loss, healthy eating, and exercise can make dramatic improvements."

When Being Big-Boned Gives You an Edge

When it comes to avoiding osteoporosis—the brittle bone disease responsible for more than a half a million bone fractures a year among American women—lean women can learn a lot from larger-size women.

"The truth is, being overweight means stronger bones," says Gordon M. Wardlaw, R.D., Ph.D., associate professor of medical dietetics at Ohio State University in Columbus. "It sounds like heresy because so many other health problems are caused by being overweight. But here's one case where bigger is better."

But the big-body–strong-bones link shouldn't give lean women the green light to pack on pounds, Dr. Wardlaw notes. "There are too many other health hazards associated with being overweight. A woman can learn from this connection to help keep her own bones sturdy regardless of her body weight," he says. Here's how.

■ Bear some weight. A large woman puts mild stress on her bones with every step, stimulating mineralization. You can get the same effect with weight-bearing fitness routines such as walking, jogging, or aerobics, Dr. Wardlaw says.

■ Eat your calcium. A large woman may not be a strict dieter and may, as a result, get more of the calcium she needs for bone health. You can bone up on calcium with low-fat and nonfat dairy products as well as foods like calcium-fortified orange juice and canned fish with small bones, notes Dr. Wardlaw.

■ Consider estrogen at menopause. A large woman's body fat produces more estrogen, a hormone that aids in bone maintenance. At menopause, consider hormone replacement therapy to counteract falling estrogen levels that can compromise bone health, Dr. Wardlaw suggests.

A Little Weight Loss Goes a Long Way

When these doctors say that you only need to lose "small amounts" of weight to gain more health, exactly how many pounds are they talking about?

Well, when a panel of 20 experts on body weight gathered for the

American Health Foundation's Roundtable on Healthy Weight, they determined that the best healthy weight-loss goals for women who are overweight ránge from 10 pounds for a woman who is 5 feet tall to 14 pounds for a woman who is 5 feet, 8 inches tall. Such a modest loss, they concluded, was enough to turn the tide from a higher risk of disease to a higher likelihood of better health.

And yet, many women often strive for big weight losses. We long to look as svelte as a Hollywood actress or a runway model—and we feel defeated when we fall short of these unrealistic ideals. In essence, we let Barbie, Twiggy, or some air-brushed image in a fashion magazine become our weight-loss coach. And what cruel and demanding coaches they are.

"When women try to lose weight just to look thinner, they often go to extremes. They may try fad diets or exercise too hard or use diet pills. They may try to reach an unrealistic weight that cannot be maintained. They may harm their health," says Kathy McManus, R.D., manager of clinical nutrition at Brigham and Women's Hospital in Boston.

But none of that is necessary.

"Even very modest losses—even 5 or 10 pounds—can have a significant, positive impact on health," notes Susan Zelitch Yanovski, M.D., an obesity expert with the National Institute of Diabetes and Digestive and Kidney Diseases at the National Institutes of Health in Bethesda, Maryland.

Let's take a look at the details of that "significant, positive impact," how losing a few pounds can improve the health of almost every organ and system in your body.

The Weight Comes Off—And the Beat Goes On

Once considered a "man's condition," heart disease is now recognized as the leading cause of death among women in the United States. Many factors raise a woman's risk for a heart attack, such as menopause, a family history of heart disease, hypertension, diabetes, and unhealthy levels of blood fats.

But overweight may outweigh them all.

When researchers working on Harvard University's landmark Nurse's Health Study tracked the health of 115,195 women for 16 years, they found a strong relationship between weight and heart disease deaths. Compared with women whose weight remained stable, those who gained 22 pounds or more since the age of 18 had more than a 150

Banish Your Belly

Whether you can barely "pinch an inch" or have trouble seeing past your tummy to your toes, abdominal fat is the body fat that poses the biggest health risks for women, according to Susan K. Fried, Ph.D., associate professor of nutritional sciences at Rutgers University in New Brunswick, New Jersey.

"Intra-abdominal fat—the fat inside the abdominal cavity around our internal organs—is responsible for health problems," says Dr. Fried, who studies upper-body obesity and its impact on health. "It's often the real problem when people are overweight. And it's the one fat women should be most concerned about."

Not dreaded hip fat. Not jiggly thigh fat. Not even the blubbery fat that collects far too easily on our buttocks. Beware of belly fat, Dr. Fried says, because it's the body's most metabolically active fat.

"Hip fat and thigh fat are quiet fat," she says. "But belly fat produces a lot of fatty acids that go into the bloodstream and directly to the liver. This has a big impact on the body and can lead to diabetes, high blood pressure, and heart disease."

How can you tell if you have it? Start by lying down and looking at your belly. "If your fat hangs to the sides, it's most likely just under the skin," Dr. Fried says. "That's not good fat, but it's not as dangerous as the fat that pops up when you lie down. That's a sign of fat packed around internal organs."

You can also check your waist/hip ratio. (For directions, see "Determine Your Waist/Hip Ratio" on page 55.) "If your waist/hip ratio is over .85, you should sort of start worrying about it," Dr. Fried says. "Have your physician regularly check your blood lipids, blood pressure, and blood glucose to see if upper-body fat is having a deleterious effect."

Happily, Dr. Fried notes that a combination of physical activity and low-fat, low-calorie eating can reduce belly fat. "Aerobic exercise, like brisk walking, seems to be the most effective," she says. "Do it for at least 30 minutes, at least three times a week, and you can start to see abdominal fat shrink."

percent higher risk of heart disease. And women who were overweight by 40 pounds or more increased their risk by 600 percent.

The Fat-to-Firm prescription? Lose excess weight—or maintain a

Beyond Burning Calories:
The Fitness Prescription

Whether you walk, swim, bike, strut your stuff in an aerobics class, or take part in any kind of regular physical activity, the benefits a woman can derive from a regular fitness routine go far beyond toning and weight loss.

Physical activity alone—without a change in diet or losing a pound—can help reduce the risk of heart disease, calm high blood pressure, and improve diabetes.

Why? "Exercise can change your body composition, reducing body fat and increasing muscle size," explains endocrinologist and physiologist Robert H. Eckel, M.D., program director for the General Clinical Research Center at the University of Colorado Health Sciences Center in Denver. "With less body fat, those health risks drop," he adds.

A regular workout also encourages your muscle cells to work much more efficiently and has a beneficial effect on your nervous system.

Here's how exercise can help.

■ Lower your heart disease risk. Regular exercise, all by itself, can reduce a woman's risk by about 20 percent. "It raises levels of high-density lipoproteins," the beneficial cholesterol that helps protect you from heart disease, Dr. Eckel says.

For best results, aim for 30 minutes of aerobic exercise three days a week.

■ Tame high blood pressure. Physical activity has a unique ability to prevent high blood pressure—and to quickly lower it, says David

healthy body weight—by revving up your physical activity and eating a low-fat diet. These may be the most powerful steps a woman can take to lower her risk of heart disease.

"By losing weight, a woman can reduce dangerously high blood levels of low-density lipoproteins (LDLs) and triglycerides," says Penny Kris-Etherton, R.D., Ph.D., professor in the department of nutrition at Pennsylvania State University in University Park. "Once she stabilizes at a lower weight, levels of "good" high-density lipoproteins (HDLs)

McCarron, M.D., head of the division of nephrology, hypertension, and clinical pharmacology at Oregon Health Sciences University in Portland.

"Often, it's really the exercise that's responsible for a drop in blood pressure when a woman loses weight," Dr. McCarron notes. Working out may soothe raging blood pressure by calming the sympathetic nervous system, which controls the tightening and relaxing of blood vessels.

Aim for 20 to 60 minutes of moderate activity, such as brisk walking, cycling, or swimming, three to five times a week.

■ Prevent or improve diabetes. Physical activity prompts your body to transport glucose into cells and use your own insulin more effectively, reducing insulin resistance.

"That means blood sugar is under better control," says certified diabetes educator Guyton Hornsby, Ph.D., associate professor of exercise physiology at West Virginia University in Morgantown. "This can help prevent the development of Type II diabetes, the most common form of diabetes. It also means someone with diabetes might need less medication."

A fitness routine that successfully maintains control of blood glucose levels can also prevent some of the serious complications that come with diabetes—such as hypertension, heart disease, kidney damage, blindness, and nerve damage. Aim for 20 to 40 minutes of exercise at least three times a week, suggests the American Diabetes Association. But first, consult your doctor.

rise. Exercise also raises HDLs. This is important news for us because low HDLs and high triglycerides are two predictors of heart disease in women." (LDL cholesterol is the "bad" kind that clogs arteries. HDL cholesterol is the "good" kind that helps banish LDLs from your body. Triglycerides are another heart-damaging blood fat.)

Now, we're not talking about achieving major shifts in levels of blood fat—we're talking about a very productive nudge. For every one-point rise in HDLs, heart disease risk drops by 3 percent. Risk also drops 2 to 3 percent for every 1-percent drop in total cholesterol. Dr. Kris-Etherton and her colleagues estimate that a woman who adopts a low-fat diet, loses weight, and exercises regularly can reduce her risk of heart disease by up to 30 percent.

While the risk of heart disease is low for most women until menopause, premenopausal women should take preventing heart disease very seriously, Dr. Cygan says. "It's never too early for prevention. It's never too early—or too late—to make a difference."

Turn Down the Pressure

High blood pressure seems a bit like gray hair—the older you get, the more likely it is to make an appearance. One in eight women between the ages of 35 and 44 has high blood pressure. That rate doubles to nearly one in four by the time women reach age 54. And by age 64, nearly half of all women have joined the club. But there's one big difference between gray hair and high blood pressure. Gray hair doesn't cause heart disease and stroke.

"High blood pressure carries a big health penalty," says David A. McCarron, M.D., head of the division of nephrology, hypertension, and clinical pharmacology at Oregon Health Sciences University in Portland. With high blood pressure, your risk of a stroke is 12 times higher than that of a woman with normal blood pressure, and your risk of a heart attack goes up sixfold. Kidney failure is also more likely.

There are many causes of high blood pressure. But one has become increasingly obvious to health scientists. "High blood pressure, and all the problems that come with it, gets worse as a woman's weight and body fat grow larger," says Dr. McCarron.

The good news is that the Fat-to-Firm Program, with its emphasis on maintaining a healthy weight, may be a woman's best defense against high blood pressure. And losing weight may be the most effective strategy to calm blood pressure that's already soaring—better, in fact, than taking blood-pressure medication as a first course of action. Up to half of the Americans who take high blood pressure medication could reduce or eliminate these drugs by losing as little as 9 to 11 pounds, Dr. McCarron says.

And changes in blood pressure levels can come quickly. "When a woman is losing weight, she may see her blood pressure start to decrease within the first two or three weeks," he says.

Diabetes: When Sugar Isn't Sweet

Overweight is a major risk factor for Type II (adult-onset) diabetes, the most common form of the disease. So, since a higher percentage of women than men are overweight, they have a higher incidence of diabetes: Of the 16 million Americans with the condition, over half are women.

"Central obesity—tummy fat and fat around internal organs—is the real culprit," says Ronald Arky, M.D., professor of medicine at Harvard Medical School and chief of the diabetes section at Brigham and Women's Hospital in Boston. "This kind of overweight," he continues, "increases insulin resistance." Insulin is the hormone that allows cells to use blood sugar for fuel. When there's insulin resistance, too much blood sugar stays in the bloodstream—and you have diabetes.

You also have low energy, and you're thirsty. Among women, diabetes quadruples the risk for heart disease. Untreated, diabetes can cause complications like blindness, kidney disease, stroke, and nerve damage.

A pregnant woman with untreated diabetes puts her child at greater risk for birth defects and infant death. And mothers with diabetes are more likely to need cesarean sections because their condition puts them at higher risk for large-birth-weight babies.

Happily, there may be a natural way to prevent and treat diabetes: Lose weight. According to the American Diabetes Association, trimming 5 to 10 percent of body weight (for a 150-pound woman, that's 7½ to 15 pounds) greatly improves the way cells use insulin.

In the Nurse's Health Study, women who lost more than 11 pounds cut their risk for diabetes by 50 percent. But women who gained 11 to 17 pounds between age 18 and middle age raised their risk by 90 percent. And women who gained between 17 and 23 pounds increased their risk by 170 percent.

So a healthy weight-loss plan like the Fat-to-Firm Program, says Dr. Arky, can help delay or prevent diabetes in women at high risk for the disease: women who are overweight; have a family history of diabetes; are predisposed to the disease, such as African-Americans, Hispanics, and Native Americans; or have a history of gestational diabetes (a temporary form of the disease that can develop during pregnancy).

"Losing weight and being physically active are the most therapeutic things you can do for Type II diabetes," Dr. Arky says. "There's nothing like a weight loss of 5, 10, or 15 pounds to improve things and to reduce the need for medication."

Problem Solved

I Hate to Exercise!

Call Diane Sallemi a fitness phobe.

At 245 pounds, Diane, 46, of Fountain Valley, California, knew she needed physical activity to help shed excess weight and control her high blood pressure. "But I had never done any exercise in my life. Zero. I barely could get started," she says.

So she concentrated on doing exactly what she liked very, very s-l-o-w-l-y.

"I decided to walk and use an exercise bike," she says. "The first day, I could barely do a total of 5 minutes."

Now, she's up to 45 minutes a day. "I walk through my neighborhood; it's nice to get out and see other people," she says. "And I usually watch TV while I use the bike. I like a shopping channel."

Today, call her a fitness fan. "I've noticed that regular exercise keeps my blood pressure down even when I eat a little extra food," she says. "And it helps in other ways. The other day, my car broke down, and I had to walk home about 2 miles. It was no big deal. I wasn't even out of breath."

And if you have Type II diabetes, says the American Diabetes Association, maintaining a 10 to 20 percent weight loss for three years or more reduces your chances of developing complications from the disease, lowering the risk as much as 40 to 60 percent for some people.

The Cancer Connection

Scientists aren't sure why extra pounds can increase a woman's risk of cancer, but the link is clear, especially for reproductive cancers. Compared with lean women, women who are 30 to 40 pounds overweight have a 1½ to 3 times higher risk of endometrial cancer. Overweight may also be associated with higher risk for ovarian cancer, as is a high-fat diet.

Rates of breast cancer are higher among postmenopausal women who are overweight, says I-Min Lee, M.D., Sc.D., assistant professor of medicine at Harvard Medical School. Women with more abdominal fat are also at higher risk. "Body fat causes greater production of the hormone estrogen, which plays a role in the development of reproductive cancers," she notes.

While overweight doesn't seem to raise breast cancer risks for younger women, the weight gain that eventually can stack the odds against women seems to begin decades before menopause, according to researchers from the H. Lee Moffitt Cancer Center and Research Institute at the University of South Florida College of Medicine in Tampa. What's the riskiest decade for weight gain? The thirties, when childbearing can increase body fat and new responsibilities whittle away the free time a woman could have used to stay fit.

Colon cancer is also more common among overweight women and is also related to lack of physical activity, a high-fat diet, and low intake of fruits and vegetables.

How can you respond to the cancer-overweight connection? "Don't gain weight," says Dr. Lee says. "That can be hard to do—American women gain about 1 to 2 pounds a year. Exercise seems promising for reducing the risk of breast cancer. And eating a low-fat diet with plenty of fruits and vegetables seems important for reducing the risks of other cancers."

A healthy weight. Regular physical activity. Lots of tasty, good-for-you fruits and vegetables. They're all cornerstones of the Fat-to-Firm Program.

Soothe the Pain of Arthritis—Or Prevent It

When arthritis strikes a woman's knees, hips, or even hands, excess pounds are often the culprit.

David T. Felson, M.D., professor of medicine and public health at Boston University School of Medicine, estimates that a woman who loses just 11 pounds cuts her risk of knee arthritis in half. And if you're already coping with the twinges, aches, and pains, weight loss can soothe knee pain. "Small losses can make a big difference," he says.

Women who are more than 40 pounds overweight have four times more arthritis of the knees than normal-weight women. It may be simply a matter of force: Knees absorb an impact equal to three to six times the weight of your body with each step, notes Dr. Felson. More pounds may eventually mean more force than your knee joints can comfortably handle.

Enter the Fat-to-Firm Program. With gentle, healthy weight loss, the ache of arthritis is likely to ease as you slenderize.

High blood pressure, high cholesterol, heart disease, stroke, diabetes, cancer, arthritis. Serious conditions—but the Fat-to-Firm Program is serious, too. Serious about improving your health.

▶

Chapter 4

Figuring Out Your True Weight-Loss Needs

**Deciding on a *realistic* new weight is
the best way to guarantee that you'll stay
thinner for the rest of your life.**

For Jill Cude, a 42-year-old engineering-company manager from Houston, the weight-loss countdown began one January.

"I wanted to lose weight in time for my 20th high school reunion, scheduled for August," she says. "The question was, how much to take off?"

Jill weighed 143 pounds but longed to return to the lithe 122 pounds she had weighed as a high school senior. "But the dietitian who was helping me suggested that we talk about a more-appropriate weight—128 pounds, a weight I could maintain and not look emaciated," she recalls. "At first, I wasn't sure I'd like it."

By August, Jill had shed 15 pounds, reaching her revised but realistic goal. On reunion night, she slipped into a size 6, red silk pantsuit with rhinestones sparkling at the shoulders and discovered that *realistic* also meant attractive. "My outfit looked fabulous," she recalls. "I got a lot of compliments."

Best of all, Jill has maintained her new weight ever since by following a healthy eating plan and fitting lots of activity into her day. Her long-term success is real proof that she had, indeed, determined her true weight-loss needs. At 128 pounds Jill looks and feels great, and she can maintain her new slim look with a comfortable amount of physical activity and with meals that don't sacrifice nutrition or the foods she really loves. As a bonus, she has also lowered her risk for a variety of health problems.

Wants, Needs, and Reality

If you've ever stood in the mirror, frowning at your hips, tummy, or thighs, or consulted an "ideal body weight" chart and found that you're pounds away from perfect, then you, like Jill, have probably dreamed about how much weight you *want* to lose.

If a doctor has ever advised you to shed pounds in order to control a medical condition like high blood cholesterol, diabetes, high blood pressure, or heart disease, then you have probably heard about the pounds you *need* to lose.

And if you've ever attempted to slim down and discovered that reaching a goal weight—or maintaining it—is more challenging than you ever expected, then it's likely you've discovered that many factors control how much weight you actually *can* lose.

That's why determining your true weight-loss needs is an essential part of the Fat-to-Firm Program. Figuring it out means that you need to balance your desires, your needs, your lifestyle, and your body's natural tendencies, according to Shiriki Kumanyika, R.D., Ph.D., professor and head of the department of human nutrition and dietetics at the University of Illinois, Chicago, and a member of the advisory committee that established the U.S. government's 1995 Dietary Guidelines for Americans.

"There's no magic number," says Dr. Kumanyika. "A woman cannot pick a goal weight off a chart. She has to factor in her own current weight and weight history, her family's health history, her personal health goals, her own eating patterns, and her level of activity. Then, she can pick a weight-reduction target that makes sense."

For women, making this highly personal decision often means stepping away from our culture's loud-and-clear message that thinner is better.

"Weight for women is a huge emotional issue," says Debbie Then, Ph.D., a psychologist in private practice in Los Angeles. "Women are valued in society for their looks, while men are more often valued for what they do. So women feel much more pressure, from within and from outside, to be thin. As a result, many women never really appreciate their own unique, beautiful bodies."

The Fat-to-Firm Program offers three ways to determine your true weight-loss needs. But first, experts suggest asking yourself a couple of key questions.

Why Do You Want to Lose Weight?

At the Duke University Diet and Fitness Center in Durham, North Carolina, program and medical director Michael Hamilton, M.D., asks a simple question of women who want to lose weight: Why?

"The best reason to lose weight is if you feel your weight is in some way negatively impacting your life," says Dr. Hamilton.

"Excessive weight could be jeopardizing your health or interfering with your ability to get up in the morning and have the energy to do the things you want to do. It could be making you feel embarrassed and unwilling to go out socially to the movies or on a hike or to parties," Dr. Hamilton says.

So ask yourself, does your weight interfere with your life—physically, socially, or psychologically? If your answer is yes, consider the reasons. Do you find yourself turning to food to calm stress or soothe difficult emotions? If so, it may be time to break the emotional eating cycle. (For more information on emotion-driven eating, see chapter 2.) Or do you simply feel too big to take part in activities you enjoy, or do you know that your weight is a health risk? Then a new eating plan and more physical activity may be all you need, says Dr. Hamilton.

Do you find yourself postponing changes you would like to make in your life, telling yourself that happiness, new relationships, new interests, or a different job must wait until you've lost weight? The real barrier may not be your weight at all, says Marcia Hutchinson, Ed.D., a psychologist in the Boston area and author of *Transforming Body Image: Learning to Love the Body You Have.*

"I like to ask women, 'Well, what would be different about your life if you were thinner—how would your relationships change, how would the way you project yourself in the world change, how would the way you care about yourself change, how would the way you feel about yourself as a sexual being change?' " Dr. Hutchinson says. "Getting rid of extra pounds won't change other parts of your life, unless you can also make a change in how you think about yourself."

Start by making a list of the things that you would like to do, or be, "if only" you were thinner, suggests Dr. Then. You may want to feel more attractive, take up a new hobby, or make a job change. Next, make an action plan for achieving those goals—which will include, but not be limited to, adopting a healthy eating plan and adding more physical activity to your day. The process may bring up fears and insecurities, but it can also be very empowering, she says.

What Kind of Shape Are You In, Really?

Often, women approach weight loss by dreaming about the number of pounds they would like to lose, rather than by having a clear picture of how their bodies actually look. If your mental image of your body shape is inaccurate—if, for example, you dislike your hips and thighs because you think they're huge when in fact they're only slightly padded—you may set an unattainable weight-loss goal.

"It's important for a woman to have a realistic sense of her body before beginning a weight-loss program," says Yasmin Mossavar-Rahmani, R.D., Ph.D., assistant clinical professor in the department of epidemiology and social medicine at Albert Einstein College of Medicine of Yeshiva University in New York City. "Otherwise, she may diet unnecessarily or try to lose too much weight."

In a study at a Brooklyn hospital, Dr. Mossavar-Rahmani and other researchers asked 150 women employees—from doctors to laundry workers—to estimate their body sizes. When the researchers compared their guesses with accurate measurements, they found that half the women had inaccurate perceptions—believing their bodies were bigger, or sometimes smaller, than they actually were. The less accurate a woman's self-perception was, researchers found, the more likely she was to diet.

One way to find out if you have a true-to-life mental picture of your own body shape is to make a life-size drawing of what you think your body looks like on an old sheet or taped-together newspaper pages. Then, lie down on the drawing and have a friend trace your true outline, suggests Dr. Hutchinson. "Women tend to overestimate their body size. I've asked women to do this in workshops, and invariably, their perception and emotional sense of themselves is bigger than they really are."

Calculate Your Body Mass Index

To find your body mass index (BMI), locate your height in the left column. Move across the chart (to the right) until you hit your approximate weight. Then follow that column down to the corresponding BMI number at the bottom of the chart.

Your ideal BMI? Between 20 and 25. But each woman's ideal

Height	Weight (lb.)						
4'10"	91	96	100	105	110	115	119
4'11"	94	99	104	109	114	119	124
5'0"	97	102	107	112	118	123	128
5'1"	100	106	111	116	122	127	132
5'2"	104	109	115	120	126	131	136
5'3"	107	113	118	124	130	135	141
5'4"	110	116	122	128	134	140	145
5'5"	114	120	126	132	138	144	150
5'6"	118	124	130	136	142	148	155
5'7"	121	127	134	140	146	153	159
5'8"	125	131	138	144	151	158	164
5'9"	128	135	142	149	155	162	169
5'10"	132	139	146	153	160	167	174
5'11"	136	143	150	157	165	172	179
6'0"	140	147	154	162	169	177	184
BMI	**19**	**20**	**21**	**22**	**23**	**24**	**25**

If, by doing this exercise, you discover that your mental image of your body is wildly inaccurate, adjust your weight-loss goals accordingly.

Body Mass Index: Better Than a Scale

You can further pin down your "real" size with a measurement tool recommended by weight-loss experts: the body mass index (BMI).

Body mass index is a single number based on a scientific formula that compares your height to your weight. (To determine your BMI, consult the chart, "Calculate Your Body Mass Index.") The result helps predict

BMI depends, in part, on her personal health risks and age. Heart disease, breast cancer, diabetes, and arthritis may all be affected by a high BMI. On the flip side, the good news for women with large BMIs is this: You can reduce health risks significantly by losing just enough weight to drop one number from your BMI.

Height				Weight (lb.)			
4'10"	124	129	134	138	143	148	153
4'11"	128	133	138	143	148	153	158
5'0"	133	138	143	148	153	158	163
5'1"	137	143	148	153	158	164	169
5'2"	142	147	153	158	164	169	174
5'3"	146	152	158	163	169	175	180
5'4"	151	157	163	169	174	180	186
5'5"	156	162	168	174	180	186	192
5'6"	161	167	173	179	186	192	198
5'7"	166	172	178	185	191	197	204
5'8"	171	177	184	190	197	203	210
5'9"	176	182	189	196	203	209	216
5'10"	181	188	195	202	207	215	222
5'11"	186	193	200	208	215	222	229
6'0"	191	199	206	213	221	228	235
BMI	**26**	**27**	**28**	**29**	**30**	**31**	**32**

whether you are at risk for weight-related health problems. Most likely your BMI will fall somewhere between 19 and 32. If you're 5 feet, 4 inches high, for example, and you weigh 122 pounds, your BMI is 21. But if you're 5 feet, 4 inches tall and weigh 157, your BMI is considerably higher—27. Dr. Hamilton says the safest range is 20 to 25.

"A BMI of 25 to 30 is overweight," says Dr. Hamilton. "Your risk for health problems like heart disease starts going up. Above 30 definitely puts somebody in the obese category."

What's your healthiest BMI? The answer depends a great deal on your personal and inherited risk for a variety of health problems, including the following.

- Heart disease: If you're at risk for heart disease, a BMI below 22 may be safest, according to Harvard University's ongoing Nurse's Health Study. Among 115,886 women studied for eight years, 605 developed coronary artery disease. Women with BMIs under 21 had no elevated risk; risk rose gradually for BMIs up to 25 and then sharply thereafter.
- Diabetes: Women with BMIs over 28 raise their risk of diabetes, according to the American Diabetes Association.
- Breast cancer: If you have a family history of breast cancer, a BMI below 27 may be safer.
- Other health conditions: With a BMI above 27, your risk rises for conditions such as arthritis, gout, and above-normal levels of cholesterol and triglycerides (blood fats that can increase heart disease risk).

As a rule, women under age 35 should aim for a BMI of 25 or lower. You may gain weight as you age, and starting with a healthy BMI helps protect you from medical problems, says Dr. Hamilton.

What if your BMI is already outside the "ideal" range? The good news is that a woman can reduce her health risks if she loses just 10 to 14 pounds—dropping from, say, a BMI of 30 to a BMI of 28—according to a panel of 20 body-weight experts who gathered for the Roundtable on Healthy Weight, a forum sponsored by the American Health Foundation, in New York City.

Through healthy, low-fat eating and a gentle fitness plan—key components of the Fat-to-Firm Program—you can reach and maintain a healthier BMI, says Dr. Hamilton.

Where's the Fat?

Where you're overweight can be just as important as how much you weigh. Women who carry extra fat at the abdomen are at higher risk for weight-related health problems, while fat packed on your hips and thighs poses much less risk (though such fat may be harder to get rid of), says Susan Fried, Ph.D., associate professor of nutritional sciences at Rutgers University in New Brunswick, New Jersey, who studies the links between health and abdominal fat.

Get a clear picture of this fat zone with another measurement tool,

Determine Your Waist/Hip Ratio

Is your weight increasing your risk for health problems? To find out, don't just step onto the bathroom scale. In addition, measure your waist and hips and use the following formula to determine your waist/hip ratio—an additional method for assessing health risks, says Michael Hamilton, M.D., program and medical director of the Duke University Diet and Fitness Center in Durham, North Carolina.

1. Measure your waist at its slimmest point.
2. Measure your hips at the widest point.
3. Divide your waist measurement by your hip measurement:
   ____(waist in inches) ÷ ____(hips in inches) =
   ____(waist/hip ratio).

If the ratio is higher than 0.8, you may be at higher risk for heart disease, stroke, diabetes, high blood pressure, and possibly even breast cancer, according to Dr. Hamilton. Going from fat to firm can help improve your waist/hip ratio and improve your health profile.

the waist/hip ratio. Find yours by measuring your waist at the smallest point and your hips at their widest point. Then divide your waist measurement by your hip measurement. (If your waist is 34 and your hips are 42, for example, your waist/hip ratio is 0.8.) For women, waist/hip ratio over 0.8 indicates an increased risk for diabetes, heart disease, and high blood pressure, says Dr. Hamilton.

Diet, aerobic exercise, and strength training—cornerstones of the Fat-to-Firm Program—all help burn that excess fat. And the best way to keep track of your progress is an old-fashioned tape measure—or your bedroom mirror, Dr. Hamilton adds.

What about using other body-fat measuring devices, such as the calipers and electronic testers available in many gyms, to chart your fat-burning progress?

"I tell women it's not worth checking unless they're simply interested," says Dr. Hamilton. "The normal body fat range for a woman is 22 to 28 percent. But most measuring devices are not accurate enough to tell you if you've really changed, so it can be frustrating to check it after a

Discover Your Healthiest Weight Range

Once you know your body mass index and your waist/hip ratio, you can combine the two to discover your healthiest weight range, with this easy-to-use chart.

To determine whether you body weight is on target or is increasing your disease risk, find your BMI on the vertical column and your waist/hip ratio on the horizontal line. Now, locate the point where they meet to see if you may need to trim some pounds or inches.

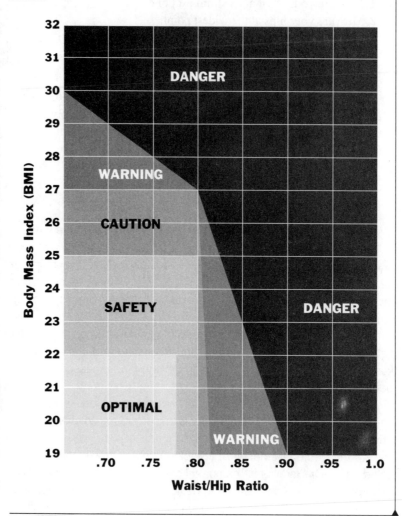

few weeks or months. It's better just to look in the mirror—if it looks like fat, it probably is fat."

What's Your Easy 'Maintenance' Weight?

You may find another important clue to your body's natural, healthy weight range by thinking back over your weight history as an adult—or by looking through the back of your closet for the clothes that once fit, says Dr. Hamilton.

Take a look at your past—and think about a weight that has seemed natural for you as an adult. Perhaps you weighed 140 for many years, then suddenly began putting on the pounds. Perhaps your "easy maintenance" weight was a bit higher than that or a bit lower. Regardless of the number, it was a weight that seemed to maintain itself, staying nearly the same whether you ate a little more or a little less or engaged in a little more or a little less physical activity.

"I like to find out what a woman weighed before she started to gain weight in adulthood," Dr. Hamilton says. "I ask if there was a weight she somehow easily maintained for a period of time. If there was, then that's probably a reasonable goal to return to."

One woman, who tipped the scales at nearly 200 pounds, told Dr. Hamilton that she wanted to slim down to 130. But when she told him that she had once maintained a weight of 160 and felt pretty good about it, he encouraged her to set a goal of 160 instead of 130.

If you've always been overweight, you may find useful clues in the weights and body sizes of your own relatives, he says.

"If both parents gained weight at a certain time in their lives, there's probably a strong genetic tendency for their children to gain weight then as well," Dr. Hamilton notes. "That simply means you have to be realistic and careful. Genes may influence 30 to 50 percent of your weight, but you can stay in control through a healthy diet and an exercise program," he adds.

What Can You Do for the Long Run?

So, look ahead. Your goal weight should be one you can maintain comfortably for years to come, one that fits into your lifestyle.

"The trick is not only losing weight but also keeping it off," says

► 57

Problem Solved

"I'm Not Fat, I Just Don't Like My Body"

Your friends and your bathroom scale tell you that your weight is just fine—yet you're still dissatisfied with how you look. What gives?

"Even normal-weight women seem to see their bodies as if they're looking in a fun-house mirror—nothing's right," says Debbie Then, Ph.D., a psychologist in private practice in Los Angeles. "It helps if a woman can gain a realistic appreciation of her body."

If your weight is fine but your self-image needs a tune-up, try these expert tips.

Think of yourself a whole person, not a collection of parts. Avoid obsessing about individual body parts and start thinking of your body as one entity, Dr. Then suggests. Play up your most attractive features and appreciate how well your body works as a whole.

Value your natural grace. Use everyday movements as an opportunity to enjoy your body's innate grace, suggests Marcia Hutchinson, Ed.D., a psychologist in the Boston area and author of *Transforming Body Image: Learning to Love the Body You Have.* "Ask yourself, 'How do I feel in my body right now?' Try this as you get up from a chair or move across the room. This can help develop a stronger internal sense of living inside your body."

Move more. If you feel clumsy or awkward, consider taking a movement class such as yoga, dance, or one of several specialized movement classes like the Feldenkrais method, Dr. Hutchinson suggests. "Many women who struggle with body image actually lack a strong sense of body awareness—they're very aware of the flaws but not aware of how well they move or can move," she says. "By taking such a class, you can develop a stronger sense of grace, of enjoying yourself as you move."

Appreciate your own uniqueness. Train yourself to appreciate your own uniqueness by appreciating it in others, Dr. Hutchinson suggests. As a first step, recall the so-called flaws of some famous, gorgeous women—such as Barbra Streisand and her prominent nose, Meryl Streep and her close-set eyes, Oprah Winfrey and her once comfortably cushioned body. "These women are not remotely perfect-looking, but they're magnetic, expressive, and attractive," she notes.

Richard L. Atkinson, M.D., professor of medicine and nutritional sciences at the University of Wisconsin in Madison and past president of the American Society for Clinical Nutrition. "To do that, you have to come up with a plan you can live with forever."

The Fat-to-Firm Program is a forever plan—not a crash diet or an extreme exercise program. It offers practical, healthy low-fat eating strategies that fit all occasions. You won't have to give up birthday cakes, ice cream in summer, or turkey and stuffing at Thanksgiving. A wealth of fitness options suit every lifestyle, budget, and schedule.

And on the Fat-to-Firm Program, you won't go hungry or miss out on important vitamins and minerals that a woman needs—and that are often missing from fad diets.

"A woman who maintains a low weight by eating few calories is probably not getting enough of the nutrients she needs for good health and protection from disease," Dr. Kumanyika says.

On the Fat-to-Firm Program, you won't find yourself roped into an exercise plan that's torture or eats up your precious time either. "If your life becomes hell, then your weight-loss goal is not workable," Dr. Hamilton notes. "When someone tells me, 'I maintained my goal weight by eating broccoli three times a day and running 6 miles every morning,' I suspect they're not going to be able to keep it up, because that doesn't sound like a workable lifestyle over the long term."

Putting It All Together: Your Fat-to-Firm Goal Weight

So there you have it: three very good ways to decide on a goal weight. You may want to lose 5 pounds or 45 pounds. You may not want to lose any weight at all but simply to lose body fat and firm up.

How can you turn your need into an easy, workable goal—one aimed at success? Consider these three ways to think about goal-setting, suggested by weight-loss experts.

First, hold the line. If you've been gaining more and more weight, your first goal might be simply to stop putting on pounds, says Dr. Kumanyika. "Ninety percent of diets are a failure," she notes. "Your best strategy might be first understanding how to hold the line, and then evaluate how and whether you can lose weight."

Set a small goal. Losing just 5 to 10 percent of your weight can dramatically improve many weight-related health problems. Small losses—10 pounds or less—can also give you a big boost of self-confidence, says Dr. Hamilton. "And within days of changing your diet, you'll feel more energetic, too."

Break a big goal into small goals. If your goal is a big one, break it down into a series of small victories, suggests Anne Dubner, R.D., a nutrition consultant in Houston and a spokesperson for the American Dietetic Association. "Don't set yourself up for unrealistic expectations," she says. "Set your sights on losing 10 pounds or less. Concentrate on that. You'll get good results." Then go to the next goal, and the next.

Chapter 5

The Age Factor: Why Was It Easier When I Was Younger?

Middle-age spread is not inevitable. In fact, as you erase the weight, you can erase the signs of aging, too.

Svelte in a midnight-black dress, 48-year-old Eileen Morgan strolled through the Philadelphia Museum of Art one spring evening with her daughter Kristen, 25. As they both admired an exhibit of French paintings, a passerby posed a surprising question. "Are you sisters?" he asked.

"I was flattered," recalls Eileen, a bank vice president from Pennsylvania. "It's nice when people think that you look younger than you are, though I think being compared with a lovely 25-year-old is a bit of a stretch."

Still, with her blonde hair, ready smile, and slender frame—at 5 feet, 8 inches, she weighs 140 pounds—Eileen exemplifies just how attractive a woman can look even as she reaches age 50.

But don't chalk up Eileen's success to luck, good genes, or regular visits to expensive spas. She credits healthy personal choices—like those recommended by experts as part of the Fat-to-Firm Program—for helping her to avoid creeping, decade-by-decade weight gain.

"I'd battled an extra 5 or 10 pounds all my life," she says. "I would diet, then re-gain the weight. Now, instead, I eat low-fat foods that I like. And every once in a while, I indulge in the high-fat foods I love—like Swiss chocolate or Häagen-Dazs ice cream."

To stay fit, Eileen sails in summer, skis in winter, works in her flower garden, and—when her busy job permits—takes aerobics classes. She also avoids the sun or slathers on protective sunscreen to shield her fair skin from wrinkle-making rays, further belying her age. "And I don't smoke cigarettes—I think that helps my skin, too," she says. In addition, Eileen chooses clothing styles that flatter her figure.

"Nobody wants to look old," she says. "And I don't think a woman has to—if she works at it a little."

The Myth of Middle-Age Spread

While sculpting a firmer, healthier, more attractive body can require new strategies as women age, "it is absolutely possible to look and feel 20 or even 30 years younger," says Miriam E. Nelson, Ph.D., an exercise physiologist in the human physiology laboratory at the U.S. Department of Agriculture Human Nutrition Research Center on Aging at Tufts University in Boston.

"It takes time. It doesn't happen overnight. It takes a commitment. But it is a miracle," Dr. Nelson says. "A woman can look fantastic. She can have that youthful spark. That bounce in her step. That firmness when she walks."

First, Dr. Nelson says, stop believing that middle-age spread is inevitable. Yes, it's true that most of us do gain weight as the birthdays roll by. According to the Centers for Disease Control and Prevention, the percentage of American women who are overweight rises dramatically with age: from one in five women in their twenties, to one in three women in their thirties and forties, to one in two women in their fifties.

But ultimately, this accumulation of extra pounds is not written in our genes, our hormones, or the laws of nature. Over the years, those factors do influence a woman's body shape, size, and her share of muscle and fat. But weight gain happens, quite simply, when we become less active, says William Evans, Ph.D., professor of applied physiology and nutrition and director of the Noll Physiological Research Center at Pennsylvania State University in University Park and author of *Biomarkers: The 10 Keys to Prolonging Vitality.*

"A sedentary lifestyle explains about 80 percent of body fatness," says Dr. Evans. "When a woman is inactive, she loses muscle mass. With less muscle mass, her body burns significantly fewer calories around the clock."

The Couch-Potato Factor

The evolution from svelte to saggy usually coincides with the onset of adult responsibilities, Dr. Evans notes.

"As people take on jobs and begin raising families, they tend to have less time for recreation than they did in their early twenties," he says. "We seem to be less likely to ride a bike or walk somewhere than we used to. We don't go out dancing or play sports—we go out to dinner or watch television. We can't go for a stroll because there are diapers to be changed or the kids need help with the homework. A lot of subtle changes take place that really add up."

Physical inactivity is a double whammy, according to Larry T. Wier, Ed.D., director of the health-related fitness program at the NASA Johnson Space Center in Houston. "Losing weight is harder if you're not in the habit of being active. You'll have less muscle strength and less functional ability, at least at the start, for physical activity. And if you've been seden-tary for a long time, you can't take advantage of the extra calorie-burning that muscle provides."

The good news is that a woman can begin reversing the couch-potato factor with as little as 2 hours and 15 minutes a week of walking, swimming, or other moderate physical activity, Dr. Wier says. And, of course, more is better. So the Fat-to-Firm Program includes moderate amounts of regular, purposeful exercise.

As the decades roll by, the benefits are significant.

"If you take a 70-year-old woman who walks or bikes or performs some moderately intense activity for 4 hours a week, and if she keeps her body fat level under control with a low-fat diet at the same time, she'll be able to handle about 30 percent more activity than a woman who is 45 years old and who doesn't get much physical activity beyond walking from her car to the office," Dr. Wier says. "That means the 70-year-old's muscles will work better. She'll feel more energetic. And she'll burn more calories."

The Motherhood Factor

Researchers are only beginning to understand the impact of preg-nancy and childbearing on a woman's weight.

How Will You Look 10 Years from Now?

Some aspects of aging are unavoidable—like the "character" lines that come with the passing years.

But other changes we associate with age, from weight gain to wrinkles caused by the sun to the ravages wrought by smoking, can be avoided, according to dermatologist Margaret A. Weiss, M.D., assistant professor of dermatology at Johns Hopkins Medical Institutions in Baltimore, and James O. Hill, Ph.D., associate director of the Center for Human Nutrition at the University of Colorado Health Sciences Center in Denver. Here's what a woman who follows the Fat-to-Firm Program can expect in her twenties, thirties, forties, and beyond if she takes age-preventive measures.

In her twenties: Thanks to regular aerobic activity and a muscle-building routine, she hasn't lost muscle or gained weight, despite responsibilities at home and work that take more and more time.

Sunscreen, protective clothing, and a hat keep sun-induced wrinkles and other skin damage to a minimum.

In her thirties: Pregnancy may leave behind unwanted pounds, and new or increased job demands may cut into her free time. While women who don't get enough exercise lose muscle and gain weight, her continued activity holds off muscle loss and all but the slightest drop in metabolism.

Facial expression lines may appear on her brow and along the inner curve of her cheeks for the first time. Since a certain amount of sun exposure is inevitable, minor skin changes associated with sunlight may be evident: She may notice small wrinkles, even white patches on the arms, hands, and legs. To minimize wrinkling, she should continue to protect her skin from the sun.

While women who smoke may show lines and wrinkles around eyes and mouth and may have less-elastic skin, not smoking avoids those problems, says Dr. Weiss. And if she does smoke, it's never too late for her to quit to forestall additional damage.

"Pregnancy has not been given enough attention by the medical community," says James O. Hill, Ph.D., associate director of the Center for Human Nutrition at the University of Colorado Health Sciences Center in Denver. "But women know it can make a big difference. They know that,

In her forties: Commitment to an active lifestyle and low-fat eating keeps pounds at bay as she approaches menopause. Metabolism continues to slow slightly, but she'll still feel—and look—young and energetic.

She may notice that her skin feels drier and fine lines appear, calling for a light moisturizer. Some sun damage appears: perhaps brown spots on the backs of hands, small wrinkles on the face, dryness of the V of skin at the neck and chest. Sun protection should continue to be a priority. Skin creams containing alpha hydroxy acids (gentle compounds derived from fruit sugar) can help smooth tiny crinkles and wrinkles and uneven pigmentation, says Dr. Weiss.

In her fifties and beyond: By now, her ovaries produce less and less estrogen and progesterone, two key female hormones. (If she has had a hysterectomy, removing the ovaries shuts off hormone production abruptly.) Menopause can also bring loss of muscle, more body fat, and a thickening waistline—but less so for the woman who is physically active and continues to perform muscle-strengthening exercises, says Dr. Hill.

Her cheeks may sag and jowls may form, signs that fat deposits under the skin are shifting in response to gravity and that her skin is losing elasticity. Skin coloring may become uneven—she may notice subtle changes as the skin thins and replenishes itself more slowly, as well as more dramatic age spots and sun damage. Avoiding sun exposure keeps more serious wrinkles and age spots at bay, says Dr. Weiss.

Regular physical activity keeps muscles toned and firm and bones stronger, helping slow the loss of bone and maintaining muscle, while other women are losing more of both. She will also feel more energetic than many of her friends.

If she is following a program of energetic activity and healthy, low-fat eating, her vitality makes her appear younger than her peers, despite the eventual "character lines" that come with maturity.

often, their bodies hold on to weight differently once they become mothers. For some women, the weight is difficult to lose."

But the extra pounds women gain during pregnancy don't have to become permanent additions to their hips, thighs, or tummies. According to the National Center for Health Statistics, 57 percent of women who were at a normal weight before pregnancy returned to within 4 pounds of their original weight 10 to 18 months after delivery.

Another 22 percent retained an extra 4 to 8 pounds, while another 20 percent were more than 8 pounds heavier. The women had each gained 25 to 35 pounds during pregnancy—the amount now recommended by experts from the National Academy of Sciences as healthier for babies than previous suggestions that women gain just 15 to 25 pounds.

Breast-feeding can help reduce a mother's post-delivery weight. But if you're well beyond the breast-feeding stage, stubborn postpartum pounds can be trimmed with a familiar formula: Get up, get going. "Physical activity, again, is very important," Dr. Wier notes. "We encourage mothers to follow their kids around, to be as active as the children are. It helps."

The Fat-to-Firm Program shows you how to build more physical activity into your daily routine, to further whittle away postpartum pounds.

The Menopause Factor

When a woman's reproductive years end at menopause, a drop in levels of the hormone estrogen can trigger changes that reshuffle her weight, her shape, and even the proportion of muscle and body fat she carries.

When researchers from the University of Vermont tracked the body compositions of 35 women for six years, they found that those who entered menopause lost 6½ pounds of what the researchers call fat-free mass—that is, muscle, bone, organs, and so forth. "We think a significant portion of what they lost was muscle mass," says researcher Michael Toth, Ph.D., a physiologist and postdoctoral fellow in the department of medicine at the University of Vermont in Burlington, who worked on the study.

The menopausal women also burned 230 fewer calories a day than the women who were approaching menopause but still premenopausal. "We think the women burned fewer calories in part because they had less muscle and in part because they were less physically active," Dr. Toth says. "That could be one of the reasons they also had more body fat. Changes in estrogen levels may have caused more of the fat to accumulate at the abdomen."

Body weight may even begin to climb within the year prior to menopause, according to a study of 577 women by researchers at the Institute of Clinical Medicine in Bologna, Italy.

Researchers firmly maintain that the menopause factor can be overcome. "Menopause may accelerate some of these weight-gain and body-composition changes, but I say, fight it," notes Eric Poehlman, Ph.D., professor of medicine at the University of Vermont.

Diet, physical activity, and muscle-building routines—all components of the Fat-to-Firm Program—can all help, say Doctors Toth and Poehlman.

Beating the Age Factor

Physical activity, the kind you enjoy. Low-fat eating, with recipes for guilt-free versions of your favorite foods. Savvy clothing choices to accentuate your best features. These components of the Fat-to-Firm Program are also the keys that experts—and women like Eileen Morgan—recommend for overcoming the factors that make us look and feel older than we would like.

Customize your age-erasing plan by targeting whatever trouble zone you feel makes you look older than you are, whether it's wide hips, a potbelly, sun-weathered skin, or an outdated wardrobe. Here's how.

Rev up your metabolism. Through easy muscle-strengthening exercises, you'll give your metabolism a push while you tone your tummy, hips, thighs, and more. "Strength training, using hand weights or exercise machines, can increase muscle strength by 5 percent every session," says Dr. Evans. More strength means more muscle mass. And more muscle mass means that you're burning more calories all the time. "In one study, women were burning 15 percent more calories every day after 13 weeks of training," he notes.

Go aerobic—and love it. Burn more calories and reduce stress with three short sessions of walking, biking, or other moderate-intensity activity a week, suggests Dr. Hill. "The most important thing is to pick an activity you like, something you can do three times a week for the next 30 years," he says. "If you don't like the gym, then don't go. Exercise should be enjoyable."

Aim to burn 300 to 400 calories each time—about what you would burn if you walked for 45 minutes to 1 hour.

Build movement into your day. You've heard it before, but it works: Take the stairs, not the elevator. Deliver messages in person, not

(continued on page 71) ▶

Remodel Your Body

Frustrated by a stubborn figure flaw? A protruding tummy that resists your most diligent dieting efforts? Wide hips that defy your efforts at overall slimming? Breasts that seem to get smaller as you get slimmer? With a savvy mix of diet, toning, and fashion, you can tame the trouble zones. Try these Fat-to-Firm remodeling strategies for the figure flaws that bother women the most, offered by women experts on nutrition, fitness, and fashion.

Tubby Tummy

Eating strategy: A healthy, low-fat diet will help shrink abdominal fat. It may also relieve bloating that can make your abdomen protrude, says Anne Dubner, R.D., a nutrition consultant in Houston and a spokesperson for the American Dietetic Association.

Toning strategy: Daily stomach crunches will tone and flatten, but be patient. While small gains come within weeks, it may take six months or longer to really tone stomach muscles, says Nancy C. Karabaic, a certified personal trainer from Wheaton, Maryland.

Clothing strategy: Focus attention on good features—like a wonderful bustline, collarbones, or face—with jewelry, scarves tied creatively around your neck or draped at your shoulders. Create an elongated look with one-color or tone-on-tone outfits in a single shade, like classic navy or gray, or a fashion color, such as champagne, suggests Clara Prezio-Henry, director of the fashion-design program at the Philadelphia College of Textiles and Science.

Wide Waist

Eating strategy: Dubner suggests a low-fat diet. It probably won't give you a cinched look, but it can help reduce body fat at the waist.

Toning strategy: Daily stomach crunches that work oblique muscles, along the sides of the abdomen, are very effective for achieving a slimmer look. Expect noticeable results in three to six months, says Karabaic.

Clothing strategy: Create the appearance of a trim waistline with dropped-waist dresses and skirts and with graceful, one-piece dresses that draw the eye away from this problem area, notes Prezio-Henry.

Hefty Hips

Eating strategy: Low-fat eating effectively reduces body fat all over the body, but in women, hip fat is often stubborn. All-over fat reduction may leave you with the same pear-shaped proportions, says Dubner.

Toning strategy: If the problem is excess weight, walking or other aerobic exercise will effectively burn fat. For toning, try sessions two to three times a week on weight machines that work the hip muscles. You can expect results in three to six months, Karabaic advises.

Clothing strategy: If you have broad pelvic bones or a genetic tendency to store fat at your hips, fashion is your best strategy, says Karabaic.

Create a long, flowing line that de-emphasizes hips with a tunic, a long cardigan, or a long jacket over a slim skirt, slim pants, or long, flowing skirt. Avoid full skirts gathered at the waist and short, cropped jackets that stop at waist or top of hip, suggests Prezio-Henry.

Large Thighs and Saddlebags

Eating strategy: Thigh fat tends to resist dietary changes, says Dubner. Nevertheless, she advocates low-fat eating and says that it is mildly to moderately effective. In other words, dieting alone won't give you perfectly svelte thighs, but it helps pare them down to some degree.

Toning strategy: Squats and lunges, performed while holding hand weights, work back and front of thighs. Even "stubbornly" big thighs will look sleeker when toned, with small results in a few weeks, more noticeable results in three to six months, Karabaic says.

Clothing strategy: Think loose and long. Straight-leg pants in crisp fabrics like gabardine, longer jackets, and slim skirts that skim the hips and thighs create slimming effects quickly. Avoid clingy or tight skirts and pants, says Prezio-Henry.

Ample Derriere

Eating strategy: Expect some reduction with a low-fat diet, Dubner notes.

(continued) ▶

Remodel Your Body—Continued

Toning strategy: Buttocks respond excellently to squats and lunges, performed while holding hand weights. Add aerobics to burn more fat. Small changes come quickly—look for a big improvement in three to six months, says Karabaic.

Clothing strategy: Choose clothes that subtly help to achieve a wedge shape—wide at the shoulder and narrow at the hemline—to make your body look tapered. (This strategy works best for taller women.) Other options: Dress in single colors and layer long tops over slim pants or skirts to create long, vertical lines, suggests Prezio-Henry.

Droopy Breasts

Eating strategy: Changing what you eat won't help, says Dubner.

Toning strategy: You can help support sagging breasts by strengthening your chest muscles. Do strength-training moves that work the pectoral muscles of the chest such as dumbbell bench presses and dumbbell flies, says Karabaic. (To learn how to do these two exercises, see pages 273 and 274.)

Clothing strategy: A well-fitting bra can smooth and lift the bustline, says Prezio-Henry. Have your bra custom-fitted at a lingerie store or better department store. Also, avoid wide belts and wide waistbands that shorten the torso, she says.

Flabby Upper Arms

Eating strategy: As with saggy breasts, changing your diet won't help underarm flab, says Dubner.

Toning strategy: Your best bet is to concentrate on toning your triceps, the muscle on the underside of your upper arm, with dumbbell exercises or resistance training machines. Also work your biceps—the top muscle—for shapely upper arms, suggests Karabaic.

Clothing strategy: Avoid sheer, tight, or short sleeves that draw the eye to this trouble zone. Lengths that fall anywhere from your elbow to wrist are best, says Prezio-Henry.

via e-mail. "When you need to find a parking space, keep in mind that all those people who parked at the closest places did you a favor. You want to park way back in the most-distant lot so that you can spend 5 to 10 minutes walking to your office and 5 to 10 minutes walking back," says Dr. Wier. "Adding more activity to all aspects of your day will burn more calories."

Slash the fat. By cutting the fat in your diet to about 25 percent of total calories, you can shed pounds, feel satisfied, and even feel more energetic. "We recommend people follow a low-fat diet as part of a plan to fight the body-fat changes that come with menopause," says Dr. Toth.

Look your best. By choosing styles that camouflage certain contours and highlight your best features—be it long legs, a slender waist, a beautiful neck, or a curvy figure—you'll look at your best, right away. Go a step further and wear styles that look modern, yet flattering. "You have to keep looking like the time period you live in," says Eileen. "You have to move on. It helps you stay young. And it's fun."

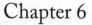

Chapter 6

Personalize Your Program

Individual solutions that meet your needs are what takes the weight off and keeps it off.

What a difference a year can make—just ask Ann or Mindy or Doris.

Ann Rinaldi still adores pizza topped with melted mozzarella cheese. Pasta with homemade red sauce remains her idea of the perfect dinner. In late afternoon she pauses for a few anisette cookies and a cup of tea at her desk. "It refreshes me," she says.

Hardly deprivation. Yet Ann, a 52-year-old customer service manager from Boston, lost more than 15 pounds in less than a year, lowering dangerously high cholesterol levels and cutting her risk for heart disease significantly.

"I've cut down the portions of high-calorie foods that I love, but I haven't cut them out entirely," she says. "I eat more fruits and vegetables. And I walk every day."

Mindy Kane still savors chocolate. And she's found a way to squeeze a workout into her busy schedule almost daily. As a result, she lost 50 pounds in a little more than a year—something fad diets never accomplished.

"I tried them all, but diets were so inflexible," says Mindy, 38, a project support manager at a Houston engineering company. "For me, flexibility was the key."

Doris Anglin, a 53-year-old mother of three, also from Houston, shed an impressive 258 pounds in 2½ years—a loss of about 100 pounds a year—after various weight-loss diets and even a stomach-shrinking operation failed. Success came with a meal strategy that met her nutritional needs and made peace with her cravings. (Doris snacks twice a day because otherwise, she says, "I'm dangerous when I'm hungry!") She added gentle workouts that fit her pace—first mall-walking, then exercising at a gym.

"It feels good to be in control—to make myself happy at the same time my weight is dropping," she says. "The secret? You have to figure out what works best for you."

Your Personalized Fat-to-Firm Road Map

As Ann, Mindy, and Doris discovered, quick weight-loss schemes or rigid eating plans won't take you from fat to firm—or help you stay there. What does? Trusting yourself and meeting your own particular needs—whether it's for an afternoon cookie, a slow-and-easy walking plan, or regular snacks to keep hunger at bay.

"The very idea of a diet is the opposite of what works," says Susan Kayman, R.D., Dr.P.H., program coordinator of regional health education for the Kaiser-Permanente Medical Group in Oakland, California, who has studied women who have successfully gone from fat to firm. "What really helps women lose weight and keep it off are very individual solutions."

Dr. Kayman found that women who successfully maintain a new, lower body weight remind her of Frank Sinatra singing, "I did it my way." "These women designed their own plans. Each had her own personal strategy that fit her life, her schedule, and her tastes," she notes. "They solved problems that stood in their way."

When you customize a program to meet your own unique needs, you'll see steady, positive changes that can last a lifetime, Dr. Kayman says. You'll learn to trust your ability to listen to your body and to firm and nourish it in your own way. More and more experts are convinced that this customized approach is the only route to achieving and maintaining a healthy body weight—and that one-size-fits-all diets are doomed to failure precisely because they don't recognize your unique needs.

That's exactly what this book can help you accomplish. The Fat-to-Firm Program is not a set of strict rules or a special weight-loss diet or a painful exercise routine. It's a set of tools you can use to design a custom-tailored firm-up plan that's perfect for you now and in years to come.

The Future You

What's in the Fat-to-Firm toolbox? The latest information and practical advice on low-fat eating, fitness, self-esteem, and looking good, from leading doctors, nutritionists, psychologists, personal trainers, and even fashion experts—with dozens of strategies for customizing the program to meet your own needs. Throughout, real women just like you share their success stories of conquered food cravings, firm-up routines wedged into time-crunched schedules, and eating plans that make room for restaurant meals and sinfully delicious treats.

You'll discover hundreds of ways to design the custom-tailored firm-up plan that's perfect for you now and in the future.

When you adapt a plan to fit your lifestyle, there's a good chance that you can follow it for years—come rain or shine, whether you're stressed-out or relaxed, busy or bored, contented or blue, notes Anne Dubner, R.D., a nutrition consultant in Houston and a spokesperson for the American Dietetic Association.

"If you want the magic in weight loss, get a mirror," Dubner says. "The person you see in the mirror is the one who will lead you to success."

Here's how the Fat-to-Firm Program can help you achieve and maintain a healthy weight—by doing it your way.

Goal #1: Lose Body Fat

The "twin engines" of fat-burning—easy aerobic workouts and healthy, low-fat eating—are the best ways to reduce body fat, says I-Min Lee, M.D., Sc.D., assistant professor of medicine at Harvard Medical School.

What to do: Customize your plan by choosing a workout you love—whether it's walking, swimming, pedaling an exercise bike in your bedroom, or jogging around the park. Follow a satisfying, low-fat, high-fiber eating plan that still includes your best-loved foods. Try recipe makeovers for your all-time favorites. And use strategies to help you cope with special situations—like meals away from home, holiday dinners, and cooking for a family that likes high-fat fare.

Together, fitness and low-fat foods can help keep a woman firm for a lifetime. "Exercise actually does more than burn calories while you're doing it," Dr. Lee says. "It motivates people to stick with a good eating plan. It gives you a psychological edge. If you've just walked 3 miles, you may be less likely to give in to a slice of cake or a candy bar."

Benefits: When you lose body fat, you look sleeker, feel more energetic, and may—if your aerobic-fitness choice is a weight-bearing exercise like walking or aerobic dance—build stronger bones, says Ralph W. Cygan, M.D., clinical professor of medicine and director of the weight-management program at the University of California, Irvine, College of Medicine. You also lower your risk for diabetes, high blood pressure, and heart disease—serious health risks for everyone, including women.

Goal #2: Gain Firmer, Trimmer Muscles

A gentle strength-training routine—at home or at the gym—at an easy pace for just 1½ hours a week will super-charge your firm-up program without building bulky, muscle-bound arms and legs, says William Evans, Ph.D., professor of applied physiology and nutrition and director of the Noll Physiological Research Center at Pennsylvania State University in University Park and author of *Biomarkers: The 10 Keys to Prolonging Vitality.*

What to do: Customize your strength-training program by working out at home or at a gym—and by choosing small barbells and dumbbells, resistance bands that look like rubber bands, or machines like Nautilus.

Benefits: Working with weights creates shapely, toned muscles and more muscle mass that burns more calories 24 hours a day, reversing the metabolic slowdown that can make women fat as they age, Dr. Evans says. Weight training also protects and strengthens bones, which is especially important after a woman reaches age 35, the period when her bones begin losing calcium.

Goal #3: Love What You Eat, Eat What You Love

The Fat-to-Firm Program is not a diet. No deprivation, ever. It calls for three meals a day, plus snacks. And room for the foods you love—

Problem Solved

Busy Women Can Eat Smart

Wondering how you can tailor a weight-loss plan to your own special needs? Here are four examples from women who found success with customized strategies.

Eat Half Now, Half Later
Ann Rinaldi, 52, of Boston, lost 15 pounds.

What she did: "I find that when I eat out, the best thing is to eat half of what I'm served," she says. "I love pizza, for example. But now, instead of having four slices, I start with a salad, then eat two slices, and take the rest home."

Why it works: In a healthy eating plan there are no forbidden foods. By controlling portion size, you can eat and enjoy virtually any food without guilt or a weight increase, says Anne Dubner, R.D., a nutrition consultant in Houston and a spokesperson for the American Dietetic Association.

A Quick Fix for Busy Nights
Jill Cude, 42, of Houston, lost 15 pounds.

What she did: "I was working full-time and going to school at night, so dinner was a problem," says Jill. "I didn't want to eat late at night when I got home, and I wanted to avoid fast food and the vending machines at the office. So I started bringing a sandwich to eat between work and school."

Why it works: Learning to identify unique trouble zones and work out custom-tailored solutions is one of the most powerful skills that a woman can use for successful weight loss and weight maintenance, says Susan Kayman, R.D., Dr.P.H., program coordinator of regional health education for the Kaiser-Permanente Medical Group in Oakland, California. "It's important to explore different solutions and not give up until you find one that works," she says.

whether it's Steak Diane, blue cheese dressing on fresh salad greens, or Ben and Jerry's New York Super Fudge Chunk Chocolate ice cream.

What to do: Customize your eating plan by eating what you like best—from snacks to dinners out, from chocolate to meat loaf. "There are no bad foods," notes nutritionist Dubner. "It's important to keep eating

The Souped-Up Solution

Diane Sallemi, 46, of Fountain Valley, California, lost 55 pounds.

What she did: "I make and eat a lot of vegetable soup," says Diane. "I really like it, it's full of vegetables and fiber that are good for me, it's really filling—and it takes time to eat, so I don't reach for other foods. It's a godsend when I come home from work really hungry."

Why it works: Foods with the fewest calories for their size and weight—like vegetables as well as fruits and grains—fill you up and provide needed nutrition without blowing your calorie budget for the day, says Dubner. Since it takes longer to fill up on vegetable soup than, say, fudge, you're less likely to overeat.

A Grab Bag of Snacks

Doris Anglin, 53, of Houston, lost 258 pounds.

What she did: "I keep safe snacks in my car—it's my emergency kit," she says. "Inside are rice cakes, fruit, and air-popped popcorn, usually. If I'm stuck somewhere and can't get a good meal or need a snack, I'll be okay. I'll also eat something from the bag before leaving the car to go to a party—to avoid high-fat snacks that will be served."

Why it works: Easy-to-transport foods, like fruits or cut-up vegetables in a plastic container, are perfect for times when you know you'll be hungry but won't have access to the healthy, low-fat foods at the center of your new eating plan, says Michael Steelman, M.D., founder of the Steelman Clinic in Oklahoma City, Oklahoma, and past president of the American Society of Bariatric Physicians.

what you really like, or you'll feel deprived. You just have to know how to do it."

Benefits: By incorporating your favorite foods into your Fat-to-Firm eating plan, you get the nutrition a woman needs to maintain strong bones, protect herself against disease, and stay alert and energetic all day. You also get the tastes and eating experience you enjoy—like birthday cake, a special night out, or a satisfying little splurge—without guilt or second-guessing.

Goal #4: Look and Feel Wonderful—Now

The Fat-to-Firm Program will help you value yourself more highly, love yourself more deeply, and take new steps toward the life you want, with expert guidance from psychologists who specialize in women, body image, and self-esteem.

What to do: Customize your plan by identifying traps that keep you from enjoying the body you have—and from presenting yourself well. Dress like a fashion pro, with detailed clothing options tailored to camouflage your trouble zones and make the most of your own best features.

Benefits: You'll gain freedom from a negative body image, freedom to enjoy looking great and feel terrific, and freedom to get on with your life and do the things you want to do.

You can stop playing the "if only..." game, too. By boosting self-esteem you can feel and look your best right away. No need to say, "If only I were skinny, then I would feel attractive or have a scintillating social life or get a new job." You can do it now.

"You don't have to lose 20 or 30 pounds in order to achieve what you want in life or have good relationships or be creative and constructive," says G. Ken Goodrick, Ph.D., assistant professor of medicine at Baylor College of Medicine and associate director of the Behavioral Medicine Research Center, both in Houston. "You can be happy and enjoy yourself now."

As Doris, the woman who lost 258 pounds says, "I may not be at my goal weight yet, but I'm taking great care of myself. Sometimes, I don't even recognize myself. At a holiday party I walked past a mirror and said to myself, 'Who's that attractive, happy woman?' I had to pinch myself—it was me."

Part 2

Eating Food
and
Loving It

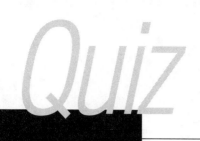

How Much Fat Do You Really Eat?

Are you making low-fat choices? What's your total fat intake? Find your "Fat I.Q." with this quiz developed by Diane Grabowski-Nepa, R.D., a nutritionist at the Pritikin Longevity Center in Santa Monica, California. Read the following statements, then rate your habits by using this scoring system.

1 = Most always   3 = Not usually
2 = Often   4 = Rarely/Never

Then, tally your score below and find new ways to cut fat out of your eating plan.

_____ **1.** To flavor bread products such as bagels, English muffins, or toast, I use nonfat cheese spreads, fruit jams, apple butter, or enjoy them plain.

_____ **2.** I use skim or low-fat milk (containing no more than 1 percent milk fat by weight).

_____ **3.** When selecting dairy products such as cheese, sour cream, cottage cheese, or cream cheese, I choose nonfat varieties.

_____ **4.** When ordering from a menu, I request my food be broiled, grilled, steamed, or baked with little or no fat.

_____ **5.** I avoid fried foods whenever possible.

_____ **6.** To sauté vegetables and other foods, I use no-stick cooking sprays, defatted broth, tomato juice, or wine in place of oils or other fats.

_____ **7.** I remove the skin from chicken or turkey before eating.

_____ **8.** When ordering a salad in a restaurant, I request it without dressing, cheese, olives, or croutons.

_____ **9.** I use nonfat condiments such as mustard or fat-free mayonnaise or salad dressing as sandwich spreads.

_____ **10.** If selecting soup in a restaurant, I favor tomato-, vegetable-, or broth-based varieties rather than creamy types.

_____ **11.** My frozen dessert choice consists of nonfat yogurt, ice cream, or sorbet.

_____ **12.** Instead of cream sauces, I choose tomato-based sauces such as pomodora or marinara to serve over pasta.

_____ **13.** I choose fish or poultry more often than beef, lamb, or pork.

_____ **14.** I include beans and lentils to create meatless meals.

_____ **15.** When preparing tuna, chicken, or potato salad, I use nonfat mayonnaise or yogurt or small amounts of low-fat mayonnaise.

_____ **16.** If choosing snacks, I select pretzels, baked tortilla chips, or fat-free potato chips.

_____ **17.** I eat several servings of fresh fruits and vegetables each day.

_____ **18.** When selecting poultry, I choose the breast meat rather than legs, thighs, or fryers.

_____ **19.** If choosing red meat, I select the leanest cuts such as round steak or top sirloin.

_____ **20.** When dressing a salad, I use low-fat salad dressings or flavored vinegars, lemon juice, or salsa.

_____ **Total Score**

Scoring: If you scored 20 to 30 points, you're a low-fat whiz. You're consuming a low-fat diet averaging below 25 percent of your calories from fat. Keep up the good work by choosing fresh fruits, vegetables, grains, nonfat dairy products, and lean protein.

If you scored 31 to 50 points, you're eating less fat than most Americans do. Your daily fat intake range is approximately 25 to 35 percent of calories from fat. Reduce fat further by substituting pasta, potatoes, vegetables, and beans for meat, cheese, and fried foods. Prepare food by steaming, baking, broiling, or sautéing with little or no added fat.

If you scored 51 to 80 points, you're eating in the high-fat zone. Your daily fat intake is greater than 35 percent of calories from fat. But small changes can bring your intake down. Try low-fat salad dressings and mayonnaise, no-stick vegetable/butter sprays, and nonfat dairy products. Substitute baked, broiled, or grilled foods for fried, battered, or crispy items.

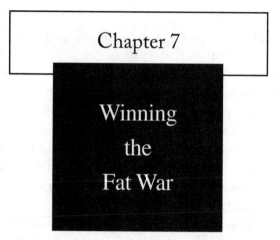

Chapter 7

Winning
the
Fat War

**Here are more than 100 easy,
effective strategies for declaring
victory over high-fat foods.**

Gwen Rutherford loved fat—in all its creamy, crunchy, rich-and-gooey glory.

There was fast fat, dripping from the cheeseburgers and french fries she grabbed at the drive-through window. Easy fat, in the chocolate bars and cream-filled snack cakes calling out to her from the office vending machine. Stealthy fat, hidden in the pork barbecue and blue cheese salad dressing she adored.

"Today, I can barely eat those things," says Gwen, 48, a computer operator from Williamsburg, Virginia. "Since I've cut back on fat, my body rebels against that stuff."

Siphoning the fat out of her meals and snacks helped Gwen lose more than 70 pounds—including more than 5 inches from each of her thighs. Today, her idea of fast food is a low-fat frozen dinner stashed in the office freezer for when she has to work late. Easy foods are the flip-top cans of fruit cocktail and the low-fat granola bars in her desk drawer. And she has devised a feel-good strategy for enjoying luscious, fat-loaded treats without overeating—or feeling remorse.

"I still eat the foods I like," Gwen notes. "But I'll have a little low-fat salad dressing now instead of gobs of the regular kind. I always ate chocolate ice cream when I had a sore throat, and now I have low-fat frozen yogurt. And once in a while, I get a snack cake from the vending machine—the raspberry Zingers are really good."

If she polishes one off, it's no disaster. "There are plenty of fat-free foods like fruit and vegetables that will fill me up the rest of the day," she notes. "And I exercise. So I know I'm burning calories, too. I never feel deprived. I'm eating just the way I want."

Eating Lean: A Woman's Number One Priority

When it comes to snack time and mealtime, reducing fat gets top priority on the Fat-to-Firm Program.

"Cutting dietary fat is a woman's single most important eating strategy for shedding excess pounds and reducing the risk of problems like heart disease, high blood pressure, diabetes, and even some types of cancer," says James J. Kenney, R.D., Ph.D., a nutrition research specialist at the Pritikin Longevity Center in Santa Monica, California. "There's plenty of evidence that it should be a woman's first priority."

What's the evidence? Consider this.

- In a Cornell University study, 13 women who ate moderately low fat meals for 11 weeks lost an average of 5½ pounds, and without going hungry—or suffering from hallucinations about chocolate brownie sundaes.

The low-fat diet got 25 to 30 percent of its calories from fat—it was not a drastic eating plan at all," says David Levitsky, Ph.D., professor of nutrition and psychology at Cornell University in Ithaca, New York, and the lead researcher on the study.

The women liked their low-fat meals and ate as much as they wanted. Still, they took in 220 fewer calories a day, compared to their calorie intake on the typical American diet.

"They were filled up," Dr. Levitsky says. "That's the really exciting lesson here: If you eat low-fat and replace the fat with fruits, vegetables, and grains, you can eat a lot. You can feel satisfied, and you can lose weight."

What would a day on the Levitsky plan taste like? For breakfast: granola, a banana muffin, and skim milk. For lunch: a turkey sandwich and blueberry yogurt. For dinner: chili with corn muffins, carrot-raisin salad, and chocolate pudding. "That's how my wife and I eat at home," he says. "We really enjoy it."

■ Low-fat eating can help break the cycle of yo-yo dieting. When researchers at Michigan State University followed the progress of 15 women and 14 men who had just completed a weight-loss program, they found that those who kept the weight off ate less fat and were more physically active.

"An eating plan that gets 20 to 30 percent of calories from fat would help a woman maintain a healthy body weight," notes researcher Sharon Hoerr, Ph.D., associate professor in the department of food science and human nutrition at Michigan State University in East Lansing. "Any woman who's lost weight and regained it would benefit. But remember," Dr. Hoerr cautions, "low-fat does not mean no fat."

"The best message is, eat five to nine servings of fruit and vegetables a day and six to 11 servings of grains, half of which should be high-fiber whole grains—not fat-free cookies, cakes, and ice cream. You need foods that will satisfy you and give you the nutrients you need," adds Dr. Hoerr.

A Healthy Bonus

A low-fat eating plan that incorporates fruits, vegetables, and whole grains is also a powerful, positive force for good health. Here's how it helps.

■ Keeps hearts healthy. Reducing saturated fat—found in meats, dairy products, and tropical oils such as coconut oil or palm oil—can reduce dangerous levels of blood cholesterol, reducing a woman's risk for heart disease, says W. Virgil Brown, M.D., director of the division of arteriosclerosis and lipid metabolism at Emory University School of Medicine in Atlanta and past president of the American Heart Association.

■ Protects against diabetes. Maintaining a healthy weight can lower your risk for diabetes, says Susan K. Fried, Ph.D., associate professor of nutritional sciences at Rutgers University in New Brunswick, New Jersey. Losing as little as 10 pounds can also help you control existing diabetes and may even reduce the need for medication.

■ Guards vision. A high-fat diet may be linked with a higher incidence of macular degeneration, the leading cause of legal blindness in the United States, experts say.

- Lowers cancer risks. A low-fat diet may reduce the risk of colon cancer, non-Hodgkin's lymphoma, and skin cancer, say experts. Maintaining a healthy weight can help reduce the risk of breast cancer after menopause and endometrial cancer. So plan a diet that forgoes chops, shakes, and buttered rolls for pasta with vegetables, hearty soups, whole-grain crackers, and fruit.

How We Really Eat

Chances are you're thinking to yourself right now, "Yes, I know that I should cut out the fat. I'm trying to cut out the fat. But I'm not losing any weight. It's a lot harder than I thought. Something's not working."

If that's the case, you're not alone. The truth is, American women are eating almost as much fat now as they did in the late 1980s, according to the United States Department of Agriculture. That's because, studies show, even though we have cut back on the percentage of calories from fat in our diets, we're eating more *total* calories. The average woman has eliminated only 6 calories of fat a day. (That's the amount in a large drop of corn oil.)

How are we getting all those extra calories? We may be overeating low-fat foods, explains Liz Marr, R.D., a nutritionist in Denver and a spokesperson for the American Dietetic Association.

We may be cutting down on obvious sources of fat, only to overeat foods laden with "stealth" fats, such as salad dressing and muffins, says Susan Nitzke, Ph.D., associate professor of nutritional sciences at the University of Wisconsin in Madison.

Or we may feel deprived of an old favorite—whether it's lasagna or gravy or ice cream—and can't give it up, she says.

We may be eating more meals away from home—and are stuck with high-fat choices at fast-food stands and in restaurants, says Dr. Levitsky. When one or more of those habits takes hold, we have entered the fat zone.

Tales from the Fat Zone

We have such an intense love-hate relationship with fat, succumbing to its charms only to discover that yesterday's bowl of Chunky

Flavor Dividends

Cheese fondue. Potatoes au gratin. Guacamole. Soufflé. When Steven Raichlen of Coconut Grove, Florida, author of *High-Flavor, Low-Fat Cooking,* serves his versions of these classic dishes, nobody misses the fat.

"My philosophy is to use intense flavorings instead of fat to make food taste delicious," Raichlen says. "To me, food has to be delicious; otherwise, who's going to eat it?"

Raichlen relies on fresh herbs, whole spices, and cooking methods and ingredients that pay big flavor dividends. "There's no room in a low-fat recipe for ingredients that don't contribute flavor," he says.

Here's how you can reap these dividends at home.

Think flavor instead of fat. Lean on delicious, low-fat ingredients to replace flavors lost to fat, Raichlen says. Here are some examples.

- Black mushrooms or shiitake mushrooms give vegetable dishes more flavor than button mushrooms.

- Oven-roasted onions add flavor to a soufflé made with egg whites and to a cheeseless potatoes "au gratin."

- Clam juice, rather than oil, adds juiciness to a seafood sauce for pasta.

- Small amounts of extra-virgin olive oil, walnut oil, or sesame oil add more flavor than the same quantity of a bland cooking oil.

- Apple cider lends depth to baked beans simmered without bacon fat and to root vegetables cooked without oil.

- Kernels of roasted corn replicate the smoky flavor of bacon fat in cornbread.

- Use a tiny bit of flavorful cheese, such as goat cheese, instead of larger amounts of mild cheese like Monterey Jack.

Monkey ice cream has become—horrors!—today's extra roll of belly flab or wider thighs. Why is fat so uniquely troublesome?

The fact is, fat is ruthless. It plays by its own rules—rules designed to make you plump. For starters, dietary fat is a caloric land mine, packing 9 calories per gram compared with 4 calories in a gram of car-

Cook in more flavor. Choose cooking methods that will bring out the flavor, Raichlen suggests. Try grilling, roasting, or stir-frying with very small amounts of oil.

Add new herb and spice flavors. The low-fat cook can experiment with new combinations of seasonings, Raichlen says. So stock your spice rack and start shaking. Here are some suggestions.

- Revive dried herbs. Chop dry herbs with fresh parsley for a burst of extra flavor.

- Make the flavor-fresh choice. Herbs like tarragon and cilantro don't dry well. If you can't find them fresh, substitute a different herb, suggests Raichlen. "Herbs that do work well when dry include basil, oregano, savory, and marjoram."

- Experiment with quantities. "Many recipes are timid in their use of spices," Raichlen says. "Start with the suggested amount, but keep tasting and don't hesitate to add more, little by little, to reach the flavor intensity you like."

- Whole spices are tastier. Buy whole cumin, mustard, and coriander seeds. "Roast the amount you need in a dry skillet for 2 to 3 minutes, then grind in a spice mill or blender," Raichlen says. "It takes an extra few minutes, but the flavor is worth it."

- Time it right. Add spices near the start of cooking. "Otherwise, they tend to have a raw taste," Raichlen says. But if you're using fresh herbs, try adding half at the beginning and half at the end to capture the natural color and freshness.

- Borrow herb-and-spice combinations from the world's most delicious cuisines. Want the taste of Italian food without the fat of lasagna or a meat-rich Bolognese sauce? Add oregano, basil, and garlic to a marinara sauce. For French cuisine, try tarragon, white wine, and garlic. For Spanish cuisine, add saffron and olives. For Mexican, try cilantro and chili peppers.

bohydrate (foods such as fruits, vegetables, and grains) or protein (foods such as meat, fish, and beans).

Once inside your body, dietary fat—whether it's butter or olive oil, lard or vegetable shortening—is fast-tracked to your fat cells. Carbohydrates, meanwhile, are burned for energy or stored in muscle as a quick fuel source called glycogen. Protein is carried off to help build and rebuild body tissues, including muscles, organs, even hair and nails.

"Dietary fat becomes body fat very efficiently," notes Dr. Kenney. "The body only uses up about 3 calories to turn 100 calories of fat into body fat. But it takes about 25 calories to turn carbohydrates into body fat. So your body actually doesn't use carbohydrates for body fat very often. In fact, I would say 95 percent of anyone's body fat comes from dietary fat."

To make matters worse, we crave fat. This impulse is partly an inborn instinct, left over from prehistoric times when fat was rare and survival uncertain. But the craving is also an acquired taste, says Richard Mattes, Ph.D., professor of nutrition at Purdue University in West Lafayette, Indiana. "Eating fat becomes a habit. The more you eat, the more you want," he says. "And there's also an emotional component. We equate fat with good times. Nobody serves raw carrots to celebrate a birthday—you have cake and ice cream."

Once eaten, fat sets off no alarms. "We have sensors all through our bodies that tell us when we have eaten enough carbohydrates, but there seem to be no fat sensors," Dr. Levitsky says. "You can eat and eat and eat fat and not feel full until your stomach is bulging."

Fat is clearly a force to be reckoned with.

Outsmarting Fat

On the Fat-to-Firm Program, you'll find more than 100 strategies for leaving the fat zone behind once and for all. You'll discover how to:

- Turn down your natural appetite for fat.
- Customize a fat-reducing plan.
- Use low-fat and nonfat foods wisely.
- Keep track of your fat intake easily.
- Use your body's natural "carbohydrate sensors" to feel full with delicious, low-fat, low-calorie, nutritious alternatives to high-fat meals.
- Enjoy moderate amounts of fat, without guilt or weight gain.

But outsmarting fat doesn't begin in your refrigerator, your kitchen, or your supermarket. It starts in your mind. "The key to low-fat eating is using your brain to look after yourself," says Laurie Meyer, R.D., a dietitian in Milwaukee, Wisconsin, and a spokesperson for the American Dietetic Association. "I tell women it's about respecting and honoring their bodies. It's being aware of what you eat, why you eat, and when you eat. And it's setting up your environment so that you can follow through on a healthy lifestyle."

Your first assignment? Determining how much fat is right for you. Here are some guidelines.

- For weight loss, strive for 20 to 30 percent of calories from fat, suggests Dr. Hoerr.

- To lower your risk of heart disease, keep your consumption of saturated fat to between 4 and 7 percent of daily calories, suggests Dr. Brown. Aim for total fat intake of no more than 20 percent of daily calories. Follow this advice if you are at higher-than-normal risk of heart disease because you have high blood cholesterol levels, elevated blood pressure, angina, an existing heart condition, a family history of heart disease, or you smoke cigarettes.

- To maintain good health and a healthy body weight, strive for 25 to 30 percent of calories from fat, Dr. Brown suggests. "For a healthy woman, a lower fat intake doesn't seem necessary."

How do you translate these recommendations into a personalized daily fat quota? If you're eating 2,000 calories a day and want to get 25 percent of those calories from fat, aim for 500 fat calories a day, says Dr. Nitzke. That's 56 grams of fat. For other goals, consult "The No-Math Fat-Gram Finder" on page 90.

Your Personal Fat Zone

Discover exactly how much fat you're eating before you start cutting back, suggests Dr. Nitzke, by becoming a fat detective for three days. Simply carry a pencil and some 3- by 5-inch cards with you. Take note of what you eat, when you eat it, and how much fat it contains. "Make it a project to read food labels," Dr. Nitzke says. "If you get something in the supermarket that doesn't have a label, such as sandwich rolls from a bin, ask for nutrition information. Supermarkets should have it handy. If you eat out, fast-food and chain restaurants usually have fat content information available. If not, ask how a dish was prepared."

The No-Math Fat-Gram Finder

Forget multiplication and long division. You can use this easy, Fat-to-Firm fat-gram finder to determine your daily fat-gram goal.

First, determine your ideal daily calorie intake. Check your height and ideal weight, then identify your activity level: low, if you don't engage in regular physical activity; moderate, if you're active for less than 3 hours a week; moderately high, if you get 3 to 5 hours

Calorie Intake

Height	Ideal Body Weight	Activity Level			
(in.)	(lb.)	low	moderate	moderately high	high
59	95	1,045	1,235	1,425	1,710
60	100	1,100	1,300	1,500	1,800
61	105	1,155	1,365	1,575	1,890
62	110	1,210	1,430	1,650	1,980
63	115	1,265	1,495	1,725	2,070
64	120	1,320	1,560	1,800	2,160
65	125	1,375	1,625	1,875	2,250
66	130	1,430	1,690	1,950	2,340
67	135	1,485	1,755	2,025	2,430
68	140	1,540	1,820	2,100	2,520
69	145	1,595	1,885	2,175	2,610
70	150	1,650	1,950	2,250	2,700
71	155	1,705	2,015	2,325	2,790
72	160	1,760	2,080	2,400	2,880

Afterward, tally your fat grams. To convert to calories, multiply the number of grams by nine. And ask yourself: Are you eating too much, too little, or just the right amount?

Then, go beyond mere numbers. Find all of your hot spots—times of the day or foods that add significantly to your daily fat intake. "Ask yourself which of these foods you can do without and which you really want to keep," Dr. Nitzke suggests. "Look for foods you hadn't realized were high in fat. These are the ones that you may want to reduce, replace, or eliminate."

of activity a week; or high, if you have a physically demanding job, engage in regular sports, or work out more than 5 hours a week.

Second, use your daily calorie intake to find your daily fat-gram quota. Remember, your goal is just a rough guideline. Some days you may eat more; some days you may eat less. Nutrition experts say it's best to balance fat intake over the course of the week.

Fat Intake

Daily Calorie Intake	Fat Grams Based on Calories from Fat		
	20%	25%	30%
1,500	33	42	50
1,600	36	44	53
1,700	38	47	57
1,800	40	50	60
1,900	42	53	63
2,000	44	56	67
2,100	47	58	70
2,200	49	61	73
2,300	51	64	77
2,400	53	67	80
2,500	56	69	83

Customize Your Fat-Subtraction Strategy

Happily, there are many paths to successful low-fat eating, Dr. Nitzke says. Here are a few strategies you can try on for size.

Give yourself a head start. Choose one fat-cutting strategy that you can easily follow all the time for automatic fat savings, suggests nutritionist Linda Gigliotti, R.D., health education coordinator for the University of California, Irvine, corporate health program and a certified diabetes expert. "Choose a change you can easily make, such as skipping butter

Dressed to Kill Your Low-Fat Eating Plan

Ah, salad—the fat-watchers dream food. After all, what's the harm in a little lettuce, a few tomato slices, a splash of dressing?

Plenty, according to the United States Department of Agriculture (USDA). When the USDA asked 1,032 American women about their daily food choices, the researchers discovered that salad dressings were the biggest source of fat in their diets, accounting for 9 percent of total fat calories—ahead of cheese and red meat.

"Salads themselves are nutritious and low in fat," notes Laurie Meyer, R.D., a dietitian in Milwaukee, Wisconsin, and a spokesperson for the American Dietetic Association. "But we forget about the dressing. Just 2 ounces can contain up to 16 grams of fat, about 25 percent of the fat a woman should eat in an entire day."

Scoop it up at a salad bar, and things could be worse: A large ladle may contain up to 6 tablespoons' worth, with 48 grams of fat and 450 calories.

Here's how to avoid the salad-dressing trap.

Switch. Most salad dressings have 6 to 7 grams of fat per tablespoon. Try lower-fat versions of your favorite dressing. "This can cut the fat in half," Meyer notes. In general, don't use dressings with more than 3 grams of fat in a 2-tablespoon serving.

Conduct your own taste test. There are dozens of low-fat and fat-free salad dressings out there. Experiment until you find one or two that you really enjoy, suggests Althea Zanecosky, R.D., a nutritionist in Philadelphia and a spokesperson for the American Dietetic Association. Buy a new one every few weeks, bring home a few at a time, or have a taste test with friends.

Toss. Dab 1 tablespoon of dressing in the bottom of your salad bowl, then add ingredients and toss to coat. "This gives you more control than if you simply dumped dressing on," notes Meyer. "If you toss, you can use half the amount of dressing."

Dip. Order your dressing on the side (or pour into a tiny bowl), then dip the tines of your fork in it before spearing lettuce. "You get a little dressing with each bite but barely any calories," Meyer says.

Dilute. Add vinegar or lemon juice to your favorite bottled dressing to dilute the fat content, Meyer suggests.

Make your own. If you dislike low-fat dressings, concoct your own using less oil and more vinegar or lemon juice, Meyer suggests.

on your bread or ordering mustard instead of mayonnaise on deli sand-wiches or having fat-free dressing on all your salads. With one or two of these, you could save hundreds of fat calories a day and never have to think twice about it. But the key is to pick small changes that you can make easily, so there's no struggle."

Use food labels. Check the fat content and serving size before you buy or eat anything, suggests Marr. "You could keep track of the fat grams with this one method or use additional information on the label to see what percentage of calories this food would represent in a 1,500-calorie diet."

Follow the 80/20 rule. About 80 percent of the food that you eat every week should be healthy and low in fat, according to Althea Zanecosky, R.D., a nutritionist in Philadelphia and a spokesperson for the American Dietetic Association. "That should include at least five servings of fruits and vegetables a day and six to 11 servings of grains, including breads," she notes. As for the other 20 percent, "it's your choice," she says. "Make it something you really like. It's important to find room for those foods, even if it's premium ice cream or brownies, so you don't feel deprived."

Aim for two out of three. Eat vegetarian at two out of three meals a day, recommends Dr. Brown. Avoid eating cheese and eggs at those vegetarian meals, too. And keep weekly meat servings to no more than seven. "If possible, have fish for two of those meat servings," he continues. "For the rest, choose small portions (less than 4 ounces) of meats that can easily be trimmed of fat, like chicken, pork, or lean beef."

Play It Fast and Flavorful

On the Fat-to-Firm Program, low-fat eating is a door to a lifetime of delicious, convenient meals and snacks. "Low-fat eating is not a prison sentence," says Marr. "It's a guideline, not something set in stone." Here's how to keep it fun, fast, and flexible.

Don't sweat the small stuff. Some days you may eat more fat than you think you should, Marr says. "You may have to go to a business lunch or dinner, celebrate a holiday, or just need a dish of ice cream," she says. "The thing to remember is that if your average fat intake over several days is where you want it, then you're on track. So if you're high one day, it's not a problem. Just try to adjust a little on another."

Take it one step at a time. Go slowly. "If a woman makes one small change, works on it for a while until it's a habit, and then makes another, she will establish habits that will last and be easy to maintain," says Dr. Nitzke.

Concentrate on flavor. Think about lower-fat foods that you enjoy—and plan easy ways to get more of them into your life, Dr. Nitzke suggests. "Studies are showing more and more that our food choices are driven in part by flavor. So take advantage of that. If you like bananas, stop at the supermarket and get some. If it's raspberries or potatoes or rye bread, go for that. Stack the odds in your favor instead of buying lower-fat foods you really don't enjoy."

Make it convenient. Think those bags of precut salad greens and prewashed baby carrots are expensive luxuries? "Not in the greater scheme of things," Dr. Nitzke says. "Think of them as fast food. If you know you don't have the time to wash and prepare a salad—or won't wash, peel, and cut up carrots—then this kind of convenience food is really your low-fat ally."

Moist, Creamy, or Crispy—Without the Fat

Crunchy "fried" fish, delicate fruit breads, thick and creamy soups. Thanks to a cook's imagination, these low-fat foods have delectable textures you would only expect from versions dripping with butter, oil, or cream.

"Texture is the most important thing to replace when you take out the fat," says Susan Massaron, nutrition manager and director of the cooking school at the Pritikin Longevity Center. "Fortunately, there are lots of ways you can replace texture at home." Here are some of her favorites.

Make moister baked goods. When the butter and oil go, or are reduced to small quantities, turn to these strategies to retain moisture.

- Replace fat with pureed peaches, pears, prunes, or sweet potatoes (try baby food if you don't want to whip up your own). "Prune is wonderful in chocolate cake recipes, but lighter-colored fruit purees, such as peach or pear, work better in less-dark cakes," Massaron says.

- Reduce fat by adding ⅓ cup pureed tofu for each cup of flour in your recipe. As an alternative, nonfat yogurt may be used instead of tofu.

- Use 1% buttermilk or skim milk instead of whole milk in low-fat recipes.

- Replace sugar with honey or mild-flavored molasses. The sticky consistency acts as an oil replacer and improve the texture of the cake.

Thicken soups, stews, and sauces without fat. Instead of stirring in cream, or butter and flour, try these alternatives.

- Simply scoop out about one-third of the soup ingredients (broth and vegetables), blend or puree, then add it back into the pot. You are thickening the soup with its own ingredients without adding any additional calories or fat.

- Add a few tablespoons of instant mashed potatoes to low-fat cream soups to thicken them.

- Mix a tablespoon or more of tomato paste into hearty soups, stews, or sauces to add heft. A little cornstarch or arrowroot, dissolved in a small amount of a cold liquid, added to sauces, will both thicken the sauce and add a shine. Be careful not to add too much or you will get a gluey consistency.

- Soak dried mushrooms in water, then cook them in the strained or filtered soaking liquid until most of it boils away. Add to the recipe. "The flavor is very intense, and the mushrooms release a natural gel that thickens other foods," Massaron says.

- Cook meats, like pork tenderloin, with prunes. "The prunes break down, taste good, and make a nice sauce. Everything looks shiny and glossy and thick," Massaron says. "The result is a real fatlike consistency."

Create creamier, richer dips and dressings. With these new approaches, you can leave the oil and sour cream behind.

- Mix apricot or peach baby food with balsamic vinegar, garlic, ginger, and mustard for a full-bodied salad dressing without the fat. "The flavor of the baby food disappears, leaving a nice, creamy texture," Massaron says. Thicken salad dressings with xanthan gum, available in health food stores.

- Replace sour cream in dip recipes with pureed white beans.

- Mix defatted chicken stock or vegetable stock with vinegar and spices for flavorful salad dressings. Use stock instead of water in sauces for the same reason.

Enjoy crispier chicken and fish, without frying. Don't give up that satisfying crunch. Here's how.

- Spritz a small amount of nonfat cooking spray into your no-stick skillet.

- Brown foods like chicken and fish before cooking them in a sauce. "Dredge the fish or chicken in a little flour first, then brown by cooking in a no-stick pan with cooking spray," Massaron says. "It works very well, without adding fat."

- Fry in the oven: Bread skinless chicken breasts, then bake for a crispy texture.

100 Ways to Subtract Fat

Some of the best fat-cutting tricks are those that the experts rely on time and again. We asked nutritionists and nutrition experts for their favorites—the ones they use at home. Here are 100 of the best.

The Low-Fat Attitude

Successful low-fat eating begins with a positive attitude. So start with these seven ways to build a healthy approach to healthy eating.

Visualize low-fat success. Ahead of time, imagine yourself making smart choices in any setting where high-fat foods abound: at the buffet of an upcoming party, at the restaurant where you'll dine this weekend, or at that wedding reception next month, suggests Edith Howard Hogan, R.D., a dietitian in Washington, D.C., and a spokesperson for the American Dietetic Association. "See yourself doing the right thing. Hear yourself saying, "I'm strong," she says.

Switch off the automatic pilot. Pay attention to why you're taking a second helping or swiping three more Christmas cookies. "Are you doing it just because the food is there? Don't put your mouth on automatic pilot—ask what the extra fat will do to your total food plan," Hogan suggests.

Be selective. Do you find yourself drinking eggnog just because 'tis the season or ladling out the creamed onions simply because they are a Thanksgiving tradition? "Especially during the holidays, we seem to eat plenty of stuff we probably wouldn't touch at other times of the year," Hogan says. "If it's high-fat and you don't love it, skip it."

Be kind to yourself. Do you find yourself reaching for chocolate bars, extra helpings, or other treats during stressful times? Head off a feeding frenzy by getting enough sleep, making time to socialize, and treating yourself well in other ways—from buying a new blouse to attending a concert. "Think of other ways to deal with stress besides reaching for a high-fat food," Hogan suggests.

Indulge without guilt. When you do have a high-fat treat—whether it's breakfast sausage or white chocolate–macadamia nut cookies—focus all your senses on the experience of eating. "I have gourmet ice cream about once a week, and I enjoy every second of it," says Zanecosky. "I don't do anything else when I'm eating it. I know that food is there for me to savor."

Take ownership. When the going gets tough, remind yourself of the reasons why you're cutting the fat. "You'll feel more in control if you remember your purpose," says Meyer. "Take ownership—you're choosing to do this. You don't have to let food control you."

Redefine the splurge. Avoid feelings of deprivation by giving yourself permission to splurge on a luxurious, low-fat treat: perhaps fresh raspberries, exotic tropical fruit from the supermarket produce aisle, or a high-quality, flavorful sorbet, suggests Meyer.

Inside the Low-Fat Kitchen

Open the drawers and cabinets of a well-stocked, low-fat kitchen, and you'll discover one of the top secrets to low-fat cooking success: great gadgets.

From sharp knives to food processors, cheese graters to microwave bowls for popcorn, these accessories are worthwhile because they enable you to save time, cut fat, and put healthy, flavorful meals on the table with a minimum of fuss, says Marr. Here are 20 of the best, as suggested by nutritionists who follow the Fat-to-Firm low-fat lifestyle at home.

Essentials

- Sharp knives. "Low-fat cooking requires a lot of slicing and dicing," notes Marr. "You'll need them to trim fat but also to do things like slicing meat thinly to present fanned out on a plate, which it makes an attractive presentation."

- No-stick sauté pan. Cooks everything from eggs to onions, pancakes to pork chops without added fat.

- Wooden or plastic spoon and spatula for no-stick pan. Protects fragile no-stick surface from scratching.

- Steamer basket. Use this to cook crisp-tender vegetables, also to steam smaller pieces of chicken or fish. Bonus: Steaming veggies retains more nutrients than boiling.

- Your refrigerator. "It's the best fat-cutting gadget in your house—if you know how to use it," says Hogan. "Use it to chill soups or gravies, then take off the layer of fat at the top. And open that hydrator drawer for the ingredients of a very good vegetable stock—throw those dried-out carrots, imperfect onions, and anything else into a stockpot with water and cook for an hour or so, then toss the vegetables out."

- Cheese grater. Produces a flavor-packed dusting of cheese for maximum flavor with minimum fat calories. Especially useful with hard, intensely flavored cheeses like Parmesan, Romano, and Pecorino.

- Roasting-pan racks. Allow the fat from meat, chicken, or meat loaf to run into the bottom of the pan instead of letting it soak into the meat.

- Blender or food processor. A small, inexpensive model will work well for chopping flavor-boosters like garlic, onions, and herbs; pureeing soups for a fat-free, creamy texture; creating low-fat fruit desserts and drinks; and more.

Nice to Have

- Fat-removing gravy pitcher or ladle. Allows you to separate fat from gravy or skim it from soup or meat drippings. "Even if you only use this at Thanksgiving, it's worth having," says Diane Quagliani, R.D., of Chicago, a spokesperson for the American Dietetic Association.

- Garlic press. "A wonderful, quick way to crush up garlic for all kinds of uses," Quagliani says. "You throw in the clove, skin and all, and it crushes out the juice and pulp."

- Microwave oven. Cooks fresh or frozen vegetables, fish, and more—quickly and with no added fat. "It's also a wonderful way to preserve vitamins and minerals," Quagliani says.

- Microwave container for popcorn. Pour kernels into this specially made bowl, cover, and pop, with no added oil. "You can just use bags of popcorn kernels this way. You don't need those packages of microwaveable popcorn with all the fat and other additives," Quagliani says.

- Microwaveable cookware. Have extra bowls and casserole pans ready, to encourage use of the microwave instead of higher-fat cooking methods.

- Yogurt strainer. Lets you prepare easy, overnight yogurt cheese. "You can also make your own using a cone-shaped coffee-filter basket and filter paper or a fine-mesh strainer and cheesecloth," Quagliani says. "Set it over a bowl, spoon in the nonfat yogurt, and refrigerate. In a few hours, the liquid drains out and you have nice, firm yogurt cheese, ready to be flavored with garlic and herbs or honey. Use it as you would cream cheese: on bagels, as a dip, in sandwiches, on baked potatoes, with fruit.

- Pressure cooker. This is a fast cooking method for all foods, including dried beans.

- Stove-top grill racks. Broil meat, fish, chicken, and veggies on a gas or electric stove. "There's a pan filled with water that catches the drippings, so there's no danger of fire, and it reduces the fat," notes Quagliani. "And you can grill year-round."

- Pastry brush. Allows you to lightly paint small amounts of oil or melted butter onto meat, baked goods, and breads.

- Kitchen shears. Scissors designed for cutting the fat from poultry and other meats—especially handy for snipping away pockets of flab that a knife can't easily reach.

- Vertical roaster. This steel device cooks a whole chicken in an upright position, instead of flat in a pan, allowing fat to drip away.

- Salad spinner. Wash lettuce, then whirl in this ingenious plastic tub to remove moisture quickly. A fast, no-fuss way to put creative, nonfat salads on the table.

Getting Ready for a Low-Fat Lifestyle

These expert-endorsed steps will help you prepare for an easy transition to low-fat cooking and eating.

Stock your pantry for low-fat success. Having quick-cooking, low-fat foods handy stacks the odds of eating low-fat in your favor, says Marr.

So, keep in the cupboard a variety of spices and vinegars in different flavors (wine vinegar and balsamic vinegar are two choices), onions, garlic, canned beans, pasta, quick-cooking grains like quick brown rice and couscous, canned low-fat soup, and canned tomato sauce, whole tomatoes, and tomato paste. In the refrigerator stock nonfat plain yogurt or nonfat sour cream, skim milk, fresh vegetables and fruit. In the freezer keep bags of frozen vegetables and boneless chicken breasts.

Make one recipe change at a time. That way, you can assess the success of a new cooking method or a new ingredient. "If you make several changes and don't like the result, you won't know which change was responsible," notes Hogan.

Don't try to cook two separate meals, one for you and one for your family. You'll wear yourself out and get discouraged.

Now, Cut the Fat

Read on for the best fat-cutting tips from the experts.

Pick your spots. Nonfat foods, from cheese to milk to lunch-meats, often work best in combination with other foods—not as stand-alones or starring ingredients, cautions Hogan. "A fat-free cream sauce may work perfectly well as a backdrop for vegetables and chicken, but it will probably be disappointing in fettuccine Alfredo, a dish that gets its appeal from fat," she says. "Use fat-free foods wisely, and you won't feel deprived or let down."

Lose your taste for fat. To trim your "fat tooth," it's important to eat low-fat foods consistently, according to Dr. Mattes. "If you switch back and forth, your mouth will stay accustomed to high-fat foods, and you won't learn to like low-fat foods."

Put your "carbohydrate sensors" to work. Concentrate on high-fiber, low-fat fruits, vegetables, and grains at meals and in-between meals, suggests Dr. Levitsky. "These foods fill you up without adding many calories or very much fat. And, they set off carbohydrate sensors in your brain and digestive system that tell when you're full."

Combine convenience foods. Create quick, low-fat, high-nutrition lunches and dinners by combining frozen and canned foods, suggests Gigliotti. "You can mix together frozen corn, stewed tomatoes, canned mushrooms, and a low-calorie frozen rice-and-chicken entrée, heat it, and you have a big, hearty stew in a hurry," she says.

Cut the butter or oil in soups. When soup and stew recipes call for sautéing onions in several tablespoons of butter or oil, reduce that to 1 or 2 teaspoons. "You'll still get a nice flavor," notes Quagliani.

Skimp on shortening. Older cookbooks call for generous amounts of butter, oil, or shortening in muffin and quick-bread recipes. You can safely cut it back by one-quarter and even as much as one-third, Quagliani says, and still have a moist product.

Ration the nuts. From fancy chicken salad to pesto to desserts, when nuts appear in the ingredients list, you can cut the amount in half or more. Chop the remaining nuts into smaller pieces—you'll still have the flavor and texture but can save 40 grams of fat or more, says Hogan. "Every little bit of savings helps."

Go light on the chips. Reducing the chocolate chips in a cookie, muffin, or cake recipe from 1 cup to ¾ cup saves about 15 grams of fat. "Cutting it back to ½ cup saves 30 grams," notes Hogan. To spread the remaining chips further, buy minichips.

Shred less coconut. Shredded coconut—a staple of desserts, Indonesian foods, and that old luncheon standby, fruit ambrosia—is a high-fat disaster. "You can safely cut the shredded coconut in a recipe in half," Hogan notes. "No one will notice."

Cheat the mix. Leave butter, oil, or margarine out of boxed rice, pilaf, and macaroni-and-cheese mixes, suggests Hogan. You won't miss it.

Conserve cheese. Use half the cheese next time you whip up a pizza at home, suggests Quagliani. And skip fatty toppings like sausage and pepperoni.

Put meat in its place. Use meat as a condiment, rather than as the focal point of the meal, suggests Gigliotti. Small pieces of beef, chicken, or fish work well in stews, soups, stir-fries, or pasta sauces, while cutting fat calories and stretching the household budget.

Say beans. Replace meat with beans in everything from soups and stews to lasagna and spaghetti sauce, suggests Gigliotti. Try red beans in tomato sauce, black beans in the lasagna, white beans in soup.

Replace meat with veggies. Substitute vegetables for some of the ground meat in meat loaf, hamburgers, or any other recipe that calls for ground meat, Gigliotti suggests. "I use shredded carrots in meat loaf—and sometimes onions, red peppers, corn kernels, and tomatoes. It cuts the caloric density of the meat."

Invite more vegetables over for lunch and dinner. Make it a habit to think about eating an extra serving of veggies at lunch and dinner, suggests Gigliotti. "Could you have a baked potato or a bowl of vegetable soup at lunch? An ear of corn with dinner? Some vegetables mixed with pasta as a main course?" she asks. "Start thinking about vegetables early in the day. Don't wait until dinnertime."

Lean on egg whites. In baking or in the breakfast skillet, replace each whole egg with two egg whites, suggests Hogan.

Get plucky. Love bacon at breakfast? Switch to turkey bacon and save 2 grams of fat per slice, says Hogan.

Examine those muffins. Muffins aren't necessarily health food, says Zanecosky. The fat content of an extra-large muffin can rival that of a doughnut.

Bid adieu to the croissant. Elegant and flaky, croissants pack a shocking amount of fat: 12 grams in a 2-ounce pastry. "The flakiness is a clue—they use butter between layers of dough to get that texture," notes Zanecosky.

Breakfast the British way. English muffins are a low-fat best bet for breakfast, says Zanecosky. "Most have about 150 calories and almost no fat at all," she says. "Yet they're tender and great with jelly."

Spread the better butter. Top bagels and toast with thick, flavorful fruit butter instead of butter, margarine, or cream cheese, suggests Quagliani. "They come in apricot, peach, pumpkin, and other flavors, and they are out of this world," she says.

Try a fruit puree. Replace fat in baked goods with ½ cup pureed prunes or applesauce, Hogan suggests. "You still get a moist texture but without the fat calories."

Choose cake flour. When preparing low-fat baked goods, use cake flour instead of all-purpose flour, Hogan says. "This works well with low-fat ingredients because it helps keep a light texture in the final product."

Concoct a new mousse. Replace the eggs in your favorite chocolate mousse recipe with gelatin to retain a satiny, full texture, Hogan suggests.

Butter, be gone. Replace the butter and sugar with dark or light corn syrup, Hogan says, to keep baked goods sweet and moist without the fat.

Hail the new Caesar. Try this fat-free twist on classic Caesar salad dressing, offered by Hogan: Mix together 6 cloves roasted garlic, ½ cup basil leaves, 3 tablespoons honey, and ¼ cup balsamic vinegar.

Toss in the guiltless crunch. Instead of using oily croutons in your salads, crumble a few flavored rice cakes, Hogan notes.

Heat up a smart sauté. When sautéing vegetables or meat, replace butter or oil with chicken broth, unsweetened pineapple juice, or wine, suggests Hogan.

Pour the skinny choice. Replace cream in recipes—and your coffee—with evaporated skim milk, Hogan suggests. It also works well in cream soups and even pumpkin pie filling.

Do the dairy switcheroo. Choosing low-fat and nonfat dairy products can save significant fat calories, while allowing a woman to get the calcium she needs, Hogan notes.

Which should you choose? Fat-free items obviously offer the best choice, calorically speaking. "But fat-free cheese does not melt as well. So if you're having a melted-cheese sandwich, use low-fat cheese instead," Hogan says. "Yet on a cold sandwich with, say, roast turkey and mustard, fat-free cheese will be perfectly tasty. It depends on how you'll use it."

Here are the savings in fat grams for low-fat and nonfat versions, compared to the same quantity of the full-fat product. Remember, every gram contains 9 calories.

- 1 cup 2% milk: saves 4.2 grams
- 1 cup skim milk: saves 8.5 grams
- 1 cup nonfat plain yogurt: saves 7 grams
- 1 tablespoon low-fat mayonnaise: saves 5.5 grams
- 1 tablespoon nonfat mayonnaise: saves 11 grams
- 2 ounces low-fat cheese: saves about 9 grams
- 2 ounces nonfat cheese: saves about 14 grams
- 1 ounce light cream cheese: saves 7.8 grams
- 1 ounce nonfat cream cheese: saves 9.8 grams
- 2 tablespoons nonfat sour cream: saves 6 grams

Lighten your toppings. You can replace sour cream with nonfat yogurt, Hogan notes.

Spritz. Use a cooking spray instead of butter, oil, or margarine when sautéing, suggests Quagliani.

Say cheese. For big cheese flavor without a lot of calories, choose strong cheeses such as blue cheese, Roquefort, Gorgonzola, Gruyère, and Parmesan, and use only a little bit, Quagliani says.

Blend a quick sauce. Create a quick, no-cook cream sauce by combining nonfat cottage cheese, a little skim milk, and herbs of your choice in the blender, Quagliani suggests. Try dill, garlic and basil, or rosemary.

Sip before you snack. Oddly, thirst is often signaled first in the stomach, leading you to think you need food and opening the door to high-fat fare. "Drink at least eight 8-ounce glasses of water a day, whether you feel like it or not," Gigliotti says. "The bonus is, staying hydrated will decrease hunger signals."

Snack time is fruit time. Whole fruit is virtually fat-free and filling, notes Gigliotti. "Think of fruit first at snack time," she says. "You may even want to switch from juice in the morning to whole fruit. The fiber will keep you satisfied, so you're less likely to reach for a high-fat snack."

The Guilt-Free Potato Chip?

Love snacks but hate the fat? Then you have probably wondered whether snack foods made with fake fat are right for you.

Chips made with the controversial fat impostor called olestra have a crunch and ever-so-slightly greasy mouthfeel that is virtually indistinguishable from regular potato chips, according to researchers at the laboratory for the study of human ingestive behavior at Pennsylvania State University in University Park. But they have none of the fat and less than half the calories. Sounds good, but experts disagree over this impostor's merits as a weight-loss tool.

When the researchers compared the fat and calorie intake of 96 women and men who ate chips made either with regular fat or with fake fat, they found that the fake-fat group took in less fat and fewer calories. If they knew they were eating fat-free chips, some people ate slightly more of them, but not enough to undermine the reductions in fat and calories.

"Fake fats could help with weight reduction, but the issue is that people have to realize that calories still count," says researcher Barbara Rolls, Ph.D., professor of nutrition at Pennsylvania State University and director of the laboratory.

Olestra is the only fake fat on the market that can be used for frying. Other fake fats on the market are used in place of butter or oil when making baked goods. Here is how the experts suggest using foods made with fake fat to the best advantage.

Samba over to salsa. At 5 calories per tablespoon, low-fat salsa isn't just for Mexican food anymore, Gigliotti notes. "You can use it on baked potatoes or mix it with nonfat sour cream for a salad dressing," she says. Try it as a sandwich topping or on vegetables, too.

Rice is nice. Big, crunchy, and available in a wide array of flavors, rice cakes make a satisfying, low-fat alternative to snack cakes and cookies, Quagliani says.

Head south of the border. Try a handful of baked tortilla chips with nonfat bean dip for a fiber-rich, low-calorie snack, Quagliani suggests. "If you keep the portions moderate, this is a great alternative to high-fat chips and dips."

Choose taste over fat. Contemplating a cherry turnover for dessert? Substitute angel food cake topped with cherry pie filling. Want a

Treat them like the regular kind. Fat-free snacks only save you calories if you eat moderate amounts, notes Dr. Rolls. If you see the words "fat-free" as a license to overeat, you could actually take in more calories.

Check your reaction. "Olestra is generally safe in snacks," says W. Virgil Brown, M.D., director of the division of arteriosclerosis and lipid metabolism at Emory University School of Medicine in Atlanta and past president of the American Heart Association. "An occasional person may experience diarrhea and cramping if he overconsumes. A little bit in potato chips is okay as long as you don't have an adverse reaction."

Don't overdo it. As olestra leaves the body, it takes with it vitamins A, D, E, and K as well as some beneficial substances called carotenoids, found in fruits and vegetables.

While the manufacturer Proctor and Gamble has fortified the olestra with the vitamins, it has not, however, added carotenoids. "Eating olestra every day is not a wise idea," according to Dr. Brown.

Consider new snacks. "The one risk I see with fake fats is that you may not lose your taste for old favorites like potato chips," Dr. Brown says. You may be better off switching to healthy, low-fat snacks like fruits and vegetables.

banana split? Half a banana, one scoop nonfat frozen yogurt, and 1 tablespoon chocolate syrup together have less than half the fat grams. "Think of creative substitutions that will satisfy your taste buds without adding fat calories," Hogan advises.

Eat exactly what you want. Indulge your desires and avoid fat by defining exactly what you want, suggests Gigliotti. "If it's chocolate, figure out if it has to be a block of chocolate, or whether a creamy pudding or a big cup of sugar-free cocoa would be satisfying," she says. "Then eat a moderate amount of whatever it is."

Cooking with Less Fat

But wait, there's more. Here are still additional ways to squeeze fat out of your menu.

Grab the measuring spoons. Measure all high-fat ingredients before you use them, recommends Quagliani. "Even a little extra oil can add a lot of calories. Get in the habit of knowing how much is in the pan."

Toss the skillet. Bake, broil, roast, or grill the foods you used to fry. "They'll taste just as good, and you save all that oil or butter," notes Hogan.

Skin that bird. Skinless chicken has half the fat of a bird with skin, Hogan says. And you get the fat savings whether you skin before or after cooking.

Moisten without adding fat. If you take the skin off chicken or turkey before cooking, use a good marinade to add moisture, Hogan advises. Or try this: Dredge the chicken in flour, then shake with bread crumbs and a little Parmesan cheese. Bake with a little chicken stock in the bottom of the pan. It's almost as crispy as fried chicken.

Pass up the self-basting bird. Self-basting chickens and turkeys contain extra fat, and that fat is often the heart-clogging saturated variety, says Meyer. "If you're concerned about fat, they're not the best choice."

Select the lightest meats. Hankering for beef? Choose a cut marked "round," "chuck," "sirloin," or "tenderloin" for the least fat, suggests Meyer. In fact, 3 ounces of top round has less fat than the same amount of dark-meat chicken without the skin. "There is still room in a low-fat diet for moderate amounts of beef, and that's good because beef is a good source of iron, which women need," she says.

Remember the ground rules. For the leanest varieties of ground beef, look for the words "loin" or "round" on the label. Also, look for dark red meat—pinker or grayer ground meats generally contain more fat. "Another clue is that low-fat ground meat, unfortunately, is usually more expensive," says Marr.

Crack the beef code. The leanest beef is marked "select," while "choice" has more fat and "prime" has the most, Meyer notes.

Reconsider the other white meat. Pork has become a fairly lean meat choice, Meyer says. "Pork breeders are coming out with lower-fat pork all the time," she notes. "If you trim visible fat and keep portions to 3 to 4 ounces, it's a great choice."

Marinate low-fat cuts. Lower-fat red meats will be less tender than high-fat varieties, Meyer says. Tenderize by soaking for several hours or overnight in an acidic marinade that includes vinegar, fruit juice, or even wine, to break down fibers. "You can even lay slices of kiwifruit on the meat for several hours," she says.

Go for game. What do buffalo, ostrich, alligator, elk, and venison have in common? They're all up-and-coming game meats that are low in fat, Meyer says. "Game meats are becoming more widely available. The taste is excellent."

Try a great impostor. Investigate low-fat versions of your favorite lunchmeats and breakfast sausages, suggests Zanecosky. Try turkey pastrami instead of the real thing, for example.

Strip out the bacon. Choose lean ham over regular bacon or turkey bacon for fat savings at breakfast and in soups or stews that call for bacon, Meyer suggests. "But avoid Virginia ham. It comes from pigs fed on peanuts. That raises the fat content."

Wash fat away. Reduce the fat in ground beef by browning it, then placing it in a colander and dousing it with boiling water. "This carries away more fat," Marr explains.

Talk turkey. When buying ground turkey, make sure the label says that the meat is all turkey breast. "Otherwise, you may be buying meat ground with turkey skin, which will be much higher in fat," Meyer says.

Select from the sea. Fish and shellfish—from trout to salmon and lobster to crab—are delicious main-dish choices that are lower in total fat and saturated fat than most cuts of beef. In fact, they're often lower than dark-meat chicken or turkey, says Meyer.

Choose a fish in water. Pick up water-packed tuna instead of the oil-packed version, says Hogan. But read the label. Occasionally, tuna packers use a higher-fat tuna in water-pack cans, boosting fat content above a fish packed in oil.

Skip the sauté step. When making spaghetti sauce, chili, soup, stew, or a casserole, don't precook chopped peppers and onions. "I just add them to the other ingredients and cook the whole dish," says Zanecosky. "You don't need the fat for the sauté that way."

Put it in the right pan. Cook pancakes and French toast in a heated, no-stick pan without any added fat, Zanecosky suggests.

Microwave the huevos. Scrambled eggs cook up light and fluffy in the microwave, with no added fat, Zanecosky says. "I just beat the eggs and add a little water."

Try a new sandwich topper. Skip the mayo and opt for relish, pickles, a little coleslaw, 1 teaspoon low-fat salad dressing, or even just lettuce and tomato on your next sandwich. "You'll be surprised at how much you don't miss mayonnaise," Zanecosky says. "If you don't like low-fat or nonfat mayo, these are good options."

Read the high-fat signals. Whether it's dinner-hour takeout or a business lunch, watch out for these words in the restaurant-menu description of an entrée: crispy, creamy, rich, sautéed, fried, and deep-fried. These are signals that the food likely contains gobs of fat, Zanecosky explains.

Stay in the low-fat zone. Safe menu choices are broiled, roasted, barbecued, baked, or steamed dishes. "But the best strategy is to ask how any dish is prepared," Zanecosky says.

Blot, blot, blot. Lay a paper napkin or two over a slice of pizza or a greasy burger and wait 30 seconds. "Any fat removed by this method may be small, but it does save some calories," Zanecosky says.

Lighten your cream sauce. Make a nonfat cream sauce by combining cornstarch and skim milk, suggests Marr. "You can also make a cheese sauce by adding nonfat cheese to this."

You say, "to-may-to." I say, "to-mah-to." Either way, use diced fresh or canned tomatoes as a flavorful base for cooking vegetables, suggests Marr.

Borrow from the past. Old-fashioned sweet-and-sour vegetables are a special nonfat change of pace, Marr says. Marinate raw or lightly steamed veggies in vinegar and sugar, adding spices if you desire. Beans or lentils can also be tossed in for a heftier side dish.

Sing sweet and low. Satisfy a sweet tooth without overloading on fat by choosing these desserts: graham crackers, angel food cake, fig bars, gingersnaps, sorbet, or nonfat ice cream or frozen yogurt, suggests Meyer.

Go exotic. The world's cuisines are a treasure trove of filling, low-fat foods, says Dr. Levitsky. So try some at home. "The foods to look for are those based on grains and vegetables, with minimal meat or no meat at all," he says. "Mexican, Italian, and Asian foods are good examples. And, they're fun to eat."

Chapter 8

Calories: Still Fattening after All These Years

Hidden calories and hefty portions can sabotage your weight-loss efforts—even if you eat low-fat foods. It's time to clear up the confusion and start losing weight.

Call her the incredible shrinking woman. In three years, Mary Smith, 33, an administrative assistant from Champaign, Illinois, lost 160 pounds. She's now a trim size 10, down from a generous size 26.

On her journey from fat to firm, Mary resisted the doughnuts and cookies left by co-workers beside the office coffeepot. She cut back on portion sizes at meals. And she stopped buying low-fat and nonfat snack foods like cookies and crackers. "I used to eat a lot of those, thinking that they were good diet foods because they're low in fat," she says. "But the reality is, there are nearly as many calories in reduced-fat foods as in the regular versions."

If your weight-loss efforts seem stalled—despite a switch to fat-free ice cream, fat-free salad dressing, fat-free cookies, fat-free lunchmeats, fat-free mayonnaise, and all the rest of the nonfat, low-fat, and reduced-fat goodies on the supermarket shelves—well, join the crowd. American women are probably more conscious of dietary fat than ever before, but they are still confused about calories. And that's sabotaging our efforts at weight loss.

▶

The truth is, we're actually eating more than ever—we're consuming 100 more calories per day than we did in the late 1980s, according to the United States Department of Agriculture. Our biggest calorie catastrophe? The new low-fat foods.

"Many people believe that if a food is low in fat, they can have as many servings as they want without gaining weight," says John Allred, Ph.D., a biochemist and professor of nutrition in the department of food science and technology at Ohio State University in Columbus and author of *Taking the Fear Out of Eating*. "But many low-fat foods are still high in calories. Ultimately, you cannot escape from one simple, age-old truth: Calories count."

Calorie Amnesia

It's hard to overdo the calories if you're dining on naturally low-fat, high-fiber, super-nutritious foods like fruits, vegetables, and whole grains, says Dr. Allred. "Those foods are low in calories and are very filling because they're full of water and fiber," he says. "Eating an extra carrot or two won't lead to weight gain. That's not the problem." It's the avalanche of low-fat and fat-free products on supermarket shelves that could be sneaking hundreds of extra calories a day—and thousands of calories a year—into your body (and onto your hips), he says.

Many of these new foods offer minuscule calorie savings because when manufacturers take out fat, they add more protein or carbohydrates, and that puts calories back in, says Constance Geiger, R.D., Ph.D., research assistant professor in the division of foods and nutrition at the University of Utah in Salt Lake City and a consultant on food labeling and nutrition. Consider these sobering facts.

- One regular fig bar has 50 calories. One fat-free fig bar also has 50 calories.
- A ½-cup serving of instant chocolate pudding, made with skim milk, has 143 calories. A ½-cup serving of the fat-free version also has 143 calories.
- Three regular chocolate chip cookies have 160 calories. Three reduced-fat chocolate chip cookies have nearly as many—150 calories.
- One cup regular chicken noodle soup has 120 calories. One cup of the reduced-fat version has 140 calories.

The Pasta Predicament

Will that plate of penne leave you pudgy? Can rotini make you rotund? In one of the oddest news flashes from the flab wars, the *New York Times,* which prides itself on accuracy, announced on its front page that "Eating Pasta Makes You Fat," a theme since repeated in many popular magazines and diet books.

What's behind this assertion? The theory is that eating carbohydrates such as pastas, breads, or even fruits and vegetables boosts levels of the hormone insulin in the bloodstream, leading to more or easier fat storage. But nutrition researchers say this hypothesis misses one basic fact: Simply put, it's calories that make you fat.

"That carbohydrate theory has been around for a while," says Paul Lachance, Ph.D., professor of food science and nutrition at Rutgers University in New Brunswick, New Jersey. "But the bottom line still is: You gain weight when you eat too many calories—whether the calories are from fat or carbohydrates. And, if you look at high-carbohydrate, low-fat diets, you see great success for weight loss and even for reversing heart disease. I think the case has been made that carbohydrates are not bad for you at all."

When it comes to weight gain, says Marion Nestle, Ph.D., professor of nutrition and chairperson of the department of nutrition and food studies at New York University in New York City, "I'm much more concerned about total calories than what those calories are made of."

So portion control is crucial. "You can't eat all the carbohydrates you want—especially calorie-dense carbohydrates like baked goods," notes Dr. Lachance. "More complex carbohydrates like fruits and vegetables are lower in calories and offer more nutrients at the same time. The trick is getting yourself to reach for those rather than fast foods like snack cakes."

But one aspect of the "beware of carbohydrates" theory is still under investigation. For people with insulin resistance, which means their cells will only take in and store blood sugar when high levels of insulin are present, a high-carbohydrate diet might indirectly raise the risk of heart disease and diabetes. Still, most members of the medical community aren't convinced that eating carbohydrates leads to medical problems.

- Nine extra-thin regular pretzels have 100 calories. Nine extra-thin fat-free pretzels also have 100 calories.
- Two tablespoons regular peanut butter contains 200 calories—the same as 2 tablespoons reduced-fat peanut butter.
- A ¼-cup serving of regular chicken gravy has 25 calories. The same quantity of fat-free chicken gravy has 15 calories.
- A regular frosted chocolate-fudge toaster pastry has 200 calories. The low-fat version has nearly as many—190 calories.

So where are the big calorie savings? "No matter how low the fat content is, you still need to check the calories," says Dr. Geiger. "You cannot assume that low-fat means low-calorie."

Yet we seem to think "low-fat" is a license to eat. When *Prevention* magazine and the Food Marketing Institute surveyed 710 female grocery shoppers and 294 male shoppers, one in three said that it was okay to eat large amounts of low-fat or fat-free foods. In the same survey seven out of 10 shoppers said that fat content influenced their food-buying decisions, while less than one in 10 mentioned calories.

That kind of "calorie amnesia" can take you quickly from firm to fat, says Marion Nestle, Ph.D., professor of nutrition and chairperson of the department of nutrition and food studies at New York University in New York City. "If you have an excess of calories from any source, you're going to be overweight. That's all there is to it."

The Eye-Mouth Gap

Overeating reduced-fat foods is just part of the story. We have lost track of portion sizes when it comes to nearly everything we eat, says Lisa Young, R.D., adjunct professor of nutrition and food studies at New York University, who researches portion-size issues.

"I happen to think that big portions are one of the causes of obesity," Young says. "If you bring portions under control, you bring calories under control. Then you can lose weight or maintain it. It doesn't mean eating teeny-tiny amounts of food. It just means taking control of what's on your plate."

Eat heaping amounts of anything, and the calorie count climbs fast. For instance, note the following:

- A heaping plate (4 cups) of fettuccine, while low in fat, could contain more than 670 calories—*before* you add the sauce.

- Drink an entire 16-ounce bottle of fruit drink—considered two servings—and you would add more than 240 extra calories to your daily total.
- Layering three 1-ounce slices of Swiss cheese—instead of one slice—on your turkey sandwich doesn't look like much extra food. Yet it would add 200 extra calories to lunch.

We can be dramatically out of touch with how many calories we take in every day. In a study from the Obesity Research Center at St. Luke's/Roosevelt Hospital Center in New York City, overweight women and men actually consumed 1,000 more calories a day than they realized. Normal-weight people ate 600 more calories a day than they realized.

Mindful Munching

You might suspect that reining in out-of-control calories will require you to subsist on microscopically small food portions or—perhaps worse—tally up every single calorie. Relax. Starvation isn't necessary. Neither is carrying a pocket calculator. Instead, Young suggests starting with mindful eating—really paying attention to what's on your plate.

"The first step is being aware of the food you're eating—both of the calories and of what a healthy portion size really looks like," she says. "Then you can make informed choices. You can balance high-calorie and low-calorie foods. You'll get the nutrition you need and still enjoy food." In fact, when you eat mindfully, you will probably enjoy food more because you'll be free of that guilty, nagging sense that you might be overeating.

So in this part of the Fat-to-Firm Program, you'll find practical ways to identify healthy portion sizes. You'll discover how to control calories and still get the nutrition a woman needs for energy, disease prevention, and healthy bones, while pleasing your taste buds and satisfying a growling stomach. And you'll learn to identify your personal high-calorie hot spots and defuse high-calorie overeating situations. So read on. And leave your calculator in your desk drawer—you won't need it.

What's on Your Plate?

Begin with an honest self-assessment of your eating, suggests Michelle Berry, R.D., a research nutritionist at the University of Pittsburgh and a nutrition counselor. Here's how.

Trust your instincts. Often, women know exactly which high-calorie foods are troublesome, Berry says.

So ask yourself about troublesome foods. And trust your instincts. The first answers that come to mind are usually the most important calorie issues to address, she says. If you suspect that portion sizes are too large, then that's an issue to address. Other common hot spots for calories include meats, cheeses, ice cream, soft drinks, and baked goods. And remember that fat-free cookies do have calories and can add up.

Find out why you overeat. Keep a food record for several days or a week, noting what you ate, how much, and when, Berry suggests. Look for patterns and trends. "This can help you clarify not just what you eat but *why* you eat it," she says.

You may find that you have splurged on high-calorie treats twice in the past week because you didn't have any quick-cooking, low-calorie foods on hand. You may tend to overeat at dinner because you had little or nothing to eat during the day, leaving you weak and famished.

"Sometimes, the reasons you overeat have nothing to do with food," Berry says. "It may be that your schedule is so busy that you can't get to the supermarket to buy healthy foods that you could cook easily at home. With a food record you can more clearly recognize the real causes for your overeating and direct your time and attention toward problem solving. You may find, for example, that better time management (including time to shop for groceries and prepare food) is the key to your success, and you can set your goals accordingly."

Never Count Calories Again

You can lose weight or maintain a healthy weight without counting calories by following the healthy lifetime eating plan of the Fat-to-Firm Program. Experts agree that these guidelines for good eating focus on foods that are naturally low in fat, high in fiber, and packed with the nutrition women need.

Happily, the high-nutrition foods that get priority on the Fat-to-Firm Program, including grains, fruits, vegetables, low-fat dairy products, and lean meats, are also low in calories. By basing your meals and snacks on these foods—it could be a chicken-and-broccoli stir-fry over rice, for example—you can control calories without counting. The trick? Simply adjust your calorie intake by adjusting the number of *servings* that you choose from each food category.

"Healthy eating comes first," says Dolores Becker, R.D., coordinator of the Weight Management Center at the Milton S. Hershey Medical Center in Hershey, Pennsylvania. "Starting out with strict rules about calories is not a healthy mind-set. It's better to think about what's in the food, to have reasons besides just calories for making food choices. That's the best way to build an eating plan that can last a lifetime."

This philosophy can help you leave the diet mentality behind once and for all. (For meal-by-meal details, see chapter 14.) Dr. Geiger says that for now, here's how to translate healthy, weight-conscious eating guidelines into calories.

- For 1,200 calories a day: Eat six servings of grains (at least three should be whole grains), three of vegetables, two of fruit, two of lean meat, three of low-fat or nonfat dairy, and limit fats, oils, and sweets.

- For approximately 1,600 calories a day: Eat eight servings of grains (at least three should be whole grains), four of vegetables, three of fruit, two of lean meat, three of low-fat or nonfat dairy, and limit fats, oils, and sweets.

- For approximately 2,200 calories a day: Eat 11 servings of grains (at least three should be whole grains), five of vegetables, four of fruit, three of lean meat, three of low-fat or nonfat dairy, and limit fats, oils, and sweets.

For calorie levels between the examples above, adjust the servings of grains and vegetables. Each serving of grains contains 80 calories; most vegetable servings have 25 calories; the starchy vegetables (potatoes, peas, corn) have 50 calories. So, to move up from 1,600 to 1,800 calories, you could add 1 cup cooked vegetables at lunch and ½ cup rice at dinner.

One caution about calories: Don't be tempted to eat less than the lowest healthy-eating recommendations or to go below 1,200 calories a day, Young says. "Below that," she says, "it's almost impossible to maintain the energy you need or to get the nutrients you need for good health and disease prevention."

Be sure to stick with recommended serving sizes, Becker adds. For grains, one serving is a slice of bread, half a bagel, half an English muffin, 1 ounce cold cereal, or ½ cup cooked cereal, rice, or pasta. For vegetables, it is 1 cup raw, leafy greens; ½ cup other vegetables; or ¾ cup vegetable juice. For fruits, one medium apple, banana, or orange; ½ cup chopped, cooked, or canned fruit; or ¾ cup juice. For dairy foods, 1 cup milk or yogurt; or 1½ ounces cheese. For meats (actually the protein

(continued on page 118)

Painless Calorie-Cutters

"There's plenty you can do to displace calories and fat and still eat a full, satisfying meal," says Constance Geiger, R.D., Ph.D., research assistant professor in the division of foods and nutrition at the University of Utah in Salt Lake City and a consultant on food labeling and nutrition. Here's a guide to getting plenty of food and plenty of taste, while leaving hip-widening calories behind.

Save 75 to 150 Calories

- Instead of 1 cup creamed corn for 184 calories, eat corn on the cob for 83 calories.
- Rather than order tropical drinks like daiquiris, piña coladas, or margaritas, order a virgin spritzer (add cranberry juice to seltzer or flavored seltzer). You'll save about 100 calories on the 1½ ounces of alcohol you forgo.
- Instead of 15 potato chips at 160 calories, have 2 cups mixed pepper strips—red, yellow, and green—for 56 calories.
- Instead of a small serving of fast-food french fries at 210 calories for 2½ ounces, have baked fries (slice potatoes, mist with nonfat cooking spray, and bake at 450°F until golden) at 110 calories for 3½ ounces.
- Instead of 1 tablespoon of margarine at 100 calories, use 2 tablespoons fat-free margarine at 10 calories.
- Instead of a 12-ounce can of cola for 151 calories, have a cup of herb tea with 1 teaspoon honey and three apricots for 75 calories.
- Instead of a candy bar for 250 calories, have a cinnamon-raisin English muffin with 2 teaspoons jam for 172 calories.
- Instead of 1 cup pineapple chunks in heavy syrup for 198 calories, have 1 cup water-packed pineapple for 78 calories.
- Instead of 1 cup coleslaw for 170 calories, have 1 cup steamed vegetables for 60 calories.

Save 150 to 250 Calories

- Instead of 2½ cups spaghetti at 490 calories, have 1 cup spaghetti mixed with 1¼ cups steamed broccoli florets and 1 cup steamed, sliced mushrooms at 265 calories.

- Instead of a fast-food quarter-pound cheeseburger at 530 calories, have a regular cheeseburger, garnished with ketchup, mustard, pickles, and onions for 320 calories.

- Instead of a small strawberry shake (about 2 cups) at 340 calories, blend together 10 frozen strawberries, half a frozen banana, and 1 cup skim milk for 3 cups strawberry smoothie at 165 calories.

- Instead of 1/2 cup potato salad for 179 calories, have 3 cups mixed greens splashed with balsamic vinegar for 27 calories.

Save More Than 250 Calories

- Instead of an appetizer of five fried mozzarella sticks for 500 calories, have 20 small steamed clams for 133 calories.

- Instead of steak fajitas with the works (four tortillas, guacamole, sour cream, pico de gallo sauce, and cheese) for 1,190 calories, have chicken fajitas with salsa and four tortillas for 865 calories.

- Instead of a baked potato loaded with cheese, butter, bacon, and sour cream for 620 calories, order a plain baked potato with 2 tablespoons salsa for 240 calories.

- Instead of a 10-ounce fudge brownie sundae for a whopping 1,130 calories, order 1/2 cup vanilla ice cream with 1/2 cup raspberries and 1 tablespoon of fudge sauce for 267 calories.

- Instead of three slices of pizza from a 12-inch pie for a total of 750 calories, order the pie with half the cheese and lots of onions, peppers, and mushrooms for about 450 calories.

- Instead of five fried onion rings for 400 calories, have eight baked onion rings for 50 calories.

- Instead of 1 cup granola for 500 calories, have 1 cup oatmeal with half a sliced banana for 200 calories.

- Instead of a three-egg omelet with 2 ounces cheese for 425 calories, use four egg whites, 1 tablespoon Parmesan, and 1/2 cup mixed onions, peppers, and tomatoes for 131 calories.

- Instead of 4 ounces turkey, two slices of Swiss cheese, and 1 tablespoon mayonnaise on two slices of whole-wheat bread for 560 calories, skip the cheese, switch to spicy brown mustard, and add tomatoes and lettuce for a 260-calorie sandwich.

group), 2 to 3 ounces cooked lean meat, poultry, or fish; ½ cup cooked beans; one egg; or 2 tablespoons peanut butter.

How much weight will you lose—and how fast? "There are 3,500 calories in each pound of body fat," says Dr. Nestle. "If you eat 500 calories less a day, you'll probably lose a pound in a week."

But an even better approach is to forget about the numbers altogether. Eat healthy and let your weight fall to its own natural, healthy level, says G. Ken Goodrick, Ph.D., assistant professor of medicine at Baylor College of Medicine and associate director of the Behavioral Medicine Research Center, both in Houston. "One of the hallmarks of people who lose weight and keep it off is that they eat and exercise for health, not for appearance," he says. "They don't think of what they eat as a diet, and so they don't go around counting calories. They are aware of low-fat foods, and they do control portions. They don't think of themselves as numbers on a scale or the value of their food as simply the number of calories it contains."

This nondiet approach has helped Ardella Bixler, 54, a hospital cook from Lancaster, Pennsylvania, finally shed 70 pounds after years of dead-end weight-loss diets. "I think in terms of food groups—I get my fruits, vegetables, protein, and grains every day," she says. "I think about portion sizes, too. Instead of having a huge plate of spaghetti, I'll have a smaller portion with some vegetables. I don't count calories, but I'm aware of them."

By the way, after a week of healthy eating, Ardella indulges in her favorite ice cream without guilt or fear. "I don't worry about the calories then," she says. "In fact, once I wrote to an ice cream company and told them how I lost all this weight while eating their ice cream."

Real-Life Weights and Measures

You know that ½ cup of your favorite premium ice cream has 175 calories. But what does ½ cup look like? Would it fill a teacup, a coffee mug, or a salad bowl? Here's the scoop: Pick the teacup. If you fill the salad bowl, you'd wind up with more than twice the calories you planned on eating.

"Women often don't know what real portion sizes look like. As a result, they're often taking in more calories than they realize," notes Young. Portion control, she says, is the key to attaining that elusive balance between eating what you love and attaining or maintaining a desirable body weight.

To help keep portions in perspective, try these suggestions.

Your At-a-Glance Guide to Portion Control

Call it portion creep. We're eating bigger and bigger portions all the time—and our hips show it.

"When women overestimate normal portion sizes, it can easily lead to eating lots of extra calories and to overweight," says nutritionist Lisa Young, R.D., a portion-size expert and adjunct professor of nutrition and food studies at New York University in New York City. "The only way to get on track is to know your portion sizes."

To help you keep your portions in perspective, here's what Young and other experts say real serving sizes of popular foods should really look like.

- 2 tablespoons peanut butter—a large walnut in the shell
- ½ cup cooked pasta—a scoop of ice cream
- ¾ cup rice—a tennis ball
- 1 cup stew, beans, or breakfast cereal—a baseball
- 1 ounce bread—a CD case
- 5 ounces wine—two-thirds of a coffee cup
- 1½ ounces hard cheese—three dominoes
- 1 teaspoon butter—the tip of your thumb
- 1½ ounces sliced, packaged cheese—about one 4- by 6-inch index card
- 2 tablespoons salad dressing—a full shot glass
- 3 ounces meat—a regular-size bar of soap
- 1 ounce potato chips or pretzels—fits in both your open, cupped palms
- 1 ounce nuts or small candies—fits in one cupped palm
- 1 tablespoon olive oil—a small coffee-creamer container

Measure it once. For foods that are easy to overdo, such as cereal, pasta, and ice cream, measure out one serving, then transfer the food into the bowl you normally use, Dr. Geiger suggests. Take note of how it looks. Next time, you'll be able to eyeball the right serving size.

Check your oil. For oils, butter, and margarine, Young says, measure a tablespoon or a teaspoon, then put it into a pan or a salad-dressing decanter or spread it on with a butter knife.

(continued on page 122)

The Totally Honest Guide to Serving Sizes

You buy a 16-ounce bottle of fruit drink. The label says that the bottle contains two servings, and that one serving is 120 calories. You drink the whole thing. There's a pint of ice cream in the freezer. The label says 1/2 cup is a serving. Is that all you eat?

For most of us, "serving size" is the size of our appetites. But if you don't keep in mind that you are doubling or tripling the calories listed under the serving size (and that those labels never tell you the calories for more than one serving), you could be setting yourself up for weight gain, says Constance Geiger, R.D., Ph.D., research assistant professor in the di-

Food	On the Food Label			Actually Consumed		
	Serving Size	Calories	Fat (g.)	Serving Size	Calories	Fat (g.)
Bottled fruit drink (16-oz. bottle)	8 oz.	120	0	16 oz.	240	0
Bran flakes with raisins breakfast cereal	1 cup	200	1.5	1 1/2 cups	250	2.3
Cheese	1 oz.	105	8.5	4 oz.	420	34
Chocolate chip cookies	3 cookies	160	8	7 cookies	373	18.7
Chocolate fudge premium ice cream	1/2 cup	290	20	1 1/2 cups	870	60
Chocolate wafers with vanilla cream filling	3 cookies	160	7	6 cookies	320	14
Cola (20-oz. bottle)	8 oz.	100	0	20 oz.	250	0

vision of foods and nutrition at the University of Utah in Salt Lake City and a consultant on food labeling and nutrition.

"Use the nutrition label on the back of the package to figure out what you're really eating," she says. "If you drink a whole bottle of fruit drink, and that's two servings, you're getting double the calories."

Sometimes the results are surprising—as the editors of *Prevention* Health Books discovered when they figured out the calories and fat in the appetite-size servings of some favorite (and frequently overeaten) foods.

Food	On the Food Label			Actually Consumed		
	Serving Size	Calories	Fat (g.)	Serving Size	Calories	Fat (g.)
Fancy vanilla cookies with dark chocolate centers	3 cookies	180	10	5 cookies	300	17
Fruit-topped packaged coffee cake	⅛ cake	110	5	¼ cake	220	10
Low-fat chocolate sandwich cookies	2 cookies	110	2.5	6 cookies	330	7.5
Potato chips	1 oz. (about 15 chips)	160	10	3 oz. (about 45 chips)	480	30
Spaghetti	2 oz. uncooked (or 1¼ cups cooked)	210	1	4 cups cooked	672	3

Weigh meats, cheeses, even big bagels. For foods with serving sizes measured by weight, such as meats and cheeses, Young suggests picking up an inexpensive kitchen scale, available for under $10. "Use it to get a sense of what a portion really looks like," she says. "You can even use it to measure store-bought bagels and muffins. Often, they're oversize and really have as many calories as five or six slices of bread."

Scale down your dinnerware. Smaller portions don't look so lonely or so tiny when served in a small bowl or on a small plate, Young says. So switch to small dessert plates and bowls, drink high-calorie drinks from smaller cups and glasses, and even consider having dinner on a salad plate, she suggests.

How to Cut Calories Your Way

Create your own calorie-cutting plan with this advice from the experts.

Eat and enjoy healthful food. Reduce your calorie intake by focusing on replacing foods instead of dwelling on deprivation. Don't waste time and energy avoiding so-called forbidden foods, Berry suggests. "When you focus on not eating a certain food, it's likely you'll find yourself thinking about it and craving it more than usual," she notes. "Instead, focus on foods to eat (healthy and delicious fruits, vegetables, whole grains, and low-fat dairy products), and you will start to visualize and desire these healthier foods more."

So, instead of promising yourself that you'll stop eating your high-calorie trouble food—perhaps it's chips at lunch—have a goal of replacing those chips with a side salad dressed with a splash of flavored vinegar.

Start the day with a plan. Choose the meal you care most about and plan the others around it, Young says. Think in terms of portions.

If you're going to an Italian restaurant for dinner, where you might easily consume 2 to 3 cups of pasta (equal to six grain servings), then concentrate on fruits, vegetables, and lean protein at breakfast and lunch. If you're having lunch at a steak house known for its gigantic steaks, don't get a deli sandwich piled with meat for dinner. Instead, design that day's breakfast and lunch around produce and grains, she suggests.

Defuse high-calorie situations. Keep low-calorie foods on hand at work and at home to get you through the times when you reach for higher-calorie fare, Berry suggests. "This could mean making time to shop for apples and baby carrots at the supermarket to eat at home after work, or taking fruit and multigrain bagels to work on Monday to last all week, so you won't need to visit the candy machine on your afternoon break," she says.

Find low-calorie versions of your favorites. Can't imagine giving up ice cream or your favorite hamburger? "Shop for lower-calorie versions of foods you eat all the time," Dr. Geiger says. "Read labels. Every week, pick one or two of your favorite foods and do a little label research. Look for a version that's lower in fat and calories and try it. If it's not to your taste, try another version."

Deploy veggies to trim your high-cal favorites. Do you love to eat big helpings of macaroni and cheese, coleslaw, or spaghetti with tomato sauce packed with ground meat? By adding veggies and using reduced-fat ingredients in these high-calorie foods, you can eat a normal-size portion and still enjoy the taste you love, while cutting calories, Dr. Geiger says.

Keep bags of frozen vegetables in the freezer and precut or grated veggies in the fridge for tricks like these: Add two 8-ounce bags of grated carrots to ½ pint coleslaw. A cup of this carrot slaw has 50 calories, compared with 200 for 1 cup regular slaw. Instead of 2 cups rice pilaf at 400 calories, mix ½ cup pilaf with 2 cups green beans, chopped red peppers, and mushrooms, for less than 200 calories.

Dress up your favorite fruit. Satisfy your sweet tooth with a smoothie, made from frozen fruit whirled in the blender with a cup of skim milk or nonfat yogurt, suggests Berry. That's dessert for less than 200 calories. Or simply blend frozen fruits like strawberries, raspberries, peaches, or blueberries with a small amount of sugar or honey for a fresh-tasting sorbet.

Whether you switch from cookies to fruit for dessert, measure portion sizes or serve up lower-calorie versions of your favorite comfort foods, perhaps the most valuable calorie-control tool of all is believing that you can do it, notes Mary, the administrative assistant who lost nine dress sizes. "Before, I never thought I could do something like this. I didn't have the mind-set to be successful," she says. "Now, I know that I can enjoy food and not gain weight. I feel free."

Chapter 9

Maximum Pleasure, Minimum Calories

**Discover the foods that truly satisfy
your appetite *and* your desire to lose weight.**

When Susanne Holt, Ph.D., a nutrition researcher with the Commonwealth Scientific and Industrial Research Corporation in Adelaide, Australia, set out to discover some of the world's most satisfying edibles, she didn't leave any of her scientific findings locked up in a laboratory.

Instead, her "super-satisfaction foods"—from apples to fish, potatoes to whole-wheat spaghetti and beyond—have starring roles when Dr. Holt sits down to a meal or grabs a quick afternoon snack. Thanks to her research, she is also extra-careful when the urge for classic "comfort foods" strikes because she has evidence that these tempting goodies actually fill us with calories, but they don't fill our stomachs with satisfaction.

"I'm very wary about chocolate, cakes, and ice cream," she says. "Now, before I indulge, I ask myself, 'Do I really need this? Do I really want to eat all those calories and not be satisfied?' Other sweet treats, such as fruits, breakfast cereals, and low-fat yogurt, are more filling and have fewer calories."

In her research, performed at the human nutrition unit of the University of Sydney, Australia, Dr. Holt and her colleagues discovered that some surprising, low-calorie foods have significantly more power to fill you up and keep you feeling satisfied for hours than do high-calorie, high-fat treats.

Choosing more of these super-satisfiers could help you save enough calories to finally lose weight or maintain the healthy weight that you have already achieved—without ever going hungry, according to Dr. Holt.

Satisfaction, Not Extra Pounds

In the University of Sydney study, students ate 240-calorie portions of 38 different foods. Then they rated their feelings of hunger or fullness every 15 minutes. At the end of 2 hours came the ultimate satisfaction test: The students were turned loose at a buffet table and allowed to eat as much food as they liked, while researchers noted how much they consumed.

When the crumbs settled, it was clear that the students who ate the most filling foods ate less food. The humble boiled potato, for example, emerged as a satisfaction superstar, rated seven times more filling than the same calorie portion of croissants.

Basing their ratings on a scale that assigned white bread an automatic score of 100, the researchers discovered that, calorie for calorie, cakes, doughnuts, candy bars, and ice cream were less satisfying than white bread.

Meanwhile, apples, oranges, whole-wheat pasta, fish, and oatmeal were two times as satisfying. Potatoes were three times as satisfying as white bread.

What gives the super-satisfiers their stomach-pleasing power, a power the researchers call satiety? "High-satiety foods were low in calories and low in fat," notes Dr. Holt. As a result, you could eat a bigger portion for the same number of calories.

Consider the potato and the croissant. Two hundred and forty calories of potato weighs in at a whopping 13 ounces—nearly an entire pound of food. But 240 calories of croissant weighs in at just over 2 ounces—one-sixth as much food. This difference relates to something called energy density, getting a lot of nutrients combined with low amounts of calories.

Super-Satisfiers

Stomach growling? Here's how foods rate when it comes to satisfying hunger pangs, according to researchers at the University of Sydney in Australia. Choosing a food from the top of the list (high-satiety index scores) can help fill you up with the fewest calories. For example, a plain potato is more than twice as satisfying as french fries and 3½ times as satisfying as potato chips.

Food	Satisfaction Rating
Potatoes	323
Fish	225
Oatmeal	209
Oranges	202
Apples	197
Pasta, whole-wheat	188
Beefsteak	176
Grapes	162
Popcorn, fat-free, air-popped	154
Cereal, bran	151
Cheese	146
Crackers, water	127
Cookies, crunchy	120
Bananas	118
French fries	116
Bread, white	100
Ice cream	96
Potato chips	91
Candy bars	70
Doughnuts	68
Cakes	65
Croissants	47

Carbohydrates: The Satisfaction Specialists

Why does energy density matter? The obvious answer is that the more weight or volume of food for a given amount of calories, the fuller you will feel and the less likely you will be to overeat, notes Barbara Rolls, Ph.D., professor of nutrition and director of the laboratory for the study of human ingestive behavior at Pennsylvania State University in University Park.

But beyond mere bulk, there are substances inside the super-satisfiers that can keep you feeling content for hours, Dr. Holt notes. Foods like potatoes, oranges, apples, and whole grains are rich in carbohydrates, which increase blood sugar levels and stimulate receptors in your body, which in turn send a loud and clear message to brain and belly that energy stores have been replenished and satisfaction has been achieved.

"We have carbohydrate sensors all over our bodies, starting in the mouth and on down through the intestines as well as in the liver and brain," says David Levitsky, Ph.D., professor of nutrition and psychol-ogy at Cornell University in Ithaca, New York. "These receptors can profoundly affect your appetite, making you feel hungry, or when you've had carbohydrates, making you feel satisfied. As long as you keep the carbohydrate sensors happy, you won't be craving more food."

In contrast, Dr. Levitsky notes, we don't have fat sensors. "Eat high-fat foods, and your body barely knows it," he says. "Nothing tells your stomach or your mouth that it's time to stop eating. So, you eat more and more."

And that's not all. Your stomach will digest the high-satisfaction superstars more slowly than the low-satisfaction duds, Dr. Holt says. The advantage here? The longer the food stays in your stomach, the longer you feel full—and won't be ransacking the refrigerator or the office vending machine for your next snack.

What's responsible for this slow digestion? In super-satisfaction meats like lean beef and fish—cooked with little or no added fat—it's the protein, Dr. Holt says.

In fruits, vegetables, and whole grains, it's complex carbohydrates not often found in refined foods, says Paul Lachance, Ph.D., professor of food science and nutrition at Rutgers University in New Brunswick, New Jersey.

"These carbohydrates are called polymers of glucose," Dr. Lachance says. "But what matters isn't the name. It's the fact that they've been shown to be more long-lasting. Digestion is slow. That's why foods like plain potatoes aren't the culprits in weight gain; a simple potato will fill you up for very few calories. In contrast, when you eat carbohydrates called simple sugars, found in refined foods like cakes and cookies, they're digested very, very quickly."

The fiber found in fruits, vegetables, and grains also lends a hand, keeping digestion slow and steady. The fiber also fills the stomach, Dr. Holt adds.

Slow-Motion Eating

Another big difference between super-satisfaction foods and low-satisfaction duds is ease of eating, Dr. Holt says.

"The bulkiness of the high-satisfaction foods means that it takes quite a bit of chewing before you can swallow them," she notes. This chewing gives your body and your brain more time to react to the food—which means you won't eat as many calories before you receive the "I feel full" message from your stomach.

But the low-satiety foods slip in quickly and quietly—"they melt in your mouth," Dr. Holt notes. "You want to eat more."

Yet our mouths may crave low-satisfaction foods, she notes. They rule the taste buds and may even release feel-good substances in the brain called opiods that produce a feeling of happiness. "These foods increase the risk of eating a lot of calories without even realizing it," she notes. "They taste so good that you still want more, even though you've already eaten quite a lot of calories."

Choosing foods like an apple or orange over a candy bar or a slice of cake can require restraint and patience, she says. "It can take effort to retrain your taste buds, but it's worthwhile," she says. "With time you come to prefer low-fat, filling foods. You should make the changes gradually, however, and allow yourself an occasional treat."

Putting Super-Satisfaction on Your Plate

On the Fat-to-Firm Program, choosing the super-satisfiers lets you stretch your calories while fitting in plenty of good taste and nutrition—without going hungry. Customize this strategy by switching the low-satisfaction foods that you eat most often for high-satisfaction alternatives. Here's how.

Take the gradual approach. First, tackle the highest-fat foods you eat on a regular basis, Dr. Holt says. The most important thing is to

Eat-Slow Snacks

Foods that are hard to eat take longer to finish, and that gives your brain more of a chance to catch up with what's in your stomach, says Michelle Berry, R.D., a research nutritionist at the University of Pittsburgh and a nutrition counselor.

"It takes 20 minutes for signals of satisfaction to reach your brain. Eat slowly and take the time to taste and enjoy food, and you will be less likely to overeat," she says. Here are some suggestions for slow-eating snacks that satisfy without overdoing the calories.

- Two big whole-grain hard pretzels. Dip each bite in mustard or barbecue sauce.

- Five low-fat crackers topped with nonfat cream cheese and vegetables. Try making up the crackers one at a time, eating one before you make the next, Berry suggests. Doing so slows you down and permits time to check for hunger and satisfaction.

- Nachos made with 15 baked tortilla chips, salsa, nonfat bean dip, and low-fat cheese. Eat while hot.

- Make-it-yourself potato wedges instead of chips. Slice a potato in slim wedges and place on a pan spritzed with no-stick spray. Sprinkle the wedges with pepper and paprika and bake at 425° to 450°F. until done (approximately 15 minutes).

- 4 cups of air-popped popcorn

- An artichoke, eaten leaf by leaf. Dip in fat-free salad dressing.

- A baked apple

- 15 frozen grapes

change the high-fat staples in your diet, including dairy and meat products, to leaner versions. If you tend to dine on high-fat meats, try a lower-fat alternative like skinless poultry, fish, or lower-fat beef. Also, if you snack on high-fat sweets like cakes, ice cream, or cookies, reach for fruit instead.

Choose "whole" foods. Reach for whole fruit, instead of fruit juice. Select whole grains—from brown rice to whole-wheat bread to whole-wheat pasta—instead of foods made with refined flour. "Look for unprocessed foods, with the fiber intact," Dr. Holt suggests.

In addition to feeling full now and for hours to come, whole foods often have more nutrients than refined versions. That includes vitamin A, for healthy skin, strong immunity, and good eyesight; vitamin C, vital for protecting cells from damage, promoting healing, and increasing iron absorption; vitamin B_{12}, for maintaining nerve tissue; iron, for carrying oxygen in the blood; and potassium, important for muscle function and energy balance.

Reach for vegetables first. High in fiber, low in fat, and super-low in calories, vegetables have all the attributes that count in a high-satisfaction food. Try for at least three servings a day—and make each serving a full cup for extra satisfaction, suggests nutritionist Linda Gigliotti, R.D., health education coordinator for the University of California, Irvine, corporate health program and a certified diabetes expert.

"Go beyond traditional images of vegetables as an iceberg lettuce salad and some canned peas," she says. "Can you add a baked potato or an ear of corn at lunch or dinner? Can you take a can of vegetable soup to work for lunch?"

Crunch, don't sip, your juice. Naturally juicy fruits and vegetables, such as watermelon, peaches, tomatoes, and peppers, have a high water content—another attribute of high-satisfaction foods. "Wholesome low-calorie foods tend to contain a lot of water, particularly fruits and vegetables," Dr. Holt says. "These whole foods require more chewing and swallowing and tend to be less palatable than the more-processed versions. These factors slow down the rate of eating, and the whole foods take up more space in your stomach. So let crunchiness and juiciness guide you to satisfying choices."

Include some protein. Beans, lentils, and low-fat meats such as fish and poultry got high marks from eaters in Dr. Holt's satisfaction study. Including moderate amounts of lean meats at lunch and dinner can help you feel more full and give more long-term satisfaction than a salad and a piece of bread ever could, Dr. Holt says.

"Many zealous dieters who have very low fat, very high carbohydrate diets try to cut all dairy products and meats out of their diets and wonder why they still feel hungry all of the time," she says. "You really need adequate, not high, amounts of low-fat protein foods in your diet to make you feel 100 percent satisfied." Consider chili made with beans and some lean ground beef, a stir-fry made with vegetables and lean meat, cooked in stock instead of oil, or a curry made with chick-peas and vegetables. Or, using nonfat chicken broth, make a soup, brimming with noodles, vegetables, and beans.

Chocolate Cures for Women Only

Sometimes, a woman needs taste-bud satisfaction, not stomach satisfaction. At a time like that, you need melt-in-your-mouth pleasure. You need—what else?—chocolate.

Nutrition experts aren't sure why women love chocolate, though one theory holds that it boosts feel-good brain chemicals. But surveys show that we do have a soft spot for treats like bonbons, fudge-ripple ice cream, and cocoa. When the Monell Chemical Senses Center in Philadelphia surveyed men's and women's food cravings, women showed a preference for chocolate, while men went for high-protein, high-fat stuff like meat.

Happily, there are more ways than ever to satisfy a chocolate urge without inhaling a 2-pound box of bittersweet truffles—and all those calories. Pinpoint your urge, then satisfy it with these chocolate cures suggested by women nutritionists.

- Cook-it-yourself chocolate pudding, made with skim milk.
- Two regular-size chocolate chip cookies. Only 6 more calories than two nonfat chocolate cookies.
- Two big and crunchy chocolate wafers
- Fat-free, low-calorie hot chocolate mix
- Homemade cocoa. Make cocoa with skim milk, according to package directions. Sweeten with a little sugar or honey.
- A snack-size candy bar
- Two individually wrapped candies—chocolate-covered cherries, peanut butter cups, chocolate mints. You can store them in the freezer and thaw them just as needed.
- Chocolate sorbet, with 1 tablespoon of chocolate syrup
- One fudge pop
- Low-fat chocolate milk

Fiber up. Maximize the fiber in meals and snacks to increase satisfaction, Dr. Holt suggests. Leave the skin on fruits like apples, pears, and peaches and on vegetables like eggplant, cucumbers, potatoes, and carrots—just scrub well before cooking and eating.

Think twice about reduced-fat fare. Refined low-fat foods, like reduced-fat and fat-free ice cream, cookies, cakes, and candies, don't have the power to fill you up.

In fact, such fare can have nearly as many calories as full-fat foods, Dr. Holt notes. Consider chocolate chip cookies: One well-known brand's regular cookie has 53 calories, while the reduced-fat version has 50 calories—a savings of a mere 3 calories. "Eating large amounts of low-fat and fat-free foods will not help people lose weight because these foods are very high in calories," she says.

Give it a little time. If you make the switch from high-fat, refined foods at meals and snacks to lower-fat, higher-fiber foods, give your taste buds about two weeks to adjust, Dr. Holt says. "If you stick with these foods, pretty soon you will find high-fat foods unpleasant."

Give yourself a break. Once you're eating super-satisfaction foods on a regular basis, an occasional indulgence won't threaten your waistline or your new eating habits. "A piece of cake or some chocolate once or twice a week won't hurt," Dr. Holt says.

Chapter 10

"I'm on a Diet, and They're Not"

Learn these smart, successful ways to cope with the 12 most common eating challenges—situations where it's hard to stick to your low-fat plan.

A toothbrush. The office fridge. A cooler chest. What could these objects possibly have in common? Each is a powerful tool that could help you stick to the Fat-to-Firm's healthy, low-fat eating plan—and lose weight.

As you'll see later in this chapter, these unlikely "tools" are part of customized solutions that real women use to overcome some of the toughest, most common obstacles to healthy eating. "When women come up with their own solutions to problems that stand in the way of losing weight or maintaining a healthy weight, they tend to be successful," notes Susan Kayman, R.D., Dr.P.H., program coordinator of regional health education for the Kaiser-Permanente Medical Group in Oakland, California.

Help yourself stick with the Fat-to-Firm eating plan by looking at your unique challenges—and then customize solutions that work for you. "Start by trying to identify the real reasons that you are making the eating choices you are making," Dr. Kayman says. "It could be that you work really hard and don't have time to shop for and prepare healthy meals or are in the midst of a family emergency that doesn't let you stick to your usual eating and exercise routines."

How can you discover your personal obstacles? Try keeping a food diary, suggests Randall Flanery, Ph.D., assistant professor in the department of community and family medicine and director of the eating disorders program at St. Louis University School of Medicine. Note what you ate, when you ate, your feelings at the time, and the circumstances, such as "standing up in the kitchen" or "a lunch appointment at work."

"Being aware will help reveal where the problem is," Dr. Flanery says. "It's a skill you can use all the time because problem solving is a continuous thing. When you're a successful problem solver, you're always fine-tuning. It's very creative."

Here are the ways real women successfully overcame a dozen of the most common challenges to healthy eating—with expert advice on how you can custom-fit solutions that address your own unique needs.

Challenge #1: "During the Holidays I Eat Like a Lumberjack"

A month before Thanksgiving, Carol Katzoff knows exactly what she's going to eat at that festive family gathering—and exactly how much.

"My husband and I practice portion control, and we don't forget about it during the holidays," says Carol, 51, of Phoenix, who has lost 50 pounds. "We'll have 4 to 6 ounces of turkey and reasonable amounts of green bean casserole, a spinach salad, baked potatoes (with a teaspoon of butter and sour cream), fruit salad, and low-fat pumpkin pie."

In years past, the feast would have been much bigger, she adds. "But we don't want to stuff ourselves. And when we told our guests about the menu this year, they all agreed it's a good idea."

Why it works: It's easy to put your mouth and your hands on automatic pilot at holiday dinners and parties because overeating has somehow become an accepted way to celebrate, notes Edith Howard Hogan, R.D., a dietitian in Washington, D.C., and a spokesperson for the American Dietetic Association.

"But it only takes an extra 500 calories a day between Thanksgiving and New Year's Day to gain 5 pounds," she notes. "And you could easily do that by mindlessly eating a few extra cookies." Considering the astronomical calorie counts of most holiday goodies—for example, a cup of eggnog has 342 calories, five sugar cookies have 360 calories, and one chocolate truffle weighs in with 59 calories—selective eating and portion control like Carol's can really pay off, Hogan says.

Try these four ways to deal with a seasonal problem food—whether it's latkes at Hanukkah, cake on your birthday, buttercream eggs at Easter, or even candy at Halloween. "You could substitute a lower-calorie item, such as hot apple cider instead of the eggnog," Hogan suggests. "You could have just a small taste. You could have a full serving but indulge infrequently, such as once or twice during a holiday season. Or you could prepare the food in a new lower-calorie way."

Challenge #2: "I Can't Stop Noshing at Night"

Meg Larsen used to eat ravenously at night, "especially after a few days of crash-dieting," she says. "I'd go for anything high-calorie, like cheeses, crackers, or cookies. Then I'd feel remorse and barely eat the next day."

Now Meg, a 46-year-old attorney and mother of two from San Francisco, who has lost 32 pounds, keeps night-eating at bay by brushing her teeth and climbing into her pajamas early in the evening. "That way, I'm not as inclined to forage in the refrigerator after dinner," she notes. Meg has also found that eating regularly throughout the day curbs her after-dark appetite.

Why it works: Nighttime eating can be a special problem for women with high-stress lives, notes Anne Dubner, R.D., a nutrition consultant in Houston and a spokesperson for the American Dietetic Association. "The first step is to avoid getting really hungry," she notes. "Eating more during the day can really help."

But if you must nosh by night, Dubner suggests trying low-fat, high-volume foods that will fill you up, not out. "Three cups of air-popped popcorn has only about 80 calories," she notes. "Or cut an apple into little pieces and really focus on eating it; don't just put food in your mouth while you watch TV or read the newspaper."

Challenge #3: "I Skip Meals to Save Calories—But It Never Seems to Help"

Doris Anglin used to skip meals all the time. "I would play games with myself," she says. "Skip breakfast to eat a huge lunch. Skip dinner to eat at a party. But it never worked. I was always overeating and eventually weighed about 500 pounds."

Doris, a 53-year-old insurance specialist from Houston, has since lost 258 pounds, and she credits her success, in part, to the fact that she no longer skips any meals. "Every morning, my son and I have breakfast. Around noon I have lunch. In the evening it's dinner," she says. "And on top of that, I have two snacks every single day. All healthy, low-fat food. This way, I'm never starving. I don't have to overeat. And it stokes my metabolism."

Why it works: Trying to limit food by skipping meals is like trying to limit your own breathing, says G. Ken Goodrick, Ph.D., assistant professor of medicine at Baylor College of Medicine and associate director of the Behavioral Medicine Research Center, both in Houston. "Sooner or later, you're going to gulp for air—or for food."

Restricting your food intake severely won't help you reach a healthy weight because it can lower your metabolic rate, so you burn fewer calories all day, and at the same time, it can actually lead to increased absorption of calories from the food you eat, Dr. Goodrick says. A better strategy is the one Doris employs: regular, low-fat meals and snacks, plus exercise.

"It can take a few weeks for a meal-skipper to feel comfortable about eating regularly, but it's worthwhile," he says. "It's good to ask friends or family for support."

Challenge #4: "I'm a Foodie. How Can I Give Up High-Fat Foods?"

Irene Hamlin has always loved good food. "From the time I was a kid, I've loved to cook," she says. "Even when I was single, I never ate a frozen dinner. I made real meals for myself."

When Irene, 46, a psychotherapist from southern California, embarked on a healthy weight-loss plan, she made some basic changes in her well-appointed kitchen. Now, she sautés with wine, broth, or fruit juice instead of butter or oil. Her rich stews are now topped with low-fat dumplings—"it's an occasional treat," she notes. And her meals have only grown more creative: "I'll top a chicken breast with roasted garlic or grated potatoes and orange–Dijon mustard sauce, then bake it. The taste is wonderful," says Irene, who has lost 20 pounds.

Why it works: Food-lovers like Irene can discover new delights, not grim restrictions, on a low-fat eating plan, says Michelle Berry, R.D., a research nutritionist at the University of Pittsburgh and a nutrition counselor. "If you think about getting variety—in flavors, in ingredients, in preparation styles—then healthy eating can be a delicious, satisfying adventure."

And food enthusiasts who experiment with new toppings, fresh herbs, beautiful garnishes, and simple, high-quality ingredients will find new creative challenges in cooking light, Berry says. "It's a new way of cooking, not a limitation," she says. "When you think of it that way, you won't be tempted to return to old ways of cooking and eating."

Challenge #5: "I'm a Charter Member of the Clean-Plate Club"

As a child, Carol Katzoff was told to eat every morsel on her plate. It was a directive she followed for 48 years, only stopping when she started a healthy weight-loss plan and learned to obey a new "stop eating" signal: her own feeling of stomach satisfaction.

"Now, if I get french fries in a restaurant, I'll only eat a few," says Carol. "I stop eating whenever I feel full. It doesn't matter how much is left on the plate. I can always save it as leftovers. It was tough at first. But it worked. I used to be a size 22. Now, I'm a size 10."

Why it works: Learning to respond to your own sense of hunger and satisfaction, as Carol has, is one of the most effective skills a woman can use on a daily basis, says Berry.

"There are many ways to start listening to your body and detecting that satisfied feeling," Berry says. "At home, try taking a smaller portion of food than usual. Eat your serving, then pause to see how you feel. If you really want more, have it. And eat slowly. It takes 20 minutes for satisfaction signals to get from your stomach to your brain."

Challenge #6: "In an Emergency, Who Can Eat Healthy? Not Me."

"I lost 160 pounds over a 2½ year period," says Mary Smith, 33, an administrative assistant from Champaign, Illinois. "Soon after I reached my goal weight, I got a telephone call that my father was seriously ill in the hospital. A week later, he passed away. Through that whole stressful time, I kept eating healthy, low-fat food. I think it really helped me."

Mary immediately devised strategies to help her stick with her plan during this family emergency. The first day, she brought a bag of fruit to the hospital. "Otherwise, I knew it would be so convenient and easy to start buying things from the candy machines," she says. When the family ate hurried meals in restaurants, she ordered vegetables and grilled chicken. "I wasn't able to exercise, so I was trying to eat fewer calories," she says. "For the first time in my life, I wasn't responding to stress by eating. I slipped up once or twice, but I didn't let it bother me."

As a result, she did not gain weight. And Mary feels that by nourishing herself, she could better withstand emotional stress.

Why it works: It's easy to reach for comfort foods or convenience foods during an emergency, whether it's a family illness, a wedding or divorce, starting a new job, or moving to a new home, says Dr. Flanery.

During tough times it's important to realize, as Mary did, that your healthy, low-fat eating plan may be disrupted—and that you may have to find new ways to keep on track. It's also vital to give yourself permission to keep taking care of your own needs, Dr. Flanery says. "Being committed to healthy eating or exercise does not mean that you're insensitive to those around you. In fact, it may make you stronger and more able to be of assistance."

It's also important to be flexible and kind to yourself. If you cannot eat healthy, low-fat food all the time, don't beat yourself up.

Challenge #7: "I'm on a Diet, and They're Not"

Meg Larsen's husband and young sons, ages 3 and 6, still miss the lasagna, homemade pizza, and bacon-wrapped meat loaf she served in the days before she began following a healthy, low-fat eating plan. "And they really loved food like McDonald's, Taco Bell, and ethnic takeout," says Meg.

But they're all adjusting. Meg has found quick recipes the whole family enjoys, such as seafood chowder with a low-fat tomato broth, low-fat pasta dishes, even steamed vegetables with rice. Sometimes, she has a low-fat entrée while her sons share a prized can of ravioli or some other "kid food." And for a treat, her husband takes their sons for fast food when Meg's working late. "My kids are picky eaters, and my husband is a hearty eater, so meeting everyone's needs has been quite a challenge," she says.

Why it works: "Everybody has the right to eat exactly as they want. And for a woman trying to reach a healthy weight, that means having the right to eat healthy food whether or not her family wants to eat the same way all the time," says Dr. Goodrick.

Meg's approach—striking a balance between healthy meals everyone likes and meeting her own needs—is a good one because she's getting on with an endeavor that's important to her without trying to please everyone else all the time. "Sometimes, you just have to do what's important and not worry about what everyone else says," Dr. Goodrick explains.

Challenge #8: "I Have No Time to Lose Weight"

When Meg Larsen takes her son to a potluck supper these days, her contribution is a savory "soup-stew" brimming with split peas, low-fat sausage, and vegetables—an easy offering that simmered all day in her slow-cooker while she worked.

On busy nights, the family enjoys low-fat burritos stuffed with beans, rice, and vegetables from a local take-out stand—one where Meg can carefully study nutrition information before ordering food.

When there's more time to cook, she concocts quick, nutritional entrées, making enough so there are leftovers for her lunch the next day. When does she do the grocery shopping? At midnight, choosing items via computer from a San Francisco–area supermarket that will deliver to her doorstep.

In the morning she grabs breakfast at a drive-through stand that carries whole-wheat bagels and nonfat caffè latte. "Time is at an absolute premium," she notes. And she has mastered the challenge, managing to reach a healthy body weight while working full-time and raising two children.

Why it works: "Planning ahead is a key attribute of people who lose weight and keep it off," says nutritionist Donna Erickson, R.D., health educator in the Weight Management Center at the Carle Clinic Association in Champaign, Illinois. Women like Meg who invest time in planning will reap the rewards when they are able to stick with a healthy eating plan despite hectic nights and whirlwind mornings.

One time-saving strategy Erickson devised is to use 3- by 5-inch cards for meal planning and shopping. "Most people have about a dozen typical meals that they serve," she says. "I suggest that as you cook each such meal, write all the dishes it includes on one side of a card—it could be chicken and rice casserole, for example, served with broccoli, pickled beets, and fruit. On the back of the card, write down every ingredient that goes into that meal."

Use the cards to plan a week's worth of meals, then take them to the store when you buy ingredients, Erickson suggests. "As the week goes along, if you find that you don't have time for Tuesday's meal, find a quicker one from the week's selections. You'll already have the ingredients on hand," she says.

Challenge #9: "My Office Is a Snack-Food Paradise"

"My office seems to be famous for co-workers bringing in food," says Mary Smith. "No matter what room you walk through, somebody has a bowl of candy. Or there's a box of cookies or doughnuts by the coffee machine."

So Mary brought in her own snacks—apples, oranges, or carrots that she stows in the office refrigerator, handy for times when the whole crowd is celebrating with high-fat treats. "This way, I feel like I'm part of the social side of eating, and I get some natural sugar from the fruit," she says. "In the past, I would have chastised people for bringing treats in. Now, I know I just have to take care of myself."

Why it works: "Office food is a major complaint of women in many jobs, including clerical workers, nurses, and teachers," says Colleen Pierre, R.D., a nutritionist in Baltimore and a spokesperson for the American Dietetic Association. "Mary's strategy is a good one because it lets her be part of celebrations. She gets to experience the emotional satisfaction of the social situation without eating high-fat, high-calorie foods that have little nutrition in them."

Mary may also be serving as a role model for other women in her office who would rather not eat the cake or cookies but feel awkward about eating something different, Pierre says.

Challenge #10: "When I Blow My Diet, I Pig Out"

"In the past, if I ate one thing that wasn't on my diet, I felt I had blown the whole day," says Mary Smith. "I thought I was a failure, so I felt bad. And when I felt bad, I would eat."

Today, Mary has a new attitude. "If I eat something that is high in fat or calories, or just have a big portion of a food like pasta, I simply say to myself, 'Well, I ate it. It's not the end of the world.' I'll try to balance it out by eating a little less over the next day or week."

Why it works: Mary has learned that there's really no good food or bad food, no one right way to eat or wrong way to eat, says Susan Moore, R.D., program manager and senior nutritionist of the obesity-management program at George Washington University in Washington, D.C. "When you overeat and have a healthy attitude about food, you respond to the situation and figure out how to deal with the extra calories. You haven't blown your eating plan. You're not a bad person."

That's a vital skill, Moore says. "Otherwise, irrational thinking takes over. You feel bad about what you've done. You get outside your comfort zone and may start eating even more. You relapse."

Mary's also smart to think in terms of how a little extra food on one day will affect her whole week's worth of calories, says Ethan Gorenstein, Ph.D., a psychologist and member of the behavioral medicine program at Columbia-Presbyterian Medical Center in New York City.

"If you consume 1,000 extra calories, as in two pieces of cake, it only amounts to an extra 142 calories a day over the course of a week," he says. Adjusting for that extra 142 calories could be as simple as skipping bread and butter with dinner each night, or forgoing a bottled soft drink each day.

Challenge #11: "He's Sabotaging My Meals"

Nicolle Hawthorne's husband wasn't really trying to wreck her healthy meal plan. But when he came home from the supermarket with fat-laden lamb chops, a pint of coleslaw, and a pint of ice cream for dinner, she felt as if her eating plan had been sabotaged.

"I did some damage control," says Nicolle, 41, a teacher from Orlando, Florida, who has lost 10 pounds and one dress size. "I had one small lamb chop, found some frozen vegetables and cooked them up instead of eating the coleslaw, and ate a tiny scoop of ice cream. It was actually good to see that I could still eat healthy and incorporate foods that I saw as dangerous. I also try now to keep more healthy foods in the house, and I ask my husband for specific foods if he does the grocery shopping."

Why it works: Sabotage, whether intended or accidental, can often be headed off at the pass with some good communication, Dr. Goodrick says. "The first step is to talk about it in a loving, assertive way," he suggests. "Tell your husband, or whoever is acting out the part of saboteur, how you feel when he brings foods you do not want to eat into the house. Then, ask for what you need and check to see that the person can and will agree."

Nicolle defused future sabotage with a combination of communication and preplanning so that she was not dependent on food brought by someone else—a good strategy for taking care of yourself, Dr. Goodrick notes.

"Sometimes, however, there are deeper issues involved," he says. "Some men don't want their wives to be too thin. They're worried about them becoming too attractive. You can try to talk this out. It's good to have a social network—friends, other family members, or a weight-loss group—to support you if that's the case."

Challenge #12: "When I Travel, My Taste Buds Rule"

Sue Dole's bags are almost always packed. As a representative of a private foundation, she's on the road at least three days a week—a lifestyle that at first caused "considerable weight gain."

"But now I've lost 32 pounds by eating carefully when I travel. And the more I do it, the easier it becomes," says Sue, 49, of St. Joseph, Illinois. "I ask a lot of questions before I order in a restaurant. I'm not afraid to make special requests—like having breadsticks that aren't brushed with butter. I always travel with reduced-fat microwave popcorn. If I'm driving, I'll bring a cooler with a sandwich, cut-up vegetables, and some fruit. If I'm flying, I bring my own snacks—like baby carrots and chopped broccoli and cauliflower, or a low-fat brownie. That keeps me away from the peanuts they always serve on board."

Why it works: Planning your food choices in advance, as Sue does, is an insurance policy that can protect you from food that you don't want to eat or from overeating when you travel, Dr. Flanery says. "The time to think about travel and eating is not when your plane is about to touch down at your destination. It's beforehand."

One planning tool is asking lots of questions, Dr. Flanery says. You might call around for a hotel with a refrigerator or kitchenette, so you can keep low-fat breakfast items and snacks handy. Or try to get one with a microwave so that you can snack on low-fat popcorn or heat up a lean frozen dinner after a busy day of business travel. For a long flight, request a low-fat meal in advance.

If you're traveling for pleasure, however, don't miss out on the local delicacies, Dr. Flanery says. Taste the chocolate, the wine, the crab cakes—whatever your destination offers. "There's little value in depriving yourself," he says. "You could end up feeling unhappy and overeat later on. It's a matter of making choices within the guidelines of your meal plan. You don't have to be a glutton to savor what a new place has to offer."

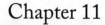

Chapter 11

Sip Your Way to Weight Loss

**From double mochas to diet sodas,
from water to wine—here's your guide
to making the most of slimming beverages
(and the least of calorie-rich drinks).**

Anne Dubner, a registered dietitian, often tells women about a magical drink guaranteed to help them lose weight.

She tells women to drink as much as they can. She tells them the liquid will fill them up so that they'll eat less, but it won't add a single calorie to their diets.

Is this a fairy tale from the Land of Weight-Loss Make-Believe?

No, the Houston nutrition consultant and spokesperson for the American Dietetic Association is telling the truth about what is probably the most underused natural weight-loss aid, water. Never had calories. Never will.

Yet when we try to lose weight, we tend to ignore water, opting instead for an array of "healthy" and "diet" drinks—beverages like fruit juice, flavored water, and diet soda.

But these drinks might actually delay our quest for a firm body. Some contain a surprising amount of calories. Some actually increase our hunger. Some make us feel sluggish or bloated. Here's how to tell the difference between truly slimming sips—and slips.

Water: All You Can Drink

Water is the number one weight-loss drink. But that's not only because it has no calories and no fat. Here are some other reasons why it's a sipping superstar.

You feel full. When water enters your stomach, it mixes with food, making you feel full more quickly and for a longer period of time, says Keith Ayoob, R.D., Ed.D., director of nutrition services at the Rose F. Kennedy Center at Albert Einstein College of Medicine of Yeshiva University in New York City.

You may mistake thirst for hunger. Drinking enough water keeps you from getting thirsty, which can also help you eat less. "People who are overweight tend to confuse hunger with thirst, so they end up eating when they should be drinking water instead," says Dr. Ayoob. If you drink enough water, you won't get thirsty—and eat.

You burn more calories. When you drink cold water (40°F or cooler), you actually burn calories, because your body has to raise the temperature of the water to 98.6°F. In the process, it burns slightly less than 1 calorie per ounce of water. So if you toss back eight glasses of cold water a day, you'll burn about 62 calories. That adds up to 430 calories a week, according to Ellington Darden, Ph.D., author of *A Flat Stomach ASAP*.

Your hands are occupied. Drinking a glass of water gives you something to do with your hands, which means that you're less likely to eat. That's particularly true at parties, where you can find yourself alone at the buffet table, stuffing chip after chip into your mouth. With a glass of water, you can sip rather than eat, says Dr. Ayoob.

Experts recommend drinking at least eight 8-ounce glasses of water a day for weight loss. Seem like an impossible task? Here are some ways to make it easier.

Turn to the bottle. If you avoid water because you don't like the taste of your tap water, opt for bottled water, says Dr. Ayoob.

Spark it with a squeeze. If you think water is bland, perk it up by adding a squeeze or two of fresh lemon or lime juice, says Dubner.

Add fruit juice for flavor. For more flavor, dilute a quarter of a glass of fruit juice with water, says Donna Weihofen, R.D., a nutritionist at the University of Wisconsin Hospital and Clinics in Madison.

Double up. Make a pact with yourself: For every nonwater beverage you consume, you'll also have a glass of water, says Dubner.

Sip all day. Purchase a large water bottle with an attached plastic straw. Keep it filled with water and take a small sip every 15 minutes.

"You'll be surprised how you can end up drinking a quart of water throughout the day and not realize you did it," says Dubner.

Make it an appetizer. Have a glass before each meal to take the edge off your hunger, says Dubner.

Put down your fork and pick up your glass. When eating, take a sip between each bite to fill up faster, says Dubner.

Diet Sodas: They Can Make You Hungry—And Thirsty

Like water, diet sodas are low in calories. But the resemblance ends there. They contain two ingredients that are weight-loss trouble: caffeine and sodium.

Sodium makes you retain water, leaving you feeling bloated and fat. Get on a scale the day after drinking a few diet sodas, and you'll actually weigh a few pounds more because your body is retaining water, says Dubner.

Caffeine boosts the secretion of insulin, a hormone that lowers your blood sugar, leaving you feeling hungry, says Dr. Ayoob. Caffeine also is a diuretic, increasing the output of urine, which makes you thirsty. Hungry and thirsty—not exactly the best combination for weight loss.

The Fat-to-Firm Program doesn't suggest that you never drink diet sodas. But you should follow these tips.

Two is the max. Keep your soda consumption to two or less a day, says Dubner.

Go for the "no." Opt for noncaffeinated sodas, says Dubner.

Water it down. Make sure to drink a glass of water with (or right after) each soda so that you flush the sodium out of your body and quench your thirst, says Dubner.

Sipper, Beware!

A number of beverages—from sparkling water to sports drinks—present themselves as healthful and slimming. But sometimes they are loaded with sugar and other ingredients that can make you fat. To avoid being fooled, try these tips.

Check the water for calories. Many clear beverages sold as "sparkling water" or "flavored water" are really sodas in disguise. "They give you the impression that they're just water because they're clear," says Dubner. "I've had people tell me they can't figure out why they aren't losing weight. I ask them to read the label on the bottled water they drink—and they discover it has more sugar and calories than cola."

Save the sports drink for a marathon. Yes, sports beverages like Gatorade are fine for football players, marathoners, and other people involved in intense and lengthy activity, replacing fluids and minerals and boosting blood sugar. But they're not necessary for the everyday exerciser—and they deliver big helpings of unneeded calories. If you exercise moderately, water is your best bet for fluid replacement, says Dubner.

Eat the fruit. Fruit juice is packed with health-boosting vitamins, but it's not the best slimming drink because ½ cup contains between 45 and 80 calories—and many people tend to drink a lot more than that for a serving.

A better beverage option is to drink water—and still eat the fruit. That way, you also get fiber, which makes the body absorb the fruit sugar more slowly, preventing a large fluctuation in energy levels and keeping you full longer, says Erica Frank, M.D., assistant professor of family and preventive medicine at Emory University School of Medicine in Atlanta.

But for those who can't bear the thought of life without juice, dilute it with sparkling water or club soda to cut down the calories, says Weihofen.

Coffee: Cream and Sugar and Calories

Too much coffee and other caffeinated beverages can hamper weight loss. As mentioned earlier, caffeine can boost the body's insulin output, making you hungry, says Dr. Ayoob. At the same time, after your caffeine rush has ended, you'll find yourself feeling very tired—and less able to make smart food choices.

Even worse are the calories. Though plain coffee alone contains a minimal amount of calories (between 5 and 15 depending on the brew), coffee's regular companions of cream, milk, sugar, syrup, chocolate, and whipped cream can easily put you well over your recommended daily intake of fat and add more calories to your diet than some desserts, says Dubner. For instance, a tall caffè mocha served at a coffee shop can pack nearly the same amount of fat as two slices of coconut custard pie.

You don't have to give up coffee entirely, but you should limit yourself to 1 to 2 cups a day, says Dubner. Also, watch what you add to your coffee so that you don't accidentally turn your drink into a dessert. Here are some tips from experts to help you keep your coffee low in fat and calories.

Ask questions. When ordering gourmet coffees, find out what will go into the cup other than coffee. You can save plenty of calories by omitting the whipped cream, heavy cream, chocolate sprinkles, syrup, and other ingredients, says Dubner. (For the calorie and fat content of some popular specialty coffees, see "The Café Calorie Count.")

Of all the ingredients added to coffee for taste, the whipped cream probably contributes the most fat and calories, says Susan Goodell, spokesperson for Starbucks, the leading U.S. retailer roaster and brand of specialty coffee, based in Seattle. "While the whipped cream is so wonderful, it's a killer," she says. For instance, the whipped cream alone in a tall mocha at Starbucks dumps 80 calories and 9 grams of fat into your system. Goodell suggests asking either for no whipped cream or for half the usual amount.

Skim yourself slim. If you ask, many coffee shops will substitute 2% or skim milk for whole, says Ted Lingle, executive director for the Specialty Coffee Association of America. For instance, Starbucks offers whole, 2% low-fat, skim, and soy milk. Asking for a drink made with skim instead of whole milk can save you anywhere from 7 to 11 grams of fat, says Goodell.

Opt for a cappy. Cappuccinos are made with foamed milk, in which air is shot into the milk, creating a frothy consistency. The air also expands the volume of the milk, meaning less milk is put into the drink as compared to other coffee beverages. So a cappuccino made with whole milk has much less fat than other coffee drinks made with whole milk, says Goodell.

Try flavored beans. To add flavor without adding calories or fat, sprinkle on some cinnamon. Or opt for coffee made from flavored beans, suggests Lingle.

Check the label. When buying flavored coffees at the supermarket, check the list of ingredients. A few flavored coffees may contain coconut oil to add a creamy taste. The oil also adds fat and calories, says Dubner. Such coffees are very different from those made with flavored beans, which contain so few extra calories that they are exempt from federal nutritional labeling laws. So they are okay.

A Toast to Slim Drinking

Women may not get huge beer bellies like men, but we know that beer, wine, and other spirits can pack on the pounds in places we don't want them.

The Café Calorie Count

Long gone are the days when you could order a cup of coffee, no questions asked. Nowadays, you have decisions to make: Mocha? Cappuccino? Latte? Whole milk? Skim? Whipped cream? Flavored syrup? Cinnamon? And those decisions can't only be based on what tastes good—you have fat and calories to think about, too.

To help ease such troublesome decisions, a group of six coffee connoisseurs sipped and sampled various coffee drinks, trying to discern which fat and calories were absolutely essential to the enjoyment of a cup of coffee and which were not. Below you'll find a compilation of those tasters' preferences and suggestions as well as the fat and calorie content of common coffee-shop drinks and their companions—milk, syrup, and whipped cream. They are arranged from most fattening to least fattening. (Beverage information comes from Starbucks, one of the most prevalent coffee shops in the country. Nutrition information is based on a 12-ounce "tall" serving.)

Coffee

Caffè Mocha
Description: a shot of espresso mixed with 1½ ounces chocolate, warm milk, and whipped cream.
Whipped cream with...
  Whole milk: 340 calories, 21 grams of fat
  2% low-fat milk: 300 calories, 16 grams of fat
  Skim milk: 260 calories, 12 grams of fat
  Soy milk: not usually served with whipped cream because people who opt for soy usually do not consume dairy beverages.
No whipped cream with...
  Whole milk: 260 calories, 12 grams of fat
  2% low-fat milk: 220 calories, 7 grams of fat
  Skim milk: 180 calories, 3 grams of fat
  Soy milk: 170 calories, 8 grams of fat
  Some of the tasters terribly missed the whipped cream, which gave the drink a sweet, rich dessertlike flavor and consistency. With whipped cream, few of the tasters found much difference between a mocha with whole milk or skim milk. The tasters offered two suggestions: If you skip the whipped cream, at least treat yourself to whole milk. Otherwise, opt for a little whipped cream with skim milk.

(continued) ▶

The Café Calorie Count—Continued

Caffè Latte
Description: a shot of espresso mixed with warm milk and ½ inch of foamed milk
Whole milk: 210 calories, 11 grams of fat
2% low-fat milk: 170 calories, 6 grams of fat
Skim milk: 120 calories, less than 1 gram of fat
Soy milk: 110 calories, 6 grams of fat
   After much sipping and contemplation, the tasters found that the latte whole milk offered a slightly creamier, heavier consistency, while the skim milk provided a stronger coffee flavor. The froth lasted longer on the latte with whole milk. A latte could easily be served with skim milk with little noticeable difference.

Cappuccino
Description: a shot of espresso, steamed milk, and foamed milk
Whole milk: 140 calories, 7 grams of fat
2% low-fat milk: 110 calories, 4 grams of fat
Skim milk: 80 calories, less than 1 gram of fat
Soy milk: 70 calories, 4 grams of fat
   Tasters found the difference between whole and skim milk even less noticeable in the cappuccino than in the latte. As with the latte, the foam did not last as long with skim milk as it did with whole. And whole milk offered a creamier consistency, while the skim milk allowed the coffee taste to come through.

Frappuccino
Description: a blended, low-fat coffee beverage, available in coffee, mocha, and espresso
Coffee flavor: 200 calories, 3 grams of fat
Other flavors: 205 to 240 calories, 3 grams of fat

Americano
Description: hot water mixed with one to four 1-ounce shots of espresso, depending on the size of the beverage
Calories: 10
Fat grams: none

Brewed/Drip Coffee

Description: regular, plain coffee
Calories: 5 to 15
Fat grams: none

Add-Ons

Whipped Cream

Amount: 1 tablespoon
Calories: 52
Fat grams: 5

Half and Half

Amount: 1 tablespoon
Calories: 20
Fat grams: 1.7

Liquid Coffee-mate Creamer

Amount: 1 tablespoon
Calories: 20
Fat grams: 1

Powdered Coffee-mate Creamer

Amount: 1 teaspoon
Calories: 10
Fat grams: 0.5

Syrup

Amount: ¾ ounce or 1½ tablespoons goes into tall 12-ounce drinks.
Calories: 50 to 60
Fat grams: none

Powders and Flavorings

Flavors: cinnamon, nutmeg, vanilla
Amount: Any amount
Calories: too few for labeling laws
Fat grams: none

A standard mixed drink delivers anywhere from 100 to more than 250 calories. (For comparisons, see "Mixed Drinks, Mixed Blessings.") Still, we sometimes think that we can compensate for the extra calories by eating less—say, skipping dinner when we go to happy hour. Unfortunately, we're usually wrong. Studies show that few of us actually cut our food intake when we drink alcohol, says Angelo Tremblay, Ph.D., professor of physiology and nutrition at Laval University in Ste. Foy, Quebec. Instead, he says, we simply add the calories we drink to the amount of calories we normally take in.

And bar foods—peanuts, nachos, wings—aren't exactly low-fat or low-sodium fare. For instance, a handful of peanuts packs 300 calories. And whoever stopped at just a handful?

The Fat-to-Firm Program isn't recommending that you become a teetotaler. Nor should you start drinking if you don't currently drink. But if you do drink, you should make smart choices so that you can toast to your health and weight-loss success. Here are some tips to help you do just that.

Limit yourself. Don't exceed one standard-size drink a day, says Dr. Ayoob.

Start with a virgin. We tend to guzzle our first drink the fastest. So start with a nonalcoholic beverage, says Natalie Payne, R.D., a dietitian at the Washington Cancer Institute and Washington Hospital Center in Washington, D.C. Then, once the low-calorie liquid has filled you up, have your alcoholic drink.

Pick a lower proof. The higher the proof of the liquor, the higher the calories. So, says Payne, if you like a particular type of drink—brandy, whiskey, or vodka—ask for the brand with the lowest proof.

Ask for a larger glass. When ordering mixed drinks, ask the bartender to put it in a tall glass and specify that you want more mixer. To prepare that kind of drink, the bartender will have to dilute it with club soda or diet ginger ale, cutting some calories. Also, the larger amount will take longer to drink, so you're less likely to order another. Similarly, when possible, add a spritz of carbonated water or club soda to wine to lower the calorie content, says Weihofen.

Go halves. Many mixed drinks are made with a shot of alcohol and club soda or seltzer. When ordering vodka and soda, scotch and soda, brandy and soda, and similar drinks, ask for half a shot of alcohol and more club soda to cut down on calories, says Payne. Just make sure that the bartender doesn't get creative by switching from club soda to calorie-rich 7Up or Sprite.

Mixed Drinks, Mixed Blessings

Mixed drinks may taste great, but the taste—often created with fruit juice and a wallop of sugar—also means plenty of extra calories. Before you order your next one, take a look at the calorie contents of some of the most popular concoctions.

Mixed Drink	Drink Size (oz.)	Calories
Piña colada (pineapple juice, rum, sugar, coconut cream)	4.5	262
Tequila sunrise (orange juice, tequila, lime juice, grenadine)	5.5	189
Screwdriver (orange juice, vodka)	7	174
Gin and tonic (tonic water, gin, lime juice)	7.5	171
Martini (gin, vermouth)	2.5	156
Manhattan (whiskey, vermouth)	2	128
Whiskey sour (lemon juice, whiskey, sugar)	3	123
Tom Collins (club soda, gin, lemon juice, sugar)	7.5	121
Bloody Mary (tomato juice, vodka, lemon juice)	5	116
Daiquiri (rum, lime juice, sugar)	2	111

Substitute skim. When ordering milk- or cream-based drinks such as Kahlúa-and-creams, toasted almonds, and White Russians, ask for skim milk instead of whole, says Payne.

Develop dry taste. Dry wines contain less sugar than sweet wines, making them less caloric, says Payne. You'll save about 15 calories a glass by drinking dry wines such as Cabernet, Merlot, and Chardonnay instead of sweet ones such as Niagara and Ravat.

Don't fear beer. Many women order dry wine rather than beer because the wine has fewer calories. But wine is also less filling, says Weihofen, and you may find yourself drinking more than one glass—and taking in far more calories—than if you had only one filling glass of beer. If you like beer, try a light or nonalcoholic beer instead of wine. (And by the way, sweet wine has as many calories as light beer.)

Be late. When going to parties where alcohol and food will be served, show up late to avoid the prime eating and drinking hour, suggests Payne. Also, whatever you do, don't stand next to the food.

Chapter 12

Mini-meals: A Small Miracle

No hunger. No bingeing. A revved-up metabolism that torches calories. Those are just three of the body-firming benefits of this powerful new style of eating.

Darla Dever's kitchen was a world of temptation. The banana cream pie called to her from the refrigerator, the cookies, from the shelves. And she usually listened—eating and eating, until way past being full.

Today, that kitchen is...just a kitchen. Darla can look at a pie and pass. Or she can have a forkful or two, wrapping up the rest for another time; she never binges. "The food doesn't have control over me anymore," says Darla, a 40-year-old married mother of two in Katy, Texas. "Now I'm in control of the food."

What made the difference for Darla? Well, the answer is so simple that it may surprise you: mini-meals.

That's right, the only thing that Darla does differently now is to eat small amounts of food whenever she's hungry, stopping as soon as she feels satisfied. She no longer skips meals. She no longer allows herself to become so hungry that she can't stand it. Mini-meals have given her new peace of mind—and a new body, free of 20 pounds of overweight.

Why You Should Eat Like There's No Tomorrow

How can something so small make such a big difference in whether or not you lose weight?

Well, mini-meals make use of a primitive and powerful biological reflex, left over from our hunter-gatherer days before menus were invented, when food could be scarce. When the stomach is empty for extended periods of time—say, if you eat only one meal a day—that reflex orders the metabolism to burn fewer calories. ("Hey, body, slow down—we might not be eating for a couple of days.") When the stomach has some food in it, that reflex tells the metabolism to speed up. ("Hey, body, get some calories while the getting is good.") So when you eat small amounts of food every 3 to 4 hours, your metabolism keeps burning extra calories—meaning that you can eat the same amount of food per day but lose more weight, says Anne Dubner, R.D., a nutrition consultant in Houston and a spokesperson for the American Dietetic Association.

Some experts theorize that mini-meals work with our stomachs in another way, by keeping it the right size. When we eat a huge meal, we overfill the 3-cup capacity of our stomachs. In fact, we stretch it out—and that larger stomach needs more food to feel full. So we eat more the next time. Mini-meals prevent all that.

Eating mini-meals also helps you avoid overeating, says Dubner. When you eat three (or fewer) meals a day, you get hungry between meals, she explains. You begin to think about food—a lot. And when you finally sit down to a meal, you tend to overeat. But when you eat small, frequent meals, you fill up every time you get close to a hunger pang. You never crave food. You are always satisfied, says Dubner.

Variety Is the Key

Okay, you're ready to try mini-meals. First, think *variety.* You want to continue to eat from all the food groups throughout the day: grains, fruits, vegetables, dairy products, and proteins. But you don't need to balance your intake of food groups at every meal as you did when you were eating three meals. Instead, you want to achieve balance over the course of an entire day, which means about six grains, two fruits, three vegetables, two dairy products, and two to three meat or protein products each day. (Be sure to take a calcium supplement for strong bones.)

Your Two Most Important Mini-meals

Imagine you are a *Jeopardy* contestant. You choose "Foods" for $500. Alex says, "The most crucial meals of the day." Your thumb feels slippery and tense on top of the buzzer. Your mind swims:

a. Breakfast, lunch, and dinner?

b. Lunch and dinner?

c. Between-meal snacks?

d. Breakfast and an after-dinner snack?

"Doo, da, doo, da, doo da doo. Doo, da, doo, da, doo, da, da, da, da, da..."

Your thumb mashes down on the buzzer as you blurt out, "What are breakfast and an after-dinner snack?"

Alex says, "Congratulations, you now have $500 more."

Why those two meals?

Remember, the main purpose of eating mini-meals is to keep your metabolism revved up so that you burn extra calories. But there's a time during every day when it's impossible to eat—when you're asleep. So you need to eat a mini-meal between dinner and bedtime to keep your calorie burners stoked, says Natalie Payne, R.D., a dietitian at the Washington Cancer Institute and Washington Hospital Center in Washington, D.C. And you need to eat your breakfast mini-meal first thing in the morning.

What to eat? Payne suggests that 1 to 2 hours before bedtime you nibble on a banana, some popcorn, or a slice of whole-wheat bread. In the morning have cereal, a bagel, or half a sandwich.

But that isn't a rigid formula, says Donna Weihofen, R.D., a nutritionist at University of Wisconsin Hospital and Clinics in Madison. You can increase or decrease servings in any category, she says—as long as you make sure to eat more grains and produce and less dairy and meat. (For an example of a week of balanced mini-meals, see page 160.)

What's the right amount of meals? It's up to you. It might be four, six, or eight. Let your body tell you what to do: Eat when you're hungry, stop when you're full, says Weihofen.

Of course, your stomach might be speaking to you, but your thoughts and feelings might drown out its messages about hunger (particularly, if you're used to denying your hunger because you're dieting). So learning to listen to your hunger might take practice, so might stopping when you're full. Here is the best advice from experts to quickly and easily adjust to mini-meals.

Keep a diary. A food diary can help you identify emotions that may trigger eating when you're not hungry, says Keith Ayoob, R.D., Ed.D., director of nutrition services at the Rose F. Kennedy Center at Albert Einstein College of Medicine of Yeshiva University in New York City. Each time you eat, write down what you ate, when you ate it, what you were doing when you ate it, and how you felt.

Make a plan. Don't wait until you're hungry to decide what to eat; hunger makes chocolate cake look like a balanced mini-meal. Plan your day's meals the night before or first thing in the morning, says Dr. Ayoob, and bring your food with you. That way, you'll have low-fat, low-calorie foods ready when the hunger hits.

Select a serving. Favor foods already portioned into individual servings, like a baked potato, a container of yogurt, or a bagel. Eating a set portion ensures that you will stop when full (or nearly full) because you will run out of food, says Michele Harvey, R.D., a diabetes educator and private nutrition consultant in Boca Raton and Delray Beach, Florida.

Slow down. Your stomach tells your brain when it's full—but it takes 20 minutes for your brain to register the message. If you eat slowly, you're more likely to realize you're full before you overeat, says Frances Oppenheimer, R.D., a dietitian at Loyola University Medical Center in Maywood, Illinois.

The best way to slow down? Have a conversation. The worst way to slow down? Watch television. People who eat while watching television tend to eat robotically, says Oppenheimer—mindlessly, quickly, and way too much.

Choose no-risk foods. As you adapt, says Dubner, choose low-calorie foods like popcorn or raw vegetables. That way, if you overeat, you'll only add a few extra calories.

Go to pieces. Mini-meals will be more satisfying if you eat them in small bites, says Dubner. So, instead of a one big rice cake, have a few of the bite-size variety. Instead of eating a big pretzel, have lots of small ones. Even take a cookie, cut it into pieces, and eat each piece.

Don't tempt yourself. If you know that you have no resistance to cookie dough, for example, stay away from it. You'll probably end up eating well beyond fullness. Choose mini-meal foods that you know you can control, says Weihofen.

Watch out for fat-free. Nonfat foods won't fill you up for very long. Also, many nonfat foods have added lots of sugary calories, says Weihofen, to make up for the loss of fat.

Schedule your meals. If you can't seem to master mini-meals, create an eating schedule with six meals a day, 3 hours apart, says Harvey. Once you get on a regular schedule, you'll more easily notice your body's hunger cues. For example, if you eat breakfast every morning at 7:00 A.M., your body will become hungry at that time.

Mealtime—Six Times a Day

Sometimes, when people first switch to mini-meals, they find they don't have the time to prepare the food—let alone time to eat it. But eating mini-meals doesn't have to be time-consuming, says Natalie Payne, R.D., a dietitian at the Washington Cancer Institute and Washington Hospital Center in Washington, D.C. Here are some time-saving strategies.

Divide and conquer. Divide your three meals in half to create six, says Dubner. If you usually eat a bagel for breakfast, for example, eat half when you get up and the other half later. If you have a sandwich for lunch, each the two halves at two different times. That way, you won't spend any more time preparing food.

Switch meals. Consider some easy-to-prepare, easy-to-eat (but somewhat unusual) choices for your meals, says Payne. For example, make a turkey sandwich the night before, grab it from the fridge on your way out the door, and eat it for breakfast when you get to work.

Keep it cold. If you work in an office where you don't have access to a refrigerator, freeze a juice box overnight and put it in the bottom of your lunch bag the following day. The frozen juice will keep easy-to-eat items such as yogurt and cheese cold, says Payne.

Stash some safe bets. At work, keep a desk drawer filled with canned fruit (in water or fruit juice), dried fruit, low-fat crackers, and other nonperishable convenience foods, suggests Payne. (And don't forget the can opener.)

Slice at night. When slicing up carrots and other raw vegetables for dinner, don't forget to slice some extras to munch on the next day while at work, suggest Payne.

A Week's Worth of Mini-meals

It can be a little daunting to figure out just what to eat when you first switch to mini-meals. So we asked Anne Dubner, R.D., a nutrition consultant in Houston and a spokesperson for the American Dietetic Association, to put together a week's worth of mini-meals. She has included suggested serving sizes, but she points out that you need to listen to your stomach when figuring out how much to eat—you should start eating when you're hungry, and you should stop when you're full. This chart also refers to recipes that appear between pages 437 and 452; each recipe makes two servings.

Monday

Breakfast
- Half a bagel with Roasted Red-Pepper Spread (see page 435), an 8-ounce glass of skim milk, and ½ cup blueberries

Midmorning Snack
- The other half of the bagel with Roasted Red-Pepper Spread

Lunch
- Half a Turkey Club Sandwich (see page 439) and a mixed garden salad with 1 tablespoon reduced-fat Russian dressing

Afternoon Snack
- The other half of the Turkey Club Sandwich

Dinner
- Pasta Primavera (see page 446) and a slice of Italian bread with 1 teaspoon diet margarine, mixed with 1 teaspoon each crushed fresh garlic and grated Parmesan cheese

Evening Snack
- An oatmeal raisin cookie

Tuesday

Breakfast
- 1 cup Easy Fruit Salad (see page 437) and an 8-ounce glass of skim milk

Midmorning Snack
- One low-fat granola bar

Lunch
- One Smoked Turkey Tortilla Roll-Up (see page 441) and ½ cup steamed broccoli

Afternoon Snack
- A handful (20 to 25) of thin pretzel sticks

Dinner
- A Mexican Tortilla Pizza (see page 448) and a mixed garden salad, topped with 1 tablespoon reduced-fat Italian dressing

Evening Snack
- 1 cup chopped raw vegetables (such as baby carrots, broccoli, and cauliflower), dipped in 2 tablespoons low-fat ranch dressing

Wednesday

Breakfast
- 1 cup cold cereal in 4 ounces skim milk, served with a 4-ounce glass of orange juice

Midmorning Snack
- A tennis-ball-size piece of fruit

Lunch
- Stuffed Belgian Endive (see page 444) with a crusty French roll topped with 1 teaspoon diet margarine

Afternoon Snack
- A nonfat flavored yogurt

Dinner
- Pasta with Quick Vegetable Sauce (see page 445) with a 1-cup serving of sliced cucumbers and carrots, mixed with 1 to 2 teaspoons low-fat Italian dressing

Evening Snack
- 3 cups popcorn

Thursday

Breakfast
- One slice of raisin bread with 1 tablespoon peanut butter

Midmorning Snack
- A reduced-fat fig bar and an 8-ounce glass of skim milk

Lunch
- Half a Chicken Salad Sandwich (see page 438) with 1 cup chopped raw vegetables (such as baby carrots and celery)

Afternoon Snack
- The other half of the Chicken Salad Sandwich

Dinner
- Cheese Quesadillas (see page 449) with ½ cup white rice, mixed with 2 tablespoons salsa

Evening Snack
- A nonfat flavored yogurt with three graham crackers

Friday

Breakfast
- Two slices of toast with a slice of low-fat cheese wedged between them and a 4-ounce glass of orange juice

Midmorning Snack
- 1 cup nonfat yogurt, mixed with ½ cup blueberries

Lunch
- Italian-Style Baked Potatoes (see page 440) with a side dish of ½ cup steamed broccoli

Afternoon Snack
- 10 fat-free tortilla chips, dipped in 2 tablespoons salsa

Dinner
- Vegetable Fried Rice (see page 447) with a side dish of scrambled eggs made from one serving of egg substitute

Evening Snack
- A flavored rice cake with 1 teaspoon peanut butter smeared on top

(continued) ▶

A Week's Worth of Mini-meals—Continued

Saturday

Breakfast
- An English muffin with scrambled egg substitute and an orange wedge, served with an 8-ounce glass of milk

Midmorning Snack
- A sandwich made with one slice of bread, half a banana, and 1 tablespoon peanut butter

Lunch
- Greek Salad (see page 442) with a slice of Italian bread

Afternoon Snack
- Six crackers with tuna, mixed with 1 tablespoon reduced-fat mayonnaise and a squirt of lemon for flavor

Dinner
- Potato Skins with Cheddar Cheese (see page 450) with ½ cup steamed broccoli

Evening Snack
- 3 cups popcorn, sprinkled with 2 teaspoons Parmesan cheese

Sunday

Breakfast
- A frozen waffle with 1 tablespoon sugar-free all-fruit spread, served with an 8-ounce glass of milk

Midmorning Snack
- A tennis-ball-size piece of fruit

Lunch
- Southwest Corn Salad (see page 443), topped with six crackers and two low-fat cheese slices

Afternoon Snack
- Eight baby carrots, dipped in 1 cup nonfat plain yogurt mixed with 1 teaspoon Dijon mustard

Dinner
- 1 ounce whole-grain French bread; 1 cup mixed garden salad; and 1 cup elbow macaroni, tossed with ¼ cup chickpeas and ¼ cup stewed tomatoes and sprinkled with 1 tablespoon Parmesan cheese

Evening Snack
- ½ cup frozen yogurt, with 1 tablespoon chocolate syrup

Dinner—Your Biggest Challenge

Dinner can be the toughest time to eat a mini-meal. If you go out to eat, you're served too much food. If you eat at home, you might linger at the table with the family—and eat more than you planned. Here are some ways to think small at dinnertime.

Have an appetizer. Have a snack ready in the fridge for when you walk in the door after work, says Dubner. After you have eaten,

Mini-meals Aren't for Everyone

True, mini-meals are a good eating plan for women trying to lose weight.

But they don't work for everyone. Some women, for instance, have runaway appetites. Once they start eating, they keep eating until they are stuffed, says Donna Weihofen, R.D., a nutritionist at University of Wisconsin Hospital and Clinics in Madison. Such women would be better off eating only a few times a day, she says.

Also, your lifestyle can make switching to mini-meals too difficult. For instance, if you work at a job where you cannot eat at your desk (like an assembly line) and you only have one lunch break, mini-meals may not be your best option, says Frances Oppenheimer, R.D., a dietitian at Loyola University Medical Center in Maywood, Illinois.

Give mini-meals a chance. But if you find that you can't make the switch, know that you are not a failure. And know that mini-meals are just one of the Fat-to-Firm Program's many options.

change into comfortable clothes, take a shower, or do whatever else you do to ready yourself for an evening meal with your family. Then spend as much time at the dinner table as you like—but you won't overeat because you won't be as hungry.

Don't stay on course. Instead, switch back and forth between courses—by alternating every bite of your main dish (say chicken or pasta) with a bite of salad. If you do that, says Dubner, your food will last as long as your family's.

Fill 'er up. Before ordering dinner at a restaurant, drink a big glass of water to quiet your appetite, says Dubner. Then take a sip of water between every bite so that you'll eat more slowly.

Hold the bread. Ask the waiter not to bring the bread. Or take one roll and send the basket back, says Harvey.

Skip the mixed drinks. Alcohol tends to wake up your appetite—and put your self-control to sleep. When eating out (or at home), don't drink alcohol before your meal, says Ralph W. Cygan, M.D., clinical professor of medicine and director of the weight-management program at the University of California, Irvine, College of Medicine.

Try a smaller portion. Ask the waiter for a smaller portion, says Harvey. For instance, you can request a meal half the size.

Don't entrée right away. When eating out, have a small bowl of noncreamy soup, such as minestrone, or a small salad before making a decision on your entrée, says Dubner. That way, you won't be as hungry when ordering.

Or don't order it at all. Instead of ordering an entrée, order an appetizer, says Harvey.

Start low, end high. Eat your vegetables first, then eat your starches, like potatoes and bread, and leave the highest-calorie and fattiest items like meat for last, says Dubner. That way you'll fill up on the lowest-calorie items and feel too full to finish the high-calorie foods.

Don't worry about detours. Every once in a while—for instance, at Thanksgiving—you will stuff yourself. Don't feel guilty. "You are not going to get lost when you take a detour—as long as you don't keep slapping yourself across the face," says Harvey. You will get lost, however, if you continually berate yourself, she says, because then you will feel so bad about yourself that you'll keep eating.

Chapter 13

Dining Out Successfully— And Realistically

Disguised fat and mega-servings make restaurants an obstacle course, but you can put weight loss (and enjoyment) back on the menu.

Sue Dole can outsmart any restaurant menu. "I eat out all the time," says Sue, 49, of St. Joseph, Illinois, who travels extensively for her job with a private foundation.

"I'm thoughtful about what I order, and it pays off—I'm losing weight," she adds.

First, she scans the menu with care. "I look for steamed vegetables, fruit plates, and simple pasta sauces that are usually low in fat," says Sue.

Then, she questions the waiter. "I ask about food preparation—whether they use butter or oil or cheese. I always ask a lot of questions," says Sue.

Finally, she orders as she pleases—perhaps an appetizer as her main course, with fruit for dessert. Breadsticks without the buttery glaze. And when she orders a salad, she requests that her dressing be on the side. "I remind myself that I'm the customer. The restaurant is there to serve me," she says. "That way, I get meals I can really enjoy without gaining weight or feeling guilty."

Why Eating Out Is In

As Sue discovered, a woman can eat out on a regular basis—whether it's for work, pleasure, or just to fuel up after a hectic day—and still successfully lose weight or maintain a healthy weight, says Hope Warshaw, R.D., a nutrition consultant in Washington, D.C., and author of *The Restaurant Companion: A Guide to Healthier Eating Out.*

"When you become menu-savvy, dining out can be healthy and enjoyable at the same time," Warshaw says.

All too often, however, eating out leads to weight gain, guilt, and that uncomfortable, stuffed-to-the-gills feeling. "The increase in overweight in America can be traced, in part, to the amount of eating we do away from home," notes Paul Lachance, Ph.D., professor of food science and nutrition at Rutgers University in New Brunswick, New Jersey. "Restaurants often give us huge meals—meals full of calories—as an indication of value for the money being spent."

But there's no retreating to the days of homemade. Due to the universal time crunch, to not wanting to cook, or simply to a preference for restaurant atmosphere and cuisine, we spend about 44 cents of every food dollar outside the home these days—up from 25 cents in 1955. To put it another way, on any given day 41 percent of American women eat out.

Happily, there's nothing inherently fattening or unhealthy about greeting the day with breakfast in a classic diner, grabbing lunch at a fast-food drive-through, or relaxing over dinner in an American-style bistro, says Warshaw. On the Fat-to-Firm Program, you'll discover surefire ways to spot hidden obstacles to healthy dining out, you'll learn strategies to overcome those obstacles, and you'll soon find that a restaurant meal can be a pure, nonfattening pleasure.

Obstacle #1: A Special Occasion—10 Times a Week

Once, restaurant meals were reserved for anniversaries, birthdays, or romantic evening dates. We dressed up and ordered fancy foods with abandon—knowing full well that tomorrow we would be back to meat loaf at the kitchen table.

Today, celebrations account for just 5 percent of meals out, according to a survey of restaurant patrons co-sponsored by the Thomas Food Industry Register. "Yet the sheer thrill of dining out never goes away completely, even if you eat out all the time," notes Janet Bukovinsky Teacher, former restaurant reviewer for *Philadelphia Magazine.*

And therein lies the first obstacle to healthy, nonfattening restaurant eating. While a good meal out can soothe us, raise our spirits, or rekindle the flame with our spouses, all too often we still order—and indulge—as if every meal were a special occasion, says Donna Erickson, R.D., health educator in the Weight Management Center at the Carle Clinic Association in Champaign, Illinois. We throw caution to the wind. "If you look at how often you eat out in a week, you may see that it isn't a special occasion at all," she says. "It's a way of life."

Obstacle #2: All That Fat

Restaurant food is loaded with fat, from the butter we spread on our bread right on through to dessert, notes Jane Freiman, a former restaurant critic for *New York Newsday* and the former underground gourmet for *New York Magazine*. "There's cream, cheese, crispy things like potato pancakes and parsnip chips, dressing on the salad, butter sauce on the tuna—and that's just in the appetizers."

If one thing unites Manhattan's fanciest eateries with hamburger joints, family restaurants, and bistros across the country, it's fat. Perhaps you have never nibbled a deep-fried parsnip chip, but did you know that a breaded and fried chicken sandwich may have 710 calories—390 of them from fat? Or that a salad in a taco bowl may have 840 calories—470 from fat? "Once you know the fat is lurking, there's plenty you can do to reduce it to limit how much of it you eat," Erickson notes. Here's how.

Grill the waiter, nicely. Learn all you can about food before you order. "Ask about the ingredients and the preparation style," Erickson says. "I ask if the food was marinated, whether oil or butter is added, whether a sauce is added after cooking." And don't worry. Polite, assertive questions won't embarrass your companions. "My husband was surprised at all my questions at first, but now he's used to it," she says. "Waiters and chefs want to please their customers, but they're thinking about taste. It's up to you to think about fat and calories."

Special requests go more smoothly if you ask for simple changes, like getting the sauce on the side or having fish broiled with wine instead of butter.

Be firm. If food arrives and is not prepared as you requested, hold your ground, Erickson adds. "Simply say, 'I'm sorry, this isn't what I ordered. Would you please exchange it?' "

Go for these "green light" cooking styles. Erickson suggests that you scan the menu for these words that signal low-fat, low-calorie

The Fat-to-Firm Fast-Food Guide

"What'll it be?" barks a scratchy voice on the intercom, as you survey the choices at your favorite fast-food drive-through. You're hankering for a burger or a shake, but will it overwhelm your healthy weight-loss plan with calories and fat?

Not necessarily, says Colleen Pierre, R.D., a nutritionist in Baltimore and a spokesperson for the American Dietetic Association. "If you choose carefully, you can have that burger or shake," she says. "In fact, a small chocolate shake and a grilled chicken salad with

Fat Choice

Food	Calories	Calories from Fat
Burger Meal		
One big burger (such as a Big Mac, Quarter Pounder, or Whopper)	430–640	190–350
Large fries	450	200
—	—	—
Regular cola (medium-size)	240	0
TOTAL	**1,120–1,330**	**390–550**
Chicken Meal		
Breaded, fried chicken sandwich	440–710	160–390
—	—	—
Large fries	450	200
Chocolate milk shake (small)	320–360	50–60
TOTAL	**1,210–1,520**	**410–650**
Mexican Fast Food		
Taco salad in edible taco shell	840	470
Half an order of nachos	155	80
Regular cola (medium-size)	240	0
TOTAL	**1,235**	**550**

cooking techniques: baked; broiled or grilled without added fat; poached; roasted; steamed; and with tomato sauce.

Be cautious about these "red light" cooking styles. Erickson says that these menu descriptions indicate high-fat, high-calorie foods that should be avoided or eaten in limited portions: au gratin, basted, braised,

low-fat dressing is a great, low-fat meal, packed with lots of calcium for strong bones but without a lot of calories. And you get your chocolate taste for the day."

Here are some ways to turn "fat" fast food into "firm" choices. Make sure that you check with a restaurant's nutrition chart before ordering, since calorie and fat content of similar dishes can vary from one fast-food chain to another, and even within a chain.

Firm Choice

Food	Calories	Calories from Fat
Burger Meal		
Small burger*	260–270	80–90
Side salad	35–60	0–25
Fat-free dressing	30–50	0
Low-fat milk	100–130	20–45
TOTAL	425–510	100–160
Chicken Meal		
Grilled chicken, no mayo (ask for extra lettuce and tomato)	310	70
Barbecue sauce	45–50	0
Small fries	210–260	90–120
Diet cola (medium-size)	0	0
TOTAL	565–620	160–190
Mexican Fast Food		
1 light chicken soft taco	180	45
1 order pinto beans and cheese	190	80
Diet cola (medium-size)	0	0
TOTAL	370	125

*Note: Don't confuse a small burger with what some chains call junior burgers, which are considerably higher in calories.

buttered, with cheese sauce, creamy, crispy, fried, gravy, hash, hollandaise, with melted cheese, pan-fried, Parmesan, prime (the grade of meat with most fat), sautéed, and scalloped.

Begin and end with starters. Appetizers, soups, and salads often include delicious, low-fat choices, says Warshaw. Consider making

The Secrets of Ordering Low-Fat Ethnic Food

Exotic and delicious, ethnic cuisine can be a treasure trove of lean choices. "But once tossed together with high-fat items like lard, cheese, and cream, these foods can be a caloric disaster," notes Hope Warshaw, R.D., a nutrition consultant in Washington, D.C., and author of *The Restaurant Companion: A Guide to Healthier Eating Out.*

Here's how to unlock the slimming secrets of ethnic foods and leave the fat and calories behind.

Mexican Food

One slimming request to make: "May I have soft flour tortillas to dip in salsa, in place of fried tortilla chips and guacamole?"

Order these: Black beans, red and green salsa, enchilada sauce, mole sauce, soft corn or flour tortillas, burritos, fajitas, soft tacos, and grilled, marinated chicken or fish.

Pass on these: Chimichangas and tacos made with fried tortillas and, usually, cheese; tortilla chips; and dishes made with sour cream, guacamole, cheese, or the Mexican sausage called chorizo.

Chinese Food

One slimming request to make: "Please cook my order with no oil or with as little oil as possible."

Order these: Steamed dumplings, wonton soup, hot-and-sour soup, shrimp with broccoli, roast pork with vegetables, beef chow mein, lo mein, spicy green beans, steamed dishes, and vegetable stir-fries.

Pass on these: Deep-fried dishes; those containing duck, cashews, and peanuts; and any type of fried rice.

Italian Food

One slimming request to make: "Could I have a tomato sauce to dip the bread into, instead of olive oil or butter?"

Order these: Clams steamed in white wine, marinated vegetables, bean and pasta soup, pasta with tomato sauce, white clam sauce, red clam sauce, veal cacciatore, chicken in wine sauce, shrimp with tomato sauce, scallops sautéed with mushrooms and marsala wine sauce.

Pass on these: Pastas with cheese stuffing, meats cooked *saltimbocca* (sautéed in butter), and anything parmigiana (fried and topped with cheese).

a meal of these, instead of having a higher-fat entrée that is an inherently larger portion. "Practice menu creativity," she advises. "Have a salad with low-fat dressing and ask the waiter to bring an appetizer as your entrée. Or have two appetizers. The possibilities are endless."

Look beyond fat and calories. Scan the menu for fruits, vegetables, and whole grains that will give you body-building nutrients, says Colleen Pierre, R.D., a nutritionist in Baltimore and a spokesperson for the American Dietetic Association. Often, they're also low-fat choices. "We need vitamins and minerals to strengthen the immune system and run all the body's hundreds of functions," she says. "Your body is regenerating all the time. It needs nutrients for that."

Find your safety zone. Track down restaurants where you can order a tasty, low-fat meal and avoid those where that's impossible such as, perhaps, a fish-and-chips spot or fried-chicken stand, Erickson says.

Create your own lower-fat fast food. If you tend to grab high-fat food on the run, look for lower-fat alternatives that you can buy at the supermarket ahead of time, suggests Warshaw. For example, you might stock up on bagels over the weekend, then eat one lightly spread with low-fat cream cheese on the way to work in place of that high-fat breakfast croissant.

Obstacle #3: Colossal Portions

At the Homer Laughlin China Company in Newell, West Virginia, one of the nation's largest suppliers of restaurant tableware—design director Jonathan Parry is observing an astonishing trend. "Restaurants are using dessert plates bigger than dinner plates. I've seen oval dinner plates 18 inches long," Parry says. "I don't know how people eat all that food."

Gargantuan portions make diners feel as if they have gotten their money's worth, notes Gordon Sinclair, operator of Chicago's upscale Gordon Restaurant, which is bucking the trend by selling all selections as half-portions "so that customers can create their own 'tasting menu.' "

Mega-portions pack in mega-calories, notes Warshaw. Since most restaurants do not offer half-portions, you'll need other strategies to limit the amount of food on your plate. "Less food in front of you means that you'll eat less," she says. "I call that out of sight, out of mouth." Here's how.

Divide and conquer. Split an entrée with a friend and order extra vegetables, rice, baked potato, or salad on the side, suggests Constance Geiger, R.D., Ph.D., research assistant professor in the division of foods

Four-Star Smarts:
How a Restaurant Critic Doesn't Gain Weight

It's a job from heaven—or weight-gain hell. Janet Bukovinsky Teacher, former restaurant critic for *Philadelphia Magazine,* dines out at least three times a week, sampling "everything everyone at my table orders—appetizers, soups and salads, main courses, and desserts."

She's devised a strategy that lets her savor each meal without jeopardizing her healthy body weight of 130 pounds. Here's how she does it.

- Eats low-fat at other times. "I love plain grains, so I might have oatmeal for breakfast or brown rice and veggies for lunch on a reviewing day," she says. "I had a salad today with a little balsamic vinaigrette."

- Snubs bad food. "If I taste something during a review that isn't good, I don't waste calories by eating more of it," she says.

- Stops eating early. "I leave a lot of food on my plate," she says. "I tend to eat the vegetables, but I might not finish my meat."

- Orders lower-fat for herself. "I'll try to choose something like fish and ask others to have heavier meats and higher-fat foods," she says.

- Skips the cocktails. "Drinks like martinis are very popular right now, but I don't order them anymore," she says. "It adds calories."

- Makes exceptions for her favorite foods. "I love cheeses. I love pâté. When they're on the menu, I'll be greedy and get them," she says. "I don't deprive myself of something I really love."

- Works out. "I go to the gym twice a week to burn off calories," she says.

and nutrition at the University of Utah in Salt Lake City and a consultant on food labeling and nutrition. "Some restaurants may charge you a little for the extra plate, but it's worth it if it keeps you from eating a whole large, high-calorie entrée."

Take half home. Ask for a take-out box (doggie bags are passé) as soon as your meal arrives, Erickson suggests. Deposit half inside and—presto—you've avoided overeating and gotten tomorrow's lunch in the bargain. "Put the food in the box right away," she says. "Otherwise, it's easy to keep on picking at something on your plate."

If the meal is very formal, you may want to quietly transfer half to your bread plate and discreetly ask a waiter to wrap it for you to take home, rather than shoveling your dinner into the box yourself.

Sup family-style. Order fewer entrées than there are people and pass the food around. Fill in the gaps with extra orders of salad and vegetables, Warshaw suggests. "People do this in Chinese restaurants all the time," she says. "But you can do it anywhere, really."

Plan ahead. "Bank" extra calories a few days before a hearty restaurant meal by exercising a little more each day, Erickson suggests. "If you walk an extra mile for five days, you'll have burned an extra 400 to 500 calories, so you could overeat a little or have dessert without having to make adjustments," she notes.

Six More Ways to Outsmart the Menu

Here are more expert tips for enjoying restaurant meals to the fullest, while sticking with a healthy eating plan.

Don't go hungry. If you starve yourself beforehand, you may be setting yourself up to overeat at the restaurant, says Erickson. So eat breakfast, lunch, and even a small snack before heading off for your night out. Good choices are vegetables, fruits, and whole grains—low-fat, high-nutrition choices often in short supply on restaurant menus.

Sidestep the bread basket. Avoid the lure of the bread basket while you wait for your entrée by ordering sparkling water, a salad with low-fat dressing on the side, or a clear soup, suggests Warshaw. Or take one piece of bread, then send the basket—and the butter or olive oil—back.

Watch the wine. Alcoholic beverages tend to induce overeating, notes Dr. Geiger. So consider ordering one glass of wine with your meal, instead of starting before the food arrives.

"Also, make sure that you have a nonalcoholic, noncaloric beverage next to the wine and use that to quench your thirst," says Warshaw.

Luxuriate. "Enjoy the whole event, not just the food," Warshaw suggests. Soak up the atmosphere. People-watch. Converse with your dining companions.

Order side vegetables à la carte. This is a great way to mix and match vegetables, making them a larger but mainly lower-calorie portion of your meal, Erickson suggests.

Have your fruit and eat it, too. Restaurants often use fruit as garnish. So even if you don't see fresh strawberries or orange slices on the menu, ask if you could have a serving made up—some restaurants will gladly accommodate you, says Erickson.

Chapter 14

Never Go Hungry Again

**Welcome to the Fat-to-Firm eating plan—
to top nutrition, mealtime fun, no hunger,
and to finally achieving (and maintaining)
your weight-loss goal.**

Annie Schneider has rekindled her love affair with food. Her refrigerator has never been more full. Open the door, and you'll see a riot of glorious colors and flavors, from tangy fruit juices to crispy vegetables, mellow low-fat cheeses to creamy yogurts. Her cabinets brim with pasta and popcorn, bagel chips and whole-grain breads. These days, she's always experimenting with new edibles. "It's great to find something new that really makes your taste buds go wild," she says. "But I still have my old favorite treats like pizza, a little chocolate, or a lamb chop from time to time."

After six months of healthy feasting—and gentle, regular physical activity—Annie has lost 40 pounds. "This new eating plan of mine is a way of life," says this 34-year-old marketing manager for a Chicago cable-television network. "This is a very different attitude from when I used to diet. If I get off-track, I don't feel like a failure now. I just get back on track and take it bite by bite."

On the Fat-to-Firm eating plan, you'll find the same ingredients that spelled success for Annie: Regular meals, plus snacks. Room for treats like cookies, lobster, frozen desserts, and even filet mignon. Healthy meal plans that satisfy stomach hunger and provide the nutrients women need, such as calcium for strong bones and iron to build blood cells. Enough variety to keep your taste buds "going wild," so you won't feel deprived. And the promise that you'll never have to eat something you don't like.

"A woman should never eat foods she doesn't like. And on this plan, she doesn't have to," says Carla Wolper, R.D., a nutritionist and clinical coordinator at the Obesity Research Center at St. Luke's/ Roosevelt Hospital Center in New York City and the expert who developed this meal plan for the Fat-to-Firm Program. "The plan is based on balance and freedom. You're free to eat what you like. And as long as you keep the portions in check, balancing higher-fat foods against lower-fat foods, you won't gain weight."

Bite by Bite: Inside the Plan

You can expect slow, steady weight loss on the Fat-to-Firm eating plan, says Wolper. Once you reach your goal, and to maintain your weight, you simply keep enjoying the same healthy, low-fat foods in the portion sizes for your final weight range. "This isn't a diet," she says. "It's the kind of nutritious plan a woman could follow for years to come." The Fat-to-Firm eating plan meets women's unique needs in three ways: her nutritional needs, her emotional needs, and her need for healthy weight loss. Here's how.

Regular meals, plus three snacks. You'll eat every 3 to 4 hours, leaving behind the hunger and deprivation associated with dead-end diets. Think of it as a physical and emotional insurance policy against overeating. "When we go for long periods of time without food, it's very hard, psychologically, not to eat too much at the next meal," says Joni Johnston, Psy.D., clinical psychologist in Del Mar, California, and author of *Appearance Obsession: Learning to Love the Way You Look.* "Eating regularly is comforting."

Variety. You'll have opportunities to substitute new foods for familiar ones that may have become old hat, giving your body a wide range of important nutrients and keeping your taste buds interested at the same time. "There are hundreds of beneficial substances in fruits, vegetables, and grains—no single food could supply all those nutrients," says Carol Boushey, R.D., Ph.D., assistant professor of food and nutrition in the department of food and nutrition at Southern Illinois University in Carbondale. "I also think that getting a variety of foods onto your plate can help with weight loss."

In other words, eating an apple every day is good. But if familiar "healthy" foods leave you longing for Ding-Dongs or Ho-Ho's, try cubes of sweet, tropical mango mixed with fresh raspberries instead; a smoothie made with blended yogurt, pineapples, and bananas; or peaches and frozen yogurt. Is your mouth watering yet?

Freedom. "You can have filet mignon, olive oil in your spaghetti sauce, or dessert, and not gain weight on this plan if you balance your food choices throughout the day," says Wolper. "I do it myself. I might have three fruit snacks after dinner, by saving snacks from earlier in the day. Or, the other night I had spaghetti sauce with olive oil in it, so I cut back on the amount of chicken breast I served to balance the calories. And I really enjoyed my meal."

A custom fit. The Fat-to-Firm eating plan offers customized menus just right for your healthy weight goal, whether it's 110, 140, 160 pounds or more—or anywhere in between. In addition, it offers suggestions for a wide range of meals—from traditional lunch sandwiches and meat-and-potatoes dinners to elegant salads and meatless meals.

Building blocks, not a rigid menu. Use the sample menus and substitution ideas on the following pages as a guide. They're based on a simple plan that lets you avoid counting calories or fat grams.

Every day, go for six to 11 servings of breads, cereals, and grains; at least two servings of fruit; three or more of vegetables; three of low-fat dairy; two of lean meat, eggs, fish, or beans; and make limited use of fats and oils, says Wolper. Use the weight range right for you to determine how large a serving—and how many servings—will meet your needs.

How to Use the Plan

Harness the Fat-to-Firm eating plan to meet your weight-loss needs by setting small goals, Wolper suggests. If you weigh 180 pounds and your healthy weight-loss goal is 145 pounds, start by aiming for 170 pounds, then 160 pounds. "Then, you may want to stay at 160 pounds for a few weeks before you try to lose more weight," she suggests. "This will give you a chance to practice maintenance skills at your new weight, plus give you a break from losing. You may regain 2 to 3 pounds. Don't be surprised or upset, it's perfectly normal. In fact, it's usually just water-weight gain. Once your weight is stable, aim for another small weight-loss target."

In every weight category, the plan suggests a range of portion sizes for many foods in each meal. For example, breakfast at the 141 to 160 weight category for the "Low-Meat Option" calls for 1¼ to 1½ cups bran flakes with ½ to 1 cup skim milk and an orange or a half a grapefruit. If your weight goal is at the high end of the category, eat the biggest portion. If it's at the low end, eat the smallest portion. For weights in between, simply eat an in-between-size portion, Wolper says.

If you get a lot of physical activity by working out or playing sports five or more times a week, you can opt for a larger portion size, Wolper says. And if you lead a sedentary lifestyle or are over 60 years old, eat toward the low end of your weight category, she advises.

If you weigh more than 200 pounds, and your weight-loss goal is above 200 pounds, fine-tune your eating plan by adding food to the highest weight category on the menus. "For every 10 pounds, add 200 calories—about the amount in a piece of fruit with a cup of nonfat plain yogurt or two pieces of bread or 2 ounces of cheese," Wolper says. "This is one time when you will have to count calories a little bit."

Breakfast: A Fat-to-Firm Eating Plan Priority

Breakfast has the power to jump-start your journey from fat to firm because it protects you from overeating later in the day. "When you force your body to run on very little fuel in the morning, you can become ravenous and justify eating anything," notes Catherine Champagne, R.D., Ph.D., associate professor for research at the Pennington Biomedical Research Center in Baton Rouge, Louisiana.

That sets up a dangerous cycle—skip breakfast, overeat later in the day, then feel guilty or not very hungry in the morning, so you skip breakfast again, Wolper adds.

"In research studies, the meal most often associated with being thin is breakfast," Wolper notes. "There's evidence that people who eat a bigger low-fat breakfast are thinner than people who eat a small low-fat breakfast. It is a constant theme. The heaviest women who come for treatment are the women who skip breakfast."

Skipping breakfast may also teach your body to be thrifty and to save more calories from later meals as fat, Dr. Champagne adds. If you've been avoiding the breakfast table for years, make a slow return, she suggests.

(continued on page 186)

The Fat-to-Firm Eating Plan

The Low-Meat Option

100 to 120 Pounds_____
Breakfast
- ½ to ¾ cup bran flakes (or another whole-grain or high-fiber cereal) with ½ cup skim milk, an orange or half a grapefruit, and coffee or tea with 2 tablespoons 1% milk and 1 tablespoon sugar

Midmorning Snack
- ½ cup nonfat plain yogurt with ½ cup berries

Lunch
- 3 to 4 ounces turkey breast on two slices of whole-wheat bread with 1 tablespoon mustard, two slices of tomato, a few arugula or spinach leaves, and one slice of red onion; and 1 cup skim milk

Afternoon Snack
- One medium apple

Dinner
- 3 cups raw vegetables (such as zucchini, eggplant, peppers, mushrooms, and onions), sliced ¼ to ½ inch thick, sprayed or brushed with 1 to 2 tablespoons olive oil and sprinkled with garlic, salt, pepper, 2 tablespoons balsamic vinegar, 1 to 2 tablespoons grated Parmesan cheese, then grilled or broiled and served over ½ cup cooked brown rice; two oatmeal cookies; and a noncaloric beverage

Evening Snack
- 1 cup nonfat fruit-flavored yogurt

121 to 140 Pounds_____
Breakfast
- ¾ to 1¼ cups bran flakes (or other whole-grain or high-fiber cereal) with ½ cup skim milk, an orange or half a grapefruit, and coffee or tea with 2 tablespoons 1% milk and 1 tablespoon sugar

Midmorning Snack
- ½ cup nonfat plain yogurt with ½ cup berries

Lunch
- 3 to 4 ounces turkey breast on two slices of whole-wheat bread with 1 tablespoon mustard, two slices of tomato, a few arugula or spinach leaves, and one slice of red onion; and 1 cup skim milk

Afternoon Snack
- One medium apple

Dinner
- 3 cups raw vegetables (such as zucchini, eggplant, peppers, mushrooms, and onions), sliced ¼ to ½ inch thick, sprayed or brushed with 2 to 3 tablespoons olive oil and sprinkled with garlic, salt, pepper, 2 table-

spoons balsamic vinegar, 1 to 2 tablespoons grated Parmesan cheese, then grilled or broiled and served over $1/2$ cup cooked brown rice; two oatmeal cookies; and a noncaloric beverage

Evening Snack

- 1 cup nonfat fruit-flavored yogurt

141 to 160 Pounds_____
Breakfast

- $1\frac{1}{4}$ to $1\frac{1}{2}$ cups bran flakes (or other whole-grain or high-fiber cereal) with $1/2$ to 1 cup skim milk, an orange or half a grapefruit, and coffee or tea with 2 tablespoons 1% milk and 1 tablespoon sugar

Midmorning Snack

- A toasted English muffin with 1 tablespoon butter or margarine or 2 tablespoons jam

Lunch

- 4 to 6 ounces turkey breast on two slices of whole-wheat bread with 1 tablespoon mustard, two slices tomato, a few arugula or spinach leaves, and one slice red onion; and 1 cup skim milk

Afternoon Snack

- One medium apple

Dinner

- 3 to 4 cups raw vegetables (such as zucchini, eggplant, peppers,

mushrooms, and onions), sliced $1/4$ to $1/2$ inch thick, sprayed or brushed with 3 to 4 tablespoons olive oil and sprinkled with garlic, salt, pepper, 2 tablespoons balsamic vinegar, 2 tablespoons grated Parmesan cheese, then grilled or broiled and served over $1/2$ cup cooked brown rice; two oatmeal cookies; and a noncaloric beverage

Evening Snack

- 1 cup nonfat fruit-flavored yogurt

161 to 180 Pounds_____
Breakfast

- $1\frac{1}{2}$ to 2 cups bran flakes (or other whole-grain or high-fiber cereal) with 1 cup skim milk, an orange or half a grapefruit, and coffee or tea with 2 tablespoons 1% milk and 1 tablespoon sugar

Midmorning Snack

- A toasted English muffin with 1 tablespoon butter or margarine or 2 tablespoons jam

Lunch

- 6 ounces turkey breast on two slices of whole-wheat bread with 1 tablespoon mustard, two slices of tomato, a few arugula or spinach leaves, and one slice

(continued) ▶

The Fat-to-Firm Eating Plan—Continued

of red onion; $1/2$ cup fresh raspberries; and 1 cup skim milk
Afternoon Snack
- One large apple
Dinner
- 3 to 4 cups raw vegetables (such as zucchini, eggplant, peppers, mushrooms, and onions), slice $1/4$ to $1/2$ inch thick, sprayed or brushed with 3 to 4 tablespoons olive oil and sprinkled with garlic, salt, pepper, 2 tablespoons balsamic vinegar, 3 tablespoons grated Parmesan cheese, then grilled or broiled and served over 1 cup cooked brown rice; three oatmeal cookies; and a noncaloric beverage
Evening Snack
- 1 cup nonfat fruit-flavored yogurt

181 to 200 Pounds
Breakfast
- $1^{1}/2$ to 2 cups bran flakes (or other whole-grain or high-fiber cereal) with 1 cup skim milk, an orange or half a grapefruit, and coffee or tea with 2 tablespoons 1% milk and 1 tablespoon sugar
Midmorning Snack
- A toasted English muffin with 1 tablespoon butter or margarine or 2 tablespoons jam
Lunch
- 6 ounces turkey breast on two slices of whole-wheat bread with 1 tablespoon mustard, two slices of tomato, a few arugula

or spinach leaves, and one slice of red onion; 1 cup green and red pepper strips; $1/2$ cup fresh raspberries; and 1 cup skim milk
Afternoon Snack
- One large apple, cut in slices and dipped in 1 tablespoon peanut butter
Dinner
- 3 to 4 cups raw vegetables (such as zucchini, eggplant, peppers, mushrooms, and onions), slice $1/4$ to $1/2$ inch thick, sprayed or brushed with 3 to 4 tablespoons olive oil and sprinkled with garlic, salt, pepper, 2 tablespoons balsamic vinegar, 3 tablespoons grated Parmesan cheese, then grilled or broiled and served over 1 cup cooked brown rice; one small roll; three oatmeal cookies; and a noncaloric beverage
Evening Snack
- 1 cup nonfat fruit-flavored yogurt

The Meat-and Potatoes Option

110 to 120 Pounds
Breakfast
- One or two small eggs (poached or scrambled in a no-stick pan) with one slice of plain whole-wheat toast, 6 ounces orange juice or one orange, and coffee or tea with 2 tablespoons 1% milk and 1 tablespoon sugar

Midmorning Snack
- ½ to 1 cup nonfat plain yogurt with ¼ cup fruit

Lunch
- 2 cups salad greens with eight to 10 medium-size cooked shrimp, dressed with 1 teaspoon olive oil and 2 tablespoons balsamic vinegar mixed with 1 teaspoon mustard and fresh pepper; one slice of bread or small roll; and 1 cup skim milk

Afternoon Snack
- 1 cup baby carrots, with ½ cup nonfat yogurt with cracked pepper, lemon juice, and herbs

Dinner
- 4 to 5 ounces grilled filet mignon, a medium baked potato with ½ tablespoon butter or margarine, ½ cup string beans, a baked apple, and water, coffee, tea, diet soda, or other noncaloric beverage

Evening Snack
- One or two small cookies and 1 cup skim milk

121 to 140 Pounds
Breakfast
- One or two medium eggs (poached or scrambled in a non-stick pan) with one or two slices of plain whole-wheat toast, 6 ounces orange juice or one orange, and coffee or tea with 2 tablespoons 1% milk and 1 tablespoon sugar

Midmorning Snack
- ½ to 1 cup nonfat plain yogurt with ¼ cup fruit

Lunch
- 2 cups salad greens with eight to 10 medium-size cooked shrimp, dressed with 1 teaspoon olive oil and 2 tablespoons balsamic vinegar mixed with 1 teaspoon mustard and fresh pepper; one slice of bread or small roll; and 1 cup skim milk

Afternoon Snack
- 1 cup baby carrots, dipped in ½ cup nonfat yogurt flavored with cracked pepper, lemon juice, and herbs

Dinner
- 5 to 7 ounces grilled filet mignon, a medium baked potato with ½ tablespoon butter or margarine, ½ cup string beans, a baked apple, and water, coffee, tea, diet soda, or other noncaloric beverage

Evening Snack
- Two or three small cookies and 1 cup skim milk

141 to 160 Pounds
Breakfast
- One or two medium eggs (poached or scrambled in a non-stick pan) with one or two slices of whole-wheat toast, 1 tablespoon jam, 6 ounces orange juice or one orange, and coffee

(continued) ▶

The Fat-to-Firm Eating Plan—Continued

or tea with 2 tablespoons 1% milk and 1 tablespoon sugar
Midmorning Snack
- 1 cup nonfat plain yogurt with 1 cup fruit

Lunch
- 2 cups salad greens with eight to 10 medium-size cooked shrimp, dressed with 1 tablespoon olive oil and 2 tablespoons balsamic vinegar mixed with 1 teaspoon mustard and fresh pepper; one slice of bread or small roll; and 1 cup skim milk

Afternoon Snack
- 1 cup baby carrots, dipped in ½ cup nonfat yogurt flavored with cracked pepper, lemon juice, and herbs

Dinner
- 5 to 6 ounces grilled filet mignon, a large baked potato with 1 tablespoon butter or margarine, ½ cup string beans, a baked apple with 2 tablespoons regular or frozen vanilla yogurt, and water, coffee, tea, diet soda, or other noncaloric beverage

Evening Snack
- Three or four small cookies and 1 cup skim milk

161 to 180 Pounds_____
Breakfast
- One or two medium eggs (poached or scrambled in a no-stick pan) with one or two slices of whole-wheat toast, 1 table-

spoon jam, 6 ounces orange juice or one orange, and coffee or tea with 2 tablespoons 1% milk and 1 tablespoon sugar
Midmorning Snack
- 1 cup nonfat plain yogurt with 1 cup fruit

Lunch
- 2 cups salad greens with eight to 10 medium-size cooked shrimp, dressed with 1 to 2 tablespoons olive oil and 2 tablespoons balsamic vinegar mixed with 1 teaspoon mustard and fresh pepper; two slices of bread or one medium-size roll; and 1 cup skim milk

Afternoon Snack
- 1 cup baby carrots, with ½ cup nonfat yogurt with cracked pepper, lemon juice, and herbs

Dinner
- 5 to 6 ounces grilled filet mignon, a large baked potato with 1 teaspoon butter or margarine, ½ cup pickled red cabbage, ½ cup string beans, a baked apple with 2 tablespoons regular or frozen vanilla yogurt, and a noncaloric beverage

Evening Snack
- Three or four small cookies and 1 cup skim milk

181 to 200 Pounds_____
Breakfast
- One or two medium eggs (poached or scrambled in a no-

stick pan) with one or two slices of whole-wheat toast, 1 tablespoon jam, 6 ounces orange juice or one orange, and coffee or tea with 2 tablespoons 1% milk and 1 tablespoon sugar

Midmorning Snack

- 1 cup nonfat plain yogurt with 1 cup fruit

Lunch

- 2 cups salad greens with 8 to 10 medium-size cooked shrimp, dressed with 1 to 2 tablespoons olive oil and 2 tablespoons balsamic vinegar, mixed with 1 teaspoon mustard and fresh pepper; two slices of bread or one medium-size roll; and 1 cup skim milk

Afternoon Snack

- 1 cup baby carrots, dipped in 1/2 cup nonfat yogurt flavored with cracked pepper, lemon juice, and herbs

Dinner

- 5 to 6 ounces grilled filet mignon, a large baked potato with 1 teaspoon butter or margarine, 1/2 cup pickled red cabbage, 1/2 cup string beans, a baked apple with 2 tablespoons regular or frozen vanilla yogurt, and a noncaloric beverage

Evening Snack

- A slice of cherry pie (3 inches wide at crust) and 1 cup skim milk

The Lobster-and-Pasta Option

121 to 140 Pounds

Breakfast

- 1/2 cup fruit salad with 1/2 to 1 cup nonfat fruit-flavored yogurt and 1 tablespoon whole-grain cereal, and coffee or tea with 2 tablespoons 1% milk and 1 tablespoon sugar

Midmorning Snack

- One slice of toast with 1 tablespoon jam or 1/2 tablespoon butter or margarine, or four small graham crackers with 1 ounce light cream cheese

Lunch

- 3/4 to 1 cup pasta with 1/2 cup tomato sauce; 1 cup leafy salad greens with 1/2 tablespoon olive oil and 2 tablespoons balsamic vinegar, mixed with 1 teaspoon mustard and fresh pepper; and water, diet soda, or other noncaloric beverage

Afternoon Snack

- 1 cup nonfat broth with 1/2 cup frozen vegetables and 1 cup skim milk

Dinner

- Steamed lobster (6 ounces lobster meat) with 1 tablespoon melted butter; 1 cup rice, cooked in nonfat broth; 1/2 cup corn and 1/2 cup cooked spinach; 1 cup cut fruit; and water, coffee, tea, diet soda, or other noncaloric beverage

(continued) ►

The Fat-to-Firm Eating Plan—Continued

Evening Snack
- 1 cup frozen nonfat yogurt

121 to 140 Pounds_____
Breakfast
- $\frac{1}{2}$ cup fruit salad with 1 cup nonfat fruit-flavored yogurt and 1 tablespoon whole-grain cereal, and coffee or tea with 2 tablespoons 1% milk and 1 tablespoon sugar

Midmorning Snack
- One slice of toast with 1 tablespoon jam or $\frac{1}{2}$ tablespoon butter or margarine, or four small graham crackers with 1 ounce light cream cheese

Lunch
- 1 to $\frac{1}{2}$ cups pasta with $\frac{1}{2}$ cup tomato sauce; 1 cup leafy salad greens with 1 tablespoon olive oil and 2 tablespoons balsamic vinegar, mixed with 1 teaspoon mustard and fresh pepper; and water, diet soda, or other noncaloric beverage

Afternoon Snack
- 1 cup nonfat broth with $\frac{1}{2}$ cup frozen vegetables and 1 cup skim milk

Dinner
- Steamed lobster (6 ounces lobster meat) with 1 tablespoon melted butter; 1 cup rice, cooked in nonfat broth; $\frac{1}{2}$ cup corn and $\frac{1}{2}$ cup cooked spinach; 1 cup cut fruit; and water, coffee, tea, diet soda, or other noncaloric beverage

Evening Snack
- 1 cup frozen nonfat yogurt

141 to 160 Pounds_____
Breakfast
- 1 cup fruit salad with 1 cup nonfat fruit-flavored yogurt and 3 to 4 tablespoons whole-grain cereal, and coffee or tea with 2 tablespoons 1% milk and 1 tablespoon sugar

Midmorning Snack
- Two slices of toast with 1 to 2 tablespoons jam or $\frac{1}{2}$ to 1 tablespoon butter or margarine, or eight small graham crackers and 1 ounce light cream cheese

Lunch
- 1$\frac{1}{2}$ to 2 cups pasta with $\frac{1}{2}$ cup tomato sauce; 1 cup leafy salad greens with 1 tablespoon olive oil and 2 tablespoons balsamic vinegar, mixed with 1 teaspoon mustard and fresh pepper; and a noncaloric beverage

Afternoon Snack
- 1 cup nonfat broth with $\frac{1}{2}$ cup frozen vegetables and 1 cup skim milk

Dinner
- Steamed lobster (6 ounces lobster meat) with 1 tablespoon melted butter; 1 to 1$\frac{1}{2}$ cups rice, cooked in nonfat broth; $\frac{1}{2}$ cup corn and $\frac{1}{2}$ cup cooked spinach; 1 cup cut fruit; and water, coffee, tea, diet soda, or another noncaloric beverage

Evening Snack
- 1 cup frozen nonfat yogurt

161 to 180 Pounds_____
Breakfast
- 1 cup fruit salad with 1 cup nonfat fruit-flavored yogurt and 4 to 6 tablespoons whole-grain cereal, and coffee or tea with 2 tablespoons 1% milk and 1 tablespoon sugar

Midmorning Snack
- Two slices of toast with 1 to 2 tablespoons jam or $1/2$ to 1 tablespoon butter or margarine, or eight small graham crackers and 1 ounce light cream cheese

Lunch
- $1 1/2$ to 2 cups pasta with $1/2$ cup tomato sauce; 1 cup leafy salad greens with 1 tablespoon olive oil and 2 tablespoons balsamic vinegar, mixed with 1 teaspoon mustard and fresh pepper; one slice of bread or a small roll; and a noncaloric beverage

Afternoon Snack
- 1 cup nonfat broth with $1/2$ cup frozen vegetables and 1 cup skim milk

Dinner
- Steamed lobster (8 to 10 ounces lobster meat) with 1 tablespoon melted butter; 1 to $1 1/2$ cups rice, cooked in nonfat broth; $1/2$ cup corn and $1/2$ cooked cup spinach; 1 cup cut fruit; and a noncaloric beverage

Evening Snack
- 1 cup frozen nonfat yogurt and two small cookies

181 to 200 Pounds_____
Breakfast
- 1 cup fruit salad with 1 cup nonfat fruit-flavored yogurt and 4 to 6 tablespoons whole-grain cereal, and coffee or tea with 2 tablespoons 1% milk and 1 tablespoon sugar

Midmorning Snack
- Two slices of toast with 1 to 2 tablespoons jam or $1/2$ to 1 tablespoon butter or margarine, or eight small graham crackers and 1 ounce light cream cheese

Lunch
- 2 to $2 1/2$ cups pasta with $3/4$ cup tomato sauce; 1 cup leafy salad greens with 1 tablespoon olive oil and 2 tablespoons balsamic vinegar, mixed with 1 teaspoon mustard and fresh pepper; one slice of bread or a small roll; and a noncaloric beverage

Afternoon Snack
- 1 cup nonfat broth with $1/2$ cup frozen vegetables and 1 cup skim milk

Dinner
- Steamed lobster (10 ounces lobster meat) with 1 tablespoon melted butter; 1 to $1 1/2$ cups rice, cooked in nonfat broth; $1/2$ cup corn and $1/2$ cup cooked spinach; 1 cup cut fruit; and a noncaloric beverage

Evening Snack
- 1 cup frozen nonfat yogurt and two small cookies

"Don't torture yourself with trying to eat a full breakfast. But eat something: toast, fruit, or nonfat yogurt. And use your midmorning snack to catch up with the rest of your morning nutrition and energy needs." Try these strategies for getting the most out of this important meal.

Say yes to protein. Count on the protein in dairy products, low-fat egg whites and even low-fat, lean meats to boost the staying power of your morning meal, says Diane Grabowski-Nepa, R.D., a nutritionist at the Pritikin Longevity Center in Santa Monica, California. You'll feel fuller longer— a good way to avoid overconsuming at midmorning or at lunch.

"Fat-free cottage cheese, an egg-white omelet, scrambled egg-whites, fat-free egg substitutes like Egg Beaters, low-fat or fat-free cream cheese, or even fat-free yogurt can satisfy you better than just having toast or an English muffin and a piece of fruit," she says. "Personally, I'm much more satisfied when I include protein."

For another protein option, try folding diced chicken or turkey breast into an egg-white omelet as your morning entrée. Beans or soy products (tofu and tempeh) can also provide protein. Or try the combination of frijoles, corn tortillas, and scrambled fat-free egg substitute, Grabowski-Nepa suggests.

If you are at low risk for heart disease, three eggs a week isn't a problem, adds Cathy Kapica, R.D., Ph.D., associate professor of nutrition and clinical dietetics at Finch University of Health Sciences/Chicago Medical School in North Chicago.

Researchers aren't sure why protein gives you longer-lasting satisfaction. It could be because protein foods stay in your stomach longer, so you feel fuller. Or it may be because protein maintains steadier blood-sugar levels than carbohydrates alone. "When you eat carbohydrates alone, blood sugar can rise quickly and then fall, as the sugar is stored in your cells," says Grabowski-Nepa. "When it falls, you feel hungry." In one Australian study, researchers found that protein foods ranked high for immediate and long-term stomach satisfaction.

Build bone at the same time. Reaching for low-fat or nonfat dairy products at breakfast gives you an added nutritional edge: calcium. Women need 1,000 to 1,500 milligrams of calcium a day to build and maintain bone strength—about the amount in three to five glasses of skim milk—but most of us fall short. Even if you take a calcium supplement, try to fit in some dairy every day, Wolper says.

Put fiber to work. Take advantage of the growing number of high-fiber cereals and breads on supermarket shelves and get a head start on your daily fiber quotient, suggests Dr. Champagne. The weight-loss advantage? Fiber fills you up—and keeps you full—longer than re-fined foods like white bread, doughnuts, or croissants. At the same time, you'll reap big health benefits.

"Not only are whole-grain breakfast foods more filling, they also pro-vide more of the nutrition that women need," Dr. Champagne says. Among those vital nutrients are the B vitamins, vitamin E, iron, and zinc. Fiber is also vital for preventing constipation and reducing high blood cholesterol levels.

Mix and match. If you're new to high-fiber cereals, try mixing a higher-fiber variety with an old favorite, gradually increasing the propor-tion of the high-fiber type, suggests Wolper. Some tasty combos that pro-vide sweetness, crunch, and fiber are: Corn Chex and Raisin Bran; corn-flakes and Frosted Mini-Wheats; and Nut and Honey Crunch and Cheerios.

Crunch, don't sip. Don't miss the weight-loss edge tucked into fresh fruit—like sliced strawberries on your cereal, a sweet chunk of can-taloupe, teamed with nonfat cottage cheese, or an apple you can munch at stoplights on the way to work. There's plenty of fiber in the peel and the pulp, notes Dr. Champagne. "Fiber is always a big benefit if you're trying to lose weight or maintain a healthy weight. Anything that fills you up, without costing a lot of calories—like fiber—is a really useful bonus."

At the same time, fruit packs powerful nutrients like vitamins A and C and beta-carotene, while the soluble fiber can help control blood cho-lesterol levels.

Eat on the run. No time for a leisurely morning repast? You can still reap the benefits of a Fat-to-Firm eating plan breakfast with these quick picks from Dr. Boushey, who has often eaten breakfast in the car. "One of my favorites is fruit smoothie," she says. "You throw a banana, some nonfat plain yogurt, other fruit you like, and some ice cubes into a blender. Blend until smooth, then pour it into a glass with a lid, and you're ready to roll. It's thick, tasty, and really rather filling. Another simple, fast breakfast is toast with fruit jam. Bring along a piece of fruit for a more filling meal."

Midmorning Snack: The Pause That Fat-Proofs Your Plan

If you experience hunger pangs, feel a little weak, or have trouble concentrating by midmorning, it's time for the perfect pick-me-up: a snack that fills you up without filling you out, says Wolper.

How can snacking on the Fat-to-Firm eating plan help you lose

(continued on page 191)

Maximum Nutrition, The Fat-to-Firm Way

Who says women can't have it all? On the Fat-to-Firm eating plan, you can lose weight—and at the same time feel confident that you're getting the vitamins, minerals, and other nutrients that are essential for fighting fatigue, bolstering bone strength, boosting immunity, and preventing disease, says Cathy Kapica, R.D., Ph.D., associate professor of nutrition and clinical dietetics at Finch University of Health Sciences/Chicago Medical School in North Chicago.

How? Consult our reference guide below. And don't worry if your daily food choices don't exactly reflect those in the guide. "You may not hit the perfect number of servings of every food category every day, and that's okay," says Dr. Kapica. "Our bodies are good at storing nutrients. As long as you're on target over the course of a week, you're doing well."

Breads, Cereals, and Grains

Nutrients: B vitamins for healthy nerves. Iron for healthy blood. Vitamin E to defend against cell damage by free radicals (compounds generated by oxidation that can lead to cancer, heart disease, eye disorders, arthritis, and a weak immune system). Zinc for maintaining the immune system, healing wounds, helping the body regulate blood pressure and energy levels.

Whole grains also provide fiber, which is important for preventing constipation and reducing the risk of heart disease and colon cancer.

Servings per day: Six to 11, including four servings of whole grains. A serving is one slice of bread or small roll, half an English muffin, ¾ cup dry cereal, ½ cup granola or cooked cereal, ½ cup cooked pasta or rice, or ¼ cup wheat germ.

Best choices: Whole-wheat bread and rolls; brown rice and other whole grains like kasha and barley; high-fiber breakfast cereals; fortified cereals; and wheat germ for vitamin E.

Nutrient booster: Get more grain goodness by topping yogurt and even pudding with a sprinkle of crunchy high-fiber cereal or wheat germ.

Dairy Products

Nutrients: Calcium for building and maintaining strong bones.

Servings per day: Three. A serving is 8 ounces milk or yogurt; 1/3 cup grated or one to two slices of cheese; 1 1/2 cups cream soup (made with low-fat or skim milk); or 1 cup low-fat or nonfat pudding.

Best choices: Low-fat or skim milk, yogurt, cottage cheese, and sliced cheeses.

Nutrient booster: Stir 1/4 cup nonfat dry milk into 1 cup skim milk for a creamier taste and to boost the calcium content from 302 milligrams to 525 milligrams per cup.

Fruits

Nutrients: Vitamin C to prevent infection, promote healing, and enhance iron absorption. Vitamin A to preserve night vision and boost immunity. Plus hundreds of phytochemicals—substances like beta-carotene, limonene, and polyphenols that seem to reduce the risk of heart disease and cancer. Whole fruit also contains plenty of fiber.

Servings per day: At least two. A serving is 1/2 cup chopped fruit, 6 ounces juice, or a whole medium-size fruit.

Best choices: Citrus fruits, strawberries, mangoes, and papayas for vitamin C. Apricots and cantaloupes for vitamin A.

Nutrient booster: Fit in more fruit by tossing raisins into your breakfast cereal, slicing half a peach into pudding, or garnishing your dinner plate with orange wedges.

Vegetables

Nutrients: Vitamins A and C. Vitamin K for bone health. Folate to maintain red blood cells, protect against cervical cancer, and prevent neural-tube defects in children. Natural substances in food known as phytochemicals, such as sulphoraphane, which may protect cells from cancer. Beta-carotene, which may protect against cancers of the colon, lungs, and possibly of the bladder, pancreas, and throat. Vegetables also provide fiber.

Servings per day: At least three. A serving is 1/2 cup cooked vegetables or 1 cup chopped raw.

(continued) ▶

Maximum Nutrition—Continued

Best choices: Tomatoes, red peppers, cabbage, and snow peas for vitamin C; carrots, pumpkin, sweet potatoes, and winter squash for vitamin A; leafy greens like spinach and collard greens for folate, vitamin K, and carotenoids; broccoli, cauliflower, turnips, and kale for cancer-fighting substances called sulphoraphanes.

Nutrient booster: Eat more vegetables, effortlessly, by tossing frozen veggies into tomato sauce, soup, and casseroles.

Lean Meat, Fish, Lean Poultry, Beans, and Nuts

Nutrients: Protein, iron, zinc, and B vitamins for the body's constant rebuilding of muscles, bones, blood, and nerve tissue. Beans also provide fiber. And fish varieties such as anchovies, canned alba-core tuna, salmon (except smoked), and swordfish are also rich in omega-3 fatty acids that may ease arthritis, reduce the risk of heart problems, and even lift your mood.

Servings per day: Go for two. A serving is 2 to 3 ounces meat, fish, or poultry; 1/2 cup canned or cooked dry beans; one egg; or 2 tablespoons peanut butter.

Best choices: Low-fat, lower-calorie options include skinless chicken and turkey breast; white-fleshed fish like flounder and haddock; cuts of beef labeled round, chuck, sirloin, or tenderloin.

Nutrient booster: Substitute beans for some or all of the meat in a soup, stew, or sauce to lower fat but retain protein. Try red or black beans in place of beef, white beans or black-eyed peas in place of chicken, or chick-peas in place of ground beef in tomato sauce.

Fats and Oils

Nutrients: Vitamin E to protect tissue.

Servings per day: Very limited. One serving is 1 teaspoon mayonnaise, margarine, or vegetable oil.

Best choices: All fats and oils are high in calories. But olive, canola, and other oils high in monounsaturated fat, in small quantities, are better for promoting heart health than are saturated fats like butter or lard.

Nutrient booster: Keep a variety of oils on hand to take advantage of different tastes and small nutritional differences. Canola oil, for instance, contains heart-healthy omega-3 fatty acids.

weight or maintain a healthy weight? "Snacks can actually keep you on track because they keep you from becoming ravenously hungry and overeating the wrong foods later on," notes Dr. Boushey.

But that's only the beginning. "Snacks are just as important as meals," Dr. Boushey says. "So they're worth thinking about and planning for." A healthy snack can provide steady, long-lasting energy, getting you off the roller-coaster ride of grabbing a sugary snack that may give you a quick burst of energy and alertness but then lets you down, leading to cravings for more sugary treats.

That doesn't mean Fat-to-Firm eating plan snacks are dull and boring. A successful snack should fill a woman's very normal need for recreational food—having something fun to eat. "If you choose a healthy snack with a wonderful flavor or texture, you fill a need for pleasure and won't feel deprived," she notes. Here's how to craft a snack strategy that meets all your needs.

Stockpile the right stuff. At work, at home, or in your car, having the right munchables on hand can spell the difference between successful snacking and overloading on empty, energy-zapping calories, says Dr. Boushey. "If you keep healthy snacks convenient, you can grab one fast. You won't be as tempted by the high-fat, high-sugar selections in the vending machine or the office cafeteria," she says.

Keep these snack items in your desk drawer, your cabinet, or even in a tote in the car, she suggests: low-fat crackers; a few apples, oranges, or other fruits that will keep for a few days; small boxes of raisins; flavored rice cakes. "Rice cakes are the biggest boon—the flavored varieties are wonderful. They can be sweet or savory, and very crunchy. Just check the label to be sure that they're low in fat," Dr. Boushey suggests.

If there's a refrigerator handy, bring in nonfat yogurt, a block of nonfat cream cheese to spread on crackers, and fruits such as grapes, strawberries, or blueberries.

Finish breakfast. Use your morning snack to fit in satisfying, high-nutrition foods that may have been missing from your breakfast, Wolper suggests. If you had fruit and yogurt at the break of dawn, then round out the picture with whole-wheat toast or an English muffin and a dab of jam. If you went for cereal and milk in the A.M., reach for a fruit snack now.

Keep it fun. Ensure the success of your new snack habit by developing a repertoire of healthy treats that you'll look forward to eating, suggests Wolper. "Nobody should eat anything they don't like," she says.

Supplements Made Simple

Nobody's perfect. Even when eating a healthy, low-fat diet is a priority, there are times you may work through lunch, grab a hamburger at the shopping mall, or indulge yourself with chocolate ice cream—instead of dinner.

That's why you may want to consider a vitamin supplement. "It's an insurance policy," notes Cathy Kapica, R.D., Ph.D., associate professor of nutrition and clinical dietetics at Finch University of Health Sciences/Chicago Medical School in North Chicago. "A vitamin supplement can't take the place of fruits, vegetables, and grains—there are beneficial substances in real food that we haven't even discovered yet, and they're present in food in the proportions your body needs. Supplements just help fill in the gaps."

Here's Dr. Kapica's advice on finding the perfect supplement that will give you the vitamins and minerals women need.

Go for 100 percent. Skip the superpotent formulas. "When shopping for a multivitamin, flip the bottle over and look for one that gives you 100 percent of the Daily Value for basic nutrients," she suggests. Look for the following.

- Vitamin A/Beta-carotene: 5,000 international units
- Vitamin D: 400 international units
- Vitamin B_6: 2 milligrams
- Folic acid (folate): 400 micrograms
- Magnesium: 400 milligrams
- Zinc: 15 milligrams
- Copper: 2 milligrams
- Chromium: 120 micrograms

Decide about iron. How much you need depends on your age. If you're premenopausal, look for no more than 18 milligrams in a

"You have to enjoy a food to stick with it." In other words, snacks should always be a pleasure.

Customize your snack strategy by experimenting with healthy pleasure foods. Ask yourself whether you prefer crunchy foods, soft foods,

multivitamin. This will help replace iron lost each month during your menstrual period. If you're postmenopausal or don't have periods, look for a supplement with little or no added iron, says Dr. Kapica.

Take solo calcium. Dr. Kapica recommends a separate calcium supplement for two reasons: It's nearly impossible to find the calcium levels you need (1,000 to 1,500 milligrams a day) in a multivitamin, and it's better to take calcium at a different time of day than your multivitamin, to enhance absorption. "If you aren't getting two to three glasses of skim milk or the equivalent in low-fat yogurt or cheese every day, you need a calcium supplement to maintain bone strength," she says.

Opt for E. On a low-fat diet, it's hard to get the daily 100 to 400 international units of vitamin E that researchers think may reduce the risk of heart disease, diabetes, and some cancers, Dr. Kapica notes. "If you're limiting fats and oils and nuts, you may be missing out on vitamin E, so consider a separate supplement," she says.

See if your breakfast bowl is fortified. On days that you wake up to a bowl of fortified breakfast flakes, you may not need a multivitamin at all, Dr. Kapica says. "Read the label. Many cereals contain the same kinds and amounts of nutrients as a multivitamin supplement, including iron."

Save with store brands. Don't be seduced by expensive brands or labels that read "stress formula" or "all natural," Dr. Kapica says. "All vitamins, no matter what their source, work the same way in the body," she says. "So ignore the claims on the front and read what's really in the tablet. If an inexpensive store brand has what you need, buy it."

One exception: natural vitamin E is more bioactive in the body than synthetic E, but the difference in potency is taken into account in the international units—the measurement for some vitamins. One hundred units of synthetic E is as potent as 100 of natural E.

sweet foods, or savory stuff. If you dislike low-fat yogurt, try low-fat cheese and crackers. If apples seem dull, investigate seasonal gems like tangerines, peaches, or berries. If raw veggies seem forbidding, try a cup of tomato juice or vegetable juice cocktail.

Lunch: Where Good Taste and Stomach Satisfaction Meet

On the Fat-to-Firm eating plan, you can craft a quick lunch that takes advantage of the delicious flavors and satisfying staying power of foods that also provide important nutrients, says Dr. Champagne. "It's true that the same kinds of foods that make up a healthy diet are the foods that can most help you lose weight or maintain a healthy weight," she says. "The good thing is that they also taste good." Try these strategies for fitting them in at midday.

Introduce vegetables. Slide a slice of red onion and a few tangy spinach or arugula leaves into your sandwich. Assemble a side salad with fresh romaine lettuce, tomato wedges, and a splash of balsamic vinegar. Or heat up a cup of vegetable soup. Lunch is the time to start adding vegetables to your day, notes Wolper. From crunchy broccoli to a soft baked sweet potato, veggies are tasty packages full of satisfying fiber and a wealth of vitamins and other nutrients vital to good health and disease prevention.

If you have never been a vegetable fan, don't despair. "If you want to fit in more vegetables—or don't really like vegetables—there are lots of ways to combine them with other foods," notes Wolper. For example, toss pre-grated carrots into chicken salad, made with nonfat mayonnaise or yogurt, or mix chopped red peppers and onions with your next low-fat tuna salad.

Go for lean protein. Sliced roast turkey, lean beef, or ham; steamed shrimp or a broiled fish fillet—they all are excellent lunch choices, Wolper says. Not only does lean protein have a unique power to fill you up and keep you feeling full, it also increases mental alertness. Eating protein actually helps release more dopamine and norepinephrine, brain chemicals that contribute to sharp, quick thinking. And when you're feeling alert, you won't feel the same need for a high-fat, high-sugar pick-me-up, Grabowski-Nepa notes.

Nutritionists recommend most women limit protein intake to 5 to 7 ounces a day—servings about the size of two decks of cards.

Say beans. A bean burrito, bowl of chili, or beans and rice are excellent ways to add lean protein that is also high in fiber, says Wolper.

Take the grain train. Diversify your grain portfolio by building your sandwich inside a pita pocket or on a whole-grain roll, suggests Wolper. Nestle your chili or a chicken breast on a bed of rice. Or have a pasta lunch, with a zingy tomato sauce and a tablespoon of zesty Parmesan cheese, and a salad on the side.

Increase fruit fascination. Fit more fruit into your day and create new taste sensations by combining small amounts with sandwich fillings and main-dish salads, Wolper suggests. How? Add grapes to chicken salad, small chunks of apple to tuna salad, sliced pears to salad greens. Every little bit packs valuable nutrients and fiber for good health and stomach satisfaction.

Flavor without fat. Cut calories without feeling hungry by limiting your use of fats as flavorings, suggests Dr. Boushey. "That means switching to fat-free spreads on bread, going with fat-free salad dressings, switching to fat-free sour cream for baked potatoes," she says. "This strategy is very effective for weight loss because over time you lose your taste for fat. So you're taking in a lot less calories, but you're really eating the same quantity of food—you'll feel just as full if your sandwich has fat-free mayonnaise as it would with the full-fat variety."

Trade fat calories for more food. If you've traded high-fat lunchables for low-fat, healthy choices, you may have saved enough calories to add more food to your midday meal, notes Dr. Champagne. So instead of a fat-laden turkey-and-cheese sandwich slathered with mayo, have roast turkey breast with fat-free mayonnaise and greens on a whole-wheat roll, and add an orange or a salad—or even a small treat. "You can definitely eat more food if you follow a low-fat meal plan," she says. "Just be cautious with packaged low-fat foods like cookies and cakes. Often, they're no lower in calories than the full-fat originals. The most filling, low-calorie way to add more food is to choose high-nutrition fruits and vegetables."

Take a real break. You could eat lunch at your desk or in your car. But sitting down to a real meal, no matter how short, could actually enhance your weight-loss efforts, notes Dr. Johnston. "When you eat and work, or eat and do anything else, it's a set-up for overeating," she notes. "You don't notice what you're eating. Or you may take more food because in some way you may be trying to make yourself feel better because you can't really stop and take a break."

Midafternoon Snack: The Movable Feast That Prevents Overeating

On the Fat-to-Firm eating plan, savvy afternoon snacking can get you safely over two weight-loss hurdles: afternoon slump and the dinner-hour binge. Here's how.

Snack on smart foods. Battle afternoon slump and candy-machine temptations with smart choices stocked in advance, suggests Dr. Boushey. How? Bring along packets of precut, prewashed vegetables such as baby carrots or mixed bags of ready-to-eat broccoli and cauli-flower to eat with a nonfat yogurt dip. Try nonfat yogurt with fruit, low-fat or nonfat cheese with whole-grain crackers, or a slice or two of low-fat lunch-meat with mustard on a piece of bread. Keep an arsenal of healthy snacks on hand, Dr. Boushey suggests.

"You may be worried that precut vegetables or nice fruit is expen-sive, but if you compare those to the price of other recreational foods like chips and snack cakes and ice cream, they're not," Dr. Boushey notes. "I think of it this way: I'd rather spend money on maintaining a healthy weight than on becoming overweight."

If you have access to a microwave, expand your snack-time hori-zons with healthy, fiber-filled instant soups or fat-free popcorn.

Fine-tune your timing. If your hungriest moments don't come at midafternoon, but strike just before dinner or later in the evening, save your snacks for when you need them most, Wolper and Dr. Boushey both suggest.

"I get hungry right before dinner, so I tend to eat a grain snack like rice cakes then," says Dr. Boushey. "It takes the edge off."

"If you're the kind of person who loses control of her eating when you get too hungry, make sure you don't get that hungry," Wolper says. "Time your snacks to meet your needs." If hunger hits during your evening commute, save your afternoon snack for the road. "Bring along pretzels or crackers in a plastic bag, a piece of fruit, or an ounce of low-fat cream cheese."

Fill up in surprising ways. Wake up your taste buds with non-traditional snack ideas like crisp strips of red pepper, sweet sugar snap peas, or a quick, comforting soup, concocted in the microwave with broth and $\frac{1}{2}$ cup frozen vegetables, Wolper suggests. The vegetables will fill you up and provide extra nutrients, while the surprisingly delicious taste will keep your palate from craving more fattening fare.

Do a calcium check. If you haven't had at least one serving of a low-fat dairy product during the day, make it your snack, suggests Wolper. "Women need at least three glasses of skim milk a day or the equivalent in other dairy foods to fill the need for calcium."

Dinner: Quick or Fancy, You Can Have It Your Way

Whether it's a fast meal between work and a movie, a Saturday night feast, or a weeknight family supper, dinner has always been a

Dear Diary: Slip-Proof Your Plan

Whether you jot the day's meals down on a little 3- by 5-inch card or track your nutritional intake with a sophisticated computer program, keeping a food diary is one of the best ways to help yourself stick with a weight-loss program over the long haul, says Catherine Champagne, R.D., Ph.D., associate professor for research at the Pennington Biomedical Research Center in Baton Rouge, Louisiana.

"You become very aware of what you're eating," Dr. Champagne says. "You get a lot of insights on food choices that are healthy and food choices that you might want to change."

Dr. Champagne's most dramatic testimonial to the power of the food diary comes from a newspaper advice column. "A woman wrote in, saying that she never understood her weight problem because she honestly believed she never ate food. One day she decided to write down everything she put in her mouth and discovered that while she didn't eat at mealtime, she was constantly munching at other times—tasting the meals she prepared, eating little bits of peas, chicken, cake, and all the other leftovers as she cleared the table," she recalls. "All that nibbling added up to overweight, until she realized what was happening—thanks to a pen and some paper."

Keep your own food journal by carrying a pen and a small, spiral-bound notebook or even a few 3- by 5-inch cards in your purse, wallet, or pocket. Start a new page, or a new card, each day. Write down what you ate and approximately how much. Record-keeping is quickest and easiest if you write down your food choices shortly after each meal or snack, Dr. Champagne suggests. Include the "extracurricular foods" like the cookies offered by a co-worker, the hunk of cheese nibbled while preparing a casserole, that second glass of orange juice at breakfast. "It takes longer to sit at the end of the day and try to remember," she says. "And you may leave out the little things that are adding up to extra calories and extra weight."

time to unwind with delicious, comforting, filling foods, and on this plan, it still is. Try these strategies to turn up the flavor and satisfaction and turn down the fat.

Pick a quicker main course. Shop strategically so that you can reach into your refrigerator for fast-cooking, lean main courses like skinless chicken breasts, veggie burgers, lean cuts of beef such as sirloin or tenderloin, or fish fillets, suggests Dr. Kapica. Then, get ready to grill, broil, or steam your choice. Beyond the fill-you-up benefits, lean protein is rich in iron, B vitamins, zinc, and more.

Start with salad. Europeans may save salad for the end, but American women can make better use of salad as a weight-loss tool at the start of dinner, says nutritionist Grabowski-Nepa. "Tossed with fla-vored vinegar or low-calorie, fat-free dressing, it's perfect for weight loss. You'll fill up and get plenty of fiber. If you save the salad till last, you might fill up on higher-calorie foods first."

Think in color. Include two vegetables at dinner, Wolper sug-gests, and try to choose those with different colors. That way, you get eye appeal, taste appeal, stomach satisfaction, and the nutritional variety your body needs. You might have mashed sweet potatoes and steamed broc-coli, both rich in the cancer-fighting substances vitamin A and beta-carotene, or brussels sprouts, for calcium and iron, and carrots, rich in vi-tamin A.

Make room for "company" foods. On the Fat-to-Firm eating plan there is even room for filet mignon because you have the freedom to balance your food choices throughout the day, leaving room for special meals. "If you know you're going to eat a higher-fat food for lunch or dinner," notes Wolper, "balance it by eating lower-fat foods from other food groups at other meals." Wolper balances the protein and bit of fat in a lobster dinner by planning a pasta-and-salad lunch, for example.

Spoon up a chunky soup. Stir chunky vegetables into home-made or canned soup for a quick, satisfying main course—just add bread and salad, Wolper suggests. "Evidence suggests that chunky soups may be more satisfying than pureed soups or even soups with vegetables chopped into small pieces," she says.

Have one helping at a time. Tame dinnertime overeating by taking a little less food than usual, while telling yourself that you can have seconds if you really are hungry, Wolper suggests. "And don't put the serving plates on the table. Leave the food on the stove or out of reach to stop impulse eating. Then if you want more, you'll have to make the deci-sion to go get it."

Afterward, resist the temptation to eat leftovers. "This is a special issue for mothers. They feel it's important not to let food from their chil-dren's plates go to waste," Wolper notes. "So instead of eating it, wrap it up and put it in the refrigerator. When you look at it later, you probably won't want it."

Make variety your ally. Discover the world of flavors in grains, produce, proteins, and even oils, suggests Dr. Boushey. "When a healthy eating plan has a big variety of flavors, you won't feel like you're missing the foods you used to eat."

Beyond rice, try quick-cooking grains like bulgur, whole-wheat couscous, or quinoa. Instead of green beans tonight, experiment with broccoli rabe—it looks like leafy broccoli stalks and has a tangy bite. Cook a cubed parsnip with potatoes for a rich, earthy flavor. Catch a new fish at the seafood counter. "In general, low-fat fish have smooth, white skins and don't smell much when you cook them—like haddock, flounder, and cod," says Wolper.

Keep several oils on hand, suggests Dr. Boushey, and take advantage of their flavors in small quantities. For example, olive oil tastes great on salads, while mild canola oil is ideal for baking.

But go slowly. Try one new food at a time, suggests Dr. Boushey. "Experimenting with new foods should be fun, not stressful. So shop for one new food when you go to the supermarket. And introduce one new food to yourself and your family at a meal."

Introduce new foods slowly by mixing them with familiar edibles, she suggests. "If you try a new grain, mix it half-and-half with rice first, to get used to it," she says. "When we first made brown rice for our children, we mixed it half-and-half with white rice, then over a number of meals, increased the amount of brown rice. They love it. We've done the same thing with vegetables—introducing a new one with a little low-fat cheese on it, then eventually eating it plain."

Make it meatless. Tempt your taste buds with grilled vegetables with a sprinkle of Parmesan cheese, white bean and spinach soup, black beans and rice, or vegetable lasagna, made with low-fat ricotta cheese. "There are a lot of benefits to not relying on meat," says Dr. Champagne. "Focusing a meal on vegetables, grains, and beans gives you lots of fiber and lots of nutrition. And if you make it low-fat, you can eat a plateful. Afterward, it stays with you. You don't feel hungry."

Finish with refreshing fruit. Try orange sections, drizzled with raspberry puree, or a perfectly ripe pear. Finishing dinner with fruit will leave your sweet tooth and your stomach satisfied, says Wolper.

Make room for a treat. If you have already fit in enough fruit during the day, enjoy a cookie or two. "No one can stay on an eating plan if it doesn't include treats," notes Wolper. "They're important." Or revive some old-fashioned desserts like pudding (made with skim milk) or angel food cake, a low-fat confection made extra-delicious with a topping of fresh fruit.

Evening Snack: Time for a Treat

Whether you're curled up with a book, catching a television movie, or relaxing before bed, it's time for a just-right nighttime snack.

Treat your bones. Wolper suggests fitting in one last serving of dairy—to "cradle" your bones through the night, helping to prevent bone loss. Good choices include a frozen yogurt pop, a cup of skim milk with a cookie, or a half-cup of frosty, frozen nonfat yogurt.

Save up for a big snack. Nighttime eaters could forgo a snack or two earlier in the day, saving calories for a larger evening treat, Wolper suggests. "That's what women I counsel do," she says. "Sometimes, they'll have three pieces of fruit after dinner. It works because they balance it against what they've had earlier. That way, they get what they need, but they don't gain weight."

Part 3

The Exercise Equation

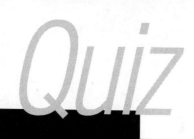

Are You Motivated to Exercise?

It's a scenario you probably know all too well: You start an exercise program with your sneakers fueled, your gym membership paid, and visions of a firmer body firmly in mind. And then you quit. Why? Exercise experts say that *motivation*—not merely wishful thinking, but practical determination—is the element most frequently lacking when people begin a new exercise program and the reason why most people quit. Motivation is a brew of many factors: your confidence in your ability to succeed, the support you receive from family and friends, your skill in thinking positively about your program, your ability to find more than one place to exercise (so it's not such a daunting task every time you do it), and your behavioral skills (like keeping a bag of exercise clothes in your car).

The quiz was developed for the Fat-to-Firm Program by Andrea L. Dunn, Ph.D., exercise psychologist and associate director of the division of epidemiology and clinical applications at the Cooper Institute for Aerobics Research in Dallas.

Read the following statements, then rate your own exercise habits by using this scoring system:

1 = Never
2 = Rarely
3 = Sometimes
4 = Often
5 = Always

_____ **1.** I am able to exercise when the weather is bad.

_____ **2.** I can find time in my busy day to exercise.

_____ **3.** If I miss an exercise session, I don't feel guilty because I know I will get back on schedule or find an alternative.

_____ **4.** I can find family or friends to talk with about my desire to exercise.

_____ **5.** I get family or friends to exercise with me as often as I like.

_____ **6.** I can find reliable and accurate sources of information about exercise whenever I have a question.

_____ **7.** I regularly record the type, time, and amount of exercise I do.

_____ **8.** I regularly set realistic short- and long-term goals to help me maintain a regular exercise routine.

_____ **9.** I try to educate myself about the benefits of physical activity and exercise.

_____ **10.** If I miss an exercise session, I think about ways to fit activity into my day in shorter (e.g., 10-minute) bouts.

_____ **11.** If I have been sick or injured, I plan how I can gradually start my exercise routine again.

_____ **12.** I can list more reasons to exercise than reasons not to exercise.

_____ **13.** I know where most of the recreation centers, gyms, and walking trails are within a 5-mile radius of my house.

_____ **14.** I regularly read the newspaper to find physical activities I might enjoy.

_____ **15.** I think of my neighborhood or neighborhood mall as a place where I can exercise.

The exercise motivation quiz you just completed assesses five motivational factors: confidence, social support, behavioral skills, positive thinking, and environmental awareness. Take a few minutes to score each of those factors using the directions below.

1. Add items 1, 2, and 3 and then fill in the following blank. This is your confidence score: _____.

2. Add items 4, 5, and 6 and then fill in the blank. This is your score for social support: _____.

(continued)

Are You Motivated to Exercise?—Continued

3. Add items 7, 8, and 9 and then fill in the blank. This is your score for behavioral skills: ____.

4. Add items 10, 11, and 12 and then fill in the blank. This is your score for positive thinking: ____.

5. Add items 13, 14, and 15 and then fill in the blank. This is your score for environmental awareness: ____.

6. Now add up all the numbers you just wrote in the previous five blanks. This is your total exercise motivation score: ____.

Scoring: After tallying your scores, read on to gain a better understanding of your motivation level.

If you scored 50 to 75 points, you are highly motivated to succeed. You have the ability to plan, carry out, and maintain a regular program of exercise and physical activity. If you follow through, you will be well on your way to achieving your goals.

If you scored 25 to 49 points, you are probably having some difficulty maintaining a regular exercise program and are still in the process of building your skills. To get more motivated, pay special attention to factors where you scored fewer than 12 points and focus on ways to bring up those scores.

If you scored less than 25 points, you have the best intentions but may not be ready for a regular routine. Think about getting short bouts of activity during the day. To get more motivated, check the factors where you scored fewer than 12 points. You'll find throughout the coming chapters tips and strategies from experts and other women for improving your motivation.

Chapter 15

The Unexpected Benefits of Getting Fit

**From an easier menopause
to harder bones, there are plenty of reasons
besides losing weight for a woman
to start exercising.**

It was morning in New York City, and Fran Kramer rolled out of bed, drank two cups of coffee, and got on her exercise bike. It was also day one of her new exercise routine—and Fran was determined to lose weight.

A few years later—and 15 pounds lighter—Fran still gets up, drinks two cups of coffee, and cycles for ½ hour most mornings. But these days, she doesn't do it to lose weight. Fran exercises because she knows it will help prevent heart disease and other major health problems. Because it makes her look and feel younger. And because it puts her in a good mood.

Fran has a lot of positive reasons for working out. And such incentives are the secret to sticking with the Fat-to-Firm exercise program.

Behind-the-Scenes Motivators

In the coming chapters you'll learn everything that you need to start exercising to lose or maintain weight. But first you need the motivation to get you going—and keep you going. And that's what this chapter is all about.

Chances are that right now, your main motivation for wanting to exercise is to help you take off extra pounds. That prompted Fran to begin. In fact, surveys show that most women rank weight loss as the number one reason why they start exercising. But when weight loss is the only reason women exercise, they set themselves up for failure, says Peggy Norwood, an exercise physiologist, president of Avalon Fitness, and former fitness director of the Duke University Diet and Fitness Center, both in Durham, North Carolina. Following a moderate exercise program and a healthy eating plan, women lose weight slowly—that is, no more than 1 to 2 pounds a week. So many get frustrated and quit well before exercise can really have an effect, Norwood explains. To stay motivated, she says, women should also focus on other reasons to exercise.

Those reasons are not hard to find. Getting in shape perked up Amy Durham, 39, of Ely, Minnesota, so much that she found herself needing less sleep—only 6 hours a night instead of 10. After she became fit, Amy no longer felt drained in the afternoon and felt more energetic throughout the day. It gave Regina Pascucci, 37, of West Trenton, New Jersey, the stamina she needed. She no longer gets tired when shopping in the mall and doing all that walking. And it helped Donna Gettings, 42, of Williamsburg, Virginia, strengthen her joints and lower her blood pressure. In fact, her doctor eventually told her she no longer needed to take her blood pressure medication. "I went for my usual checkup, and for the first time in my life, my doctor said that I was as healthy as a person can be," says Donna, who swims regularly.

Better sleep. More energy. Lower blood pressure. Keep reading to discover the facts about these and all the other unexpected benefits of getting fit.

Exercise: The All-Purpose, Feel-Better Medicine

When you begin the Fat-to-Firm exercise program, your life will improve in a lot of ways. Most important, you'll lose weight, and you'll look and feel better. But, as previously mentioned, you may have to wait a while for these benefits to kick in, especially if you have a substantial amount of weight to lose. But other benefits show up a lot sooner. So when the going seems a little slow, focus on the following exercise bonuses.

Exercise boosts energy. Not too long ago, Donna was walking around Washington, D.C., with a group of friends. Then it occurred to her: For the first time, she wasn't worrying about whether she could keep up with these women. For the first time she could remember, she hadn't circled streets like a vulture, in search of a parking space within sight of where she was meeting her friends.

Donna realized that walking did not tire her out like it used to. It occurred to her that for the first time in her life, she was fit.

"I like being able to move around," says Donna, who lost 111 pounds once she added exercise to her weight-loss program. "That's probably my greatest motivation to keep going, more so than looking good."

Like many women who begin exercise programs after years of avoiding any physical activity, Donna worried that she wouldn't have the stamina to exercise. But she found that exercise gave her more energy than before. "The cycle goes: If you don't exercise, you feel lousy. If you feel lousy, you don't want to exercise," says Donna. "If you exercise, it makes you feel good. And you'll want to exercise again. Basically, if I don't exercise, I can feel myself getting sluggish."

Donna is not alone. Woman after woman interviewed for this book who used exercise to lose weight said that working out gave them more energy than they ever had before. "I can do more now than I could 20 years ago. I don't get tired as quickly," says Marilyn Knight, 42, of Lewisburg, Kentucky, who walks regularly.

And it all makes sense, medically speaking. Exercise improves the way we breathe. That keeps us from getting winded. It builds muscle. That makes groceries easier to carry, jars easier to open, and babies easier to hoist. It makes walking easier. It makes stair climbing easier. It even makes pushing a vacuum cleaner easier.

When you don't exercise, your body slowly deteriorates. And eventually, everyday tasks become difficult. And you get tired more easily. "We have folks who get exhausted just doing housework. They can't even push a vacuum cleaner around one room," says Norwood. All that changes once they start to exercise.

Exercise turns bad moods into good ones. When psychotherapist Darlene Pearson, 59, of Seattle, quit smoking years ago, she soon realized that exercise was an effective antidote to nicotine withdrawal. She would walk whenever she got the urge to smoke. It reduced her anxiety.

Today, she often walks with women who consult her for depression

(continued on page 211) ►

There's No Excuse Not to Exercise

You know exercise is good for you. But you still don't do it.
Maybe you:

a. Don't have time.
b. Have too many family responsibilities.
c. Don't feel like it.

If you choose any or all of the above, you can rest assured that
you are not alone. These are some of the top reasons nonexercisers
gave when the Sporting Goods Manufacturers Association quizzed
people to find out who exercised and who didn't—and why. Though
excuses may be popular, they shouldn't thwart your exercise program.
Here are some tips for overcoming these barriers to working out.

No Time?

Make exercise a priority. Time is only a problem if you make
it one, says Susan W. Butterworth, Ph.D., director of wellness services for the occupational health program at Oregon Health Sciences
University in Portland. "We all have things that we need to get done.
We end up doing what's important to us. If you consider grooming
important, then you take a half-hour. If you like to get your nails
done, you make time for it. It's the same with exercise," she says.

To help make exercise a priority, talk with family, friends, and
your physician about why exercise is important. Make a list of the advantages of exercising. "Writing down the benefits sometimes helps.
In order to find time, you have to choose to make time," says Dr.
Butterworth.

Fit in what you can. The Fat-to-Firm Exercise Program takes
about 40 to 50 minutes of your time, three days a week. But this isn't
an all-or-nothing program. Start with as much time as you can spare,
suggests Dr. Butterworth. "As little as 10 minutes a day helps," she
says. Once exercise becomes a habit, chances are that you'll find
more time to do it.

Make an appointment with yourself. Write your workout in
your date book. "You don't have to tell your secretary or business
associates what the appointment is for. It's just an appointment.
And you treat it the same way as you would a business appointment," says Dr. Butterworth.

Use weekends wisely. You want to exercise at least three days a week. And weekends usually offer more time than weekdays. So go for Saturday, Sunday, plus one day during the week. On that weekday, get to work a bit earlier and then take a longer-than-normal lunch break and use it to exercise, suggests Dr. Butterworth.

Family Foiling Your Fitness Routine?

Talk about it. Sit down with your family members and explain that exercise is important. Then ask them to help you fit it in. Ask them to brainstorm ways to overcome your barriers, says Dr. Butterworth. For instance, maybe your husband or kids can cook dinner on your exercise nights.

Make it a family thing. You don't need to strap running shoes on your five-year-old and drag him along for a couple of miles. But you can have him ride his bike alongside as you jog. Or you can involve him in a gym activity such as karate while you take aerobics, says Dr. Butterworth. Try to schedule family fitness hours, with the entire family doing something active, such as walking at the zoo or tossing a Frisbee, she says.

Lost Your Motivation?

Break it up. Researchers have found that exercising in 10-minute bouts several times throughout the day is as good for cardiovascular improvement as exercising in one 30-minute session. Getting physically fit improves your fat metabolism, which helps you lose weight, and it may decrease boredom. "Some people can tolerate riding a stationary bike for 10 minutes. But after 10 minutes, they get bored. So they're willing to do 10 minutes, a couple of times a day. It's tolerable," says John M. Jakicic, Ph.D., research assistant professor in psychiatry at the University of Pittsburgh.

Make a deal. Eliana Escalanti, 35, of Orlando, Florida, used every excuse in the book: "It's too cold." "I don't have time." "I'm too tired." "I have to cook dinner for the kids." But it all came down to one central theme: Part of her really wanted to run; another part of her dreaded it.

So she made a pact with herself. On the days that she really didn't feel like running, she would walk. "Eventually, once I got out

(continued) ▶

There's No Excuse Not to Exercise—Continued

and walked a little bit, I would feel better. Then I would jog a little bit. That would get me going," Eliana says.

Distract yourself. Studies show that fast, upbeat music can help motivate you to exercise and keep you going longer. But you don't have to spend hours shopping for tapes and making your selections. The right kind is whatever kind you enjoy, says Hy Levasseur, an exercise physiologist and director of health education and fitness at the U.S. Department of Transportation in Washington, D.C. "Whatever kind of music turns you on is what you ought to listen to. It makes your workout more fun."

Other than listening to music, try watching television or reading while working out on stationary equipment. "Tying exercise to another activity helps people to take their minds off what they are doing. It takes your mind off the laborious part of it," explains Levasseur.

Get a partner. Two exercisers are better than one. "It always seems to make it easier when you share the effort. Working out with a partner keeps you both going on the days you might cop out. One motivates the other," says Levasseur.

Take baby steps. Donna J. Kinoshita, 48, of Lafayette, Colorado, couldn't imagine how she would be able to get her body to move. "I told my doctor, 'I'm so fat. I know everything would be easier and I wouldn't get so winded if I wasn't so grossly obese.' He said, 'So let's lose a pound.' I said, 'I need to lose 50.' He said, 'Concentrate on losing 1 pound.' It was baby steps. When you say, 'Oh, my God, I have to lose 50 pounds,' you never get started because it's such a humongous task," says Donna.

Set small interim goals. Make small challenges for yourself. For instance, if you start out walking 5 minutes a day, make a short-term goal to up the time to 10 minutes. And when you do that, reward yourself. Buy a new dress. Buy a pair of gym socks. Whatever. Just make sure that you have an incentive to keep going, says Roseanne Welsh Strull, 48, a certified personal trainer and lifestyle counselor in Beaverton, Oregon, and co-author of *Thinner Winners*. Then set your next goal. Try to make the goals something that you will be able to achieve within a couple weeks. That way, you'll constantly be having small successes, she says.

and other psychological problems. It helps lift their spirits, says Darlene, who's also a certified walking instructor.

She and the women she counsels aren't the only ones to discover the emotional benefits of exercise. In fact, according to one survey, exercise is one of the 10 most popular techniques people use to shake off a bad mood—and it's the most effective. Another study found that college students who exercise tended to be less shy and lonely than those who did not.

When you first start to exercise, you'll also notice that it helps relieve stress. If you have just had a run-in with your boss, for instance, a brisk walk can help you recover from the stressful encounter. Performed regularly, exercise will help keep your moods from swinging dramatically when stressful events do occur, says Norwood. "In the short term, you can burn up some of your stress. In the long run, you notice that you aren't as reactive to stress," she says.

Research suggests that exercise regulates mood in a variety of ways. For example, exercise seems to trigger the release of endorphins, opiate-like brain chemicals that act as a natural mood elevator, making you feel good all over.

Exercise relieves premenstrual discomfort. If you wanted to breed a female rat, you would take away her running wheel, confine her to a small pen where she couldn't move, and feed her too much. Under these conditions, the rat's sex hormones would surge, making her estrogen levels higher than normal.

And if that rat could talk, she would complain of some vicious symptoms. Like bloating. Breast tenderness. Moodiness. Sound familiar?

"Overeating and inactivity overstimulate the reproductive system. Being sedentary isn't healthy," says Jerilynn C. Prior, M.D., professor of medicine and endocrinology at the University of British Columbia in Vancouver.

Exercise tames those surging hormones, especially estrogen, and reduces associated discomfort such as breast tenderness, bloating, and anxiety, says Dr. Prior. And though doctors have not documented that exercise eases menstrual cramps, plenty of anecdotal evidence suggests that it does, she adds.

You'll need more than one exercise session to ease premenstrual symptoms. It takes about three months of regular aerobic exercise—on a walking or mild jogging program—for bloating and breast tenderness to abate. And six months after starting the program, anxiety and depression will subside, says Dr. Prior.

Problem Solved

For These Women, Solo Exercise Is the Key

Amy Durham, 39, of Ely, Minnesota, was self-conscious of the slightest pinkness in her cheeks. She knew exercise was the key to losing and maintaining weight. But she couldn't imagine herself in an aerobics class with sweat dripping off her nose. So she decided to exercise on a cross-country ski machine in her bedroom where no one could see her. After she started, she learned that there is nothing wrong with a good sweat.

The same solution worked for Fran Kramer, of New York City. At first, she was an aerobics-class dropout. She would attend a class for a few weeks. Then she would quit. A year later, she would try again. Then she'd quit again. She was intimidated. It seemed that all the other women had better leotards, more equipment, and better bodies. And when she saw herself in the mirrors that lined the room, she felt out of place.

"Sometimes in Manhattan you're not seeing anyone who is overweight. You're seeing workout animals," Fran says. Her solution? She got an exercise bike and began working out at home. Then she could wear whatever she wanted, didn't need to see herself in a mirror, and had no one else around to compare herself to.

When associated with stress and weight loss, however, too much exercise can bring hormone levels too low, creating haphazard ovulation and irregular or absent periods. The Fat-to-Firm Program recommends mild to moderate exercise. If you stick to building your fitness level gradually, you shouldn't have problems with sporadic ovulation or menstruation, says Dr. Prior.

Exercise eases menopause. Experts aren't exactly sure why exercise makes "the change" less of a change. But they do know that it works.

When Christina Lee, Ph.D., and her colleagues at the University of Newcastle in Australia studied menopausal women, they found that those who exercised moderately on a regular basis had more energy. The women also experienced less moodiness, anxiety, depression, sleep difficulties, sexual difficulties, night sweats, and hot flashes than those who did not. Even after one exercise session, the women felt better than they did before exercising, says Dr. Lee, a professor of psychology.

More studies are needed to pinpoint how exercise relieves menopausal discomfort. Dr. Lee suspects it may help balance out the hormonal fluctuation that occurs during menopause. But other possible explanations abound. Exercise may stimulate the release of endorphins, which mask pain, mollify anxiety, and contribute to feelings of enhanced well-being. Or exercise could simply provide a stress break from our day-to-day life as well as give us a sense of achievement and well-being, she explains.

Exercise strengthens bones. As our bones age, they lose calcium and other minerals, a process known as osteoporosis. The slow-down in estrogen production that occurs at menopause can accelerate this process. The mineral loss makes the bones more porous. And porous bones break more easily. Hip and wrist fractures are hallmarks of osteoporosis, as is a curved spine.

Exercise helps maintain and stimulate bone development and growth, which could help prevent or forestall the development of osteoporosis, says Michael Pollock, Ph.D., professor of medicine and exercise science at the University of Florida in Gainesville. "Walking and strength training are two weight-bearing activities that will help stimulate bone growth," he says. "In tennis players, the arm they use to swing the racket has denser bones than the other arm."

The earlier you start to exercise, the better. Bone growth peaks in our teens and twenties. Studies done by Dorothy Teegarden, Ph.D., assistant professor of foods in the department of Food and Nutrition at Purdue University in West Lafayette, Indiana, and her colleagues, show that high school girls who exercise can increase the density of their hip and back bones, some of the bones most likely to break in later years. "If you can maximize the amount of bone that you have at a young age, you essentially have more bone to lose," she says. "So it's going to hopefully keep you out of the fracture range when you get older."

Once past your twenties, you can't build bone mass. But you can slow its decline, adds Dr. Teegarden. If you are past age 20 and have never exercised, it's not too late to start. Exercise still may help you preserve the bone mass that you do have, she says.

Exercise protects against disease. If you want to protect your health and live longer, exercise is part of the prescription. It can help pre-

Customized Solutions to Common Problems

How can you persuade yourself to exercise on days when you just don't feel like it? The trick is to find the right incentive to get you going. Here's what some women have found works for them.

Take a monthly photo. Donna Gettings, 42, of Williamsburg, Virginia, can't forget what exercise has done for her. She has before and after photos to remind her. While she was losing weight, she took a picture of herself every month. Then she would compare the picture to the one from the month before and gleam at the difference. "Now I look at them and think, 'Daggone! I can't believe I was ever like that,' " she says.

Think happy thoughts. When you do trip up and skip a day of exercise, don't beat yourself up over it, says Roseanne Welsh Strull, 48, of Beaverton, Oregon, who lost 140 pounds and went on to become a personal trainer. "I focus on the positive. I know that sounds like a cliché. But if you think negative, you will feel negative," she says.

"If your best friend called you up and said, 'I ate 12 bagels today,' would you say, 'Well, you fat pig! Why don't you get off your butt and do something about it?' " asks Roseanne. "We would never say that to a friend. But that's what we say to ourselves. We tell ourselves that we are horrible and weak-willed. We need to start treating ourselves like our own best friends."

Make exercise equipment part of the furnishings. Amy Durham, 39, of Ely, Minnesota, made sure to put her cross-country ski machine in her bedroom. "It's the first thing I see when I get out of bed in the morning. I had to make exercise as easy as possible. If I had to go downstairs to a separate room, that would just be one thing that makes it a little bit harder," she says.

---

vent common diseases, including the following, that have been linked to premature death among women.

- Breast cancer. According to one study, one in three cases of this form of cancer could be prevented if women exercised more. Breast cancer—as well as cancers of the ovaries and endometrium—seem to be caused in part by a higher-than-average level of estrogen throughout life. Because exercise controls estrogen, it reduces the risk of those cancers.

Troubleshoot it. Before starting her exercise program, Amy thought about what excuses she might make that could sabotage it. She realized that if she exercised at a gym, she might talk herself out of going on the days when she was strapped for time. And if she exercised outside, she might cop out on the days that no one could watch her kids. So she chose to exercise at home, indoors.

Set rules. Fran Kramer of New York City gives herself options—except for the option not to exercise. She usually works out in the morning, after she's had her two cups of coffee. But if she has an early appointment, she allows herself to change routines and exercise in the evening instead. But she knows that she won't exercise after 6:30 P.M. So if she doesn't think that she can get home that early, she chooses to get up earlier and stick with the morning session. "If it means getting up before 6:00 A.M. just one day to do it, then that's what I do," Fran says.

Always remember how it makes you feel. When Donna isn't in the mood to do her mile-long swim, she tells herself that it will make her feel good. "A couple of times I had to stop swimming because of surgery, and I felt lousy," she says.

Make a symbol of your progress. When Donna lost 100 pounds, she rewarded herself by having a picture of a flying bluebird tattooed on the inside of her left ankle. "If I have any doubts about what I am doing, I just take a peek at it and I smile. It's my little gift to myself for having lost the 100," she says. If a tattoo isn't your style, reward yourself in some other way—perhaps a necklace, an office decoration, or even a refrigerator magnet—to symbolize your accomplishment.

- Heart disease. Exercise reduces the risk of heart disease by making the heart stronger, by increasing the amount of artery-protecting high-density lipoproteins, and by lowering blood pressure.

- Diabetes. Exercise improves the body's ability to use insulin, the hormone that helps controls blood sugar levels. And uncontrolled blood sugar doesn't only mean diabetes—it also means possible kidney damage and high cholesterol.

(continued on page 218)

The Anatomy of the Fat-to-Firm Exercise Program

You'll start seeing results in just the first six months of the Fat-to-Firm Program, according to experts. The accompanying diagram shows what will happen to your body and when. Information contained in this illustration is based on results that an average woman, age 35 to 45, might expect. You may see results more—or less—quickly.

Two weeks: Excitement. You think, "Hey, I'm doing it. I'm really doing it."

Four weeks: Sigh. Excitement wanes. Now you are most susceptible to falling prey to excuses. You struggle to make exercise a new habit.

Eight weeks:

• You lose an inch around your waist.
• You lose 3½ pounds of fat and gain 2 pounds of muscle.
• You burn about 70 more calories a day at rest.
• You exercise regularly with few exceptions.
• You begin adding time and intensity to your workouts.

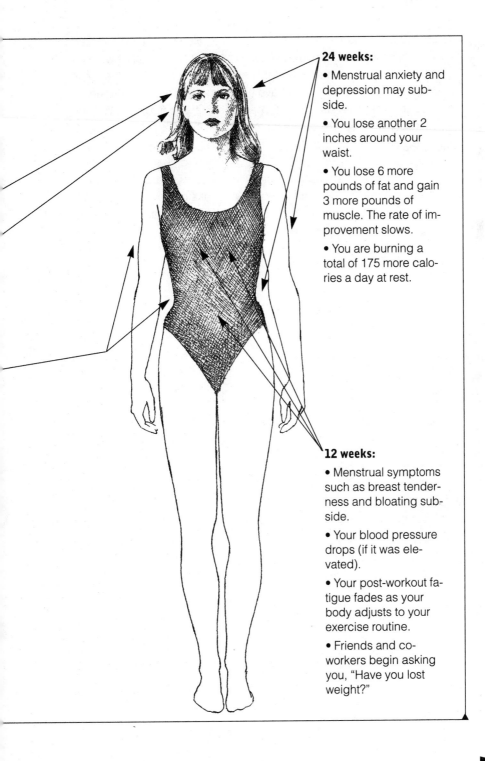

24 weeks:

• Menstrual anxiety and depression may subside.

• You lose another 2 inches around your waist.

• You lose 6 more pounds of fat and gain 3 more pounds of muscle. The rate of improvement slows.

• You are burning a total of 175 more calories a day at rest.

12 weeks:

• Menstrual symptoms such as breast tenderness and bloating subside.

• Your blood pressure drops (if it was elevated).

• Your post-workout fatigue fades as your body adjusts to your exercise routine.

• Friends and co-workers begin asking you, "Have you lost weight?"

Exercise helps ward off plenty of other diseases, too, such as arthritis. Not only does that make women live longer, it also makes women live better, by improving quality of life. The sedentary person is more likely than the physically active one to have trouble getting around or to need nursing care during the last 10 to 15 years of her life, according to William Joel Wilkinson, M.D., medical director of the division of epidemiology and clinical applications at the Cooper Institute for Aerobics Research in Dallas.

"I don't want to spend the last 10 years of my life with someone having to shampoo my hair and dress me and take me to the bathroom," says Norwood. "I exercise because I want the rest of my life to be good. I want to have fun. I want to enjoy myself."

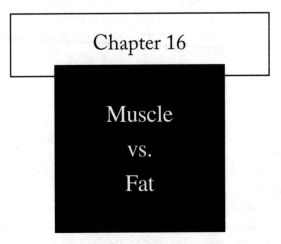

Chapter 16

Muscle vs. Fat

**Muscle burns lots of calories;
fat burns few. So how do you get
more muscle? Read on.**

Just for a moment, let's play make-believe. Pretend that two 150-pound women lie on a couch for 24 hours. Pretend that one woman is made entirely of fat, the other made entirely of muscle.

The woman made of fat would burn about 300 calories during that long, lazy day. The woman made only of muscle would burn about 5,250 calories.

Obviously, then, when it comes to weight loss, fat is not your friend.

Granted, no one is made entirely of fat or muscle. There are also bones to consider as well as various body parts, such as the brain and liver. And lots of water. So the hypothetical example of two women, above, serves only to illustrate a point: Muscle burns many more calories than fat. A pound of muscle burns at least 35 calories a day; a pound of fat burns about 2.

"The more muscle you have, the more calories you burn," says Robert Girandola, Ed.D., associate professor of exercise science at the University of Southern California in Los Angeles.

Calorie-Hungry Muscles

Muscle burns so many calories because muscle works so hard. Every time we move, we use muscle. Muscle moves our skeletons, allowing us to walk. Muscle opens and closes our jaws, letting us chew. Muscle makes our throats contract and expand so we can swallow. Muscle even makes our hearts beat and blood vessels constrict and expand. At any given time of the day, we use plenty of muscle. During a game of thumb wrestling, for example, your thumb alone works at least nine muscles.

And even while we sleep, muscle stays busy. Muscle continuously rebuilds itself by replacing and synthesizing protein, says Wayne Westcott, Ph.D., strength-training consultant in Quincy, Massachusetts, for the national YMCA.

Fat, on the other hand, burns so few calories because it does so little. Fat sits there. It sits on the backs of our arms, on our rear ends, along our stomachs, even along our ankles. It sits. It rests. And it waits. It waits for some day when some muscle complains, "I'm hungry. Feed me!" And then fat sacrifices itself. It breaks down into fatty acids and travels through blood to the hungry muscle or organ. Fat is food in a human piggy bank.

The Problem with Fat

We do need some fat. The body uses fat to make cell membranes, to keep us warm, to transport vitamins, and to run the nervous system, menstrual cycle, and reproductive system. In fact, at least 15 percent of our bodies should be fat.

The problem is that many women carry too much fat—30 percent or more. For health and weight maintenance, women should aim to keep their fat levels ideally between 20 and 25 percent, says Katherine T. Thomas, Ph.D., assistant professor of exercise science and physical education at Arizona State University in Tempe. The other 70-plus percent of the body would then be made up of what experts call lean body mass: muscles, bones, organs, and water.

Unless they exercise, keeping their fat levels between 20 and 25 percent becomes a losing battle for most women. A combination of the natural aging process and inactivity causes women, on average, to lose about 5 pounds of muscle every decade. That's 175 fewer calories a day that a woman burns each decade after adulthood. That may not sound like much, but it adds up. By the time we hit our forties, we're burning 350 fewer calories a day than we did when in our twenties. And by our sixties, we use 700 fewer calories.

Less muscle means more fat. The slower metabolism caused by less muscle then makes the average woman gain about 10 pounds of fat per decade. Ten pounds of fat takes up more space than 10 pounds of muscle. Compare a pound of shortening (pure fat) to a pound of fillet of beef (pure muscle), for example. The pound of shortening is larger. A body that loses muscle and gains fat gets larger and larger and larger, says Dr. Thomas.

More Muscle, Less Fat

Fortunately, the Fat-to-Firm Program reverses the tendency that women have to lose muscle and gain fat. The program involves three types of activity: aerobic exercise, resistance training, and lifestyle changes.

To fulfill the exercise equation of the Fat-to-Firm Program, you will:

- Spend a minimum of about ½ hour, three days a week, doing some form of aerobic activity. It will help you burn off about 10 calories a minute, or 300 calories each ½-hour exercise session.

- Use resistance training to build muscle, which will increase your metabolism and help burn off fat.

- Begin planning "functional fitness" activities on most days of the week, where you burn more calories by turning everyday activities like watching your children and talking on the phone into mini-exercise sessions.

All three aspects of the exercise equation are important to weight loss. The resistance-training program will build about a pound of muscle every month, says Dr. Westcott. After two months, your body will burn 70 more calories a day, he adds. That's 490 more calories a week. Aerobic exercise burns 300 calories a day, or if exercising three times a week, that's another 900 calories or so a week. And your functional fitness time you will burn off about 750 calories a week, he says. So all totaled, you will burn about 2,140 additional calories per week after two months on the program. Any lifestyle changes you make will add to the total calories burned. For example, these changes could include gardening, snow shoveling, parking your car farther away from the entrance to the mall, or taking the stairs instead of the elevator. And as you stay with the program, you burn more and more calories as your body builds muscle.

Though it aids weight loss, the exercise equation of the Fat-to-Firm Program is much more important for weight maintenance. It curbs the 1 pound of fat that the average woman gains each year due to muscle loss. And because the program requires a permanent change, once pounds are off, they stay off. Studies show that few women who lose weight by dieting alone actually keep the weight off. But weight that's lost while on a program containing an exercise component is most likely to stay off, says William Joel Wilkinson, M.D., medical director of the division of epidemiology and clinical applications at the Cooper Institute for Aerobics Research in Dallas.

Aerobic Exercise: Weight Loss for the Long Run

If you have ever stopped to add up the numbers of calories burned, you might falsely conclude that aerobic exercise does little for weight loss. A half-hour of moderate aerobic exercise will probably burn what seems like a measly 300 calories. Yet, you need to burn 3,500 calories to get rid of a pound of fat.

If you exercise three times a week, you burn 900 calories. So, you must exercise for 3½ weeks to burn just 1 pound.

By comparison, eliminating nearly 1,000 calories a day by cutting back on food would seem faster and easier than trying to burn the same amount through exercise. By severely limiting the calories you take in, you can lose 2 pounds or more in one week instead of in seven. And, in fact, that's what a lot of women try to do, says Dr. Wilkinson.

But in the long run, crash dieting doesn't work. Losing more than 2 pounds a week will peel off muscle as well as fat. That slows your metabolism, which will eventually result in a weight-loss plateau—you'll stop losing weight, despite your efforts, says Dr. Wilkinson. And you can't starve yourself forever. Once food intake resumes, the body adjusts and the pounds return.

Slow weight loss, on the other hand, conserves your muscle. And when combined with aerobic exercise, the exercise stimulates your muscles to develop and grow. So your metabolism stays the same.

If you made no other lifestyle changes, your three-day-a-week aerobic program would permanently take off 15 pounds or more in one year. That's still faster than the rate that most women put on weight—1 pound a year.

Other than conserving muscle and burning calories, the Fat-to-Firm aerobic exercise program helps you lose weight in three more ways.

■ Aerobic exercise helps you stick to the Fat-to-Firm eating plan. Scientific studies that look at the amount of calories burned by aerobic exercisers show an unusual result: Those exercisers lose more pounds than can be accounted for by the burned calories.

It turns out that aerobic exercisers eat less than nonexercisers do. Why? One theory is that exercise reduces anxiety and depression, which cause some women to overeat. (For complete details on the nutrition component of the Fat-to-Firm Program, see part 2, beginning on page 79.)

■ Though experts can't pin down the exact number of extra calories burned, they do know that aerobic exercise elevates your metabolism for a few hours after exercise, helping you to burn more calories when you are doing your everyday activities, says Dr. Wilkinson.

■ Aerobic exercise helps condition your heart, lungs, and other body parts so that you have more stamina to adhere to the third component of the exercise equation: achieving a more active lifestyle.

"Every good study of long-term weight loss has found that people who lose weight and keep it off have one thing in common: a regular aerobic exercise program," explains Robert McMurray, Ph.D., professor of sports science and nutrition at the University of North Carolina at Chapel Hill.

The Right Exercise at the Right Pace

In the Fat-to-Firm Program, the aerobic part of the exercise equation includes walking, swimming, cycling, and other options. (For details, see chapters 17 and 18.) To make aerobic exercise work for you, experts offer the following caveats.

Less pain means more gain. Many women have the misconception that aerobic exercise has to be hard, says Dr. Wilkinson. After all, we do refer to it as working out. Those misconceptions date to the 1970s when the popular phrase "no pain, no gain" was thrown around with

Two Fat-Burning Myths to Ignore

Two myths tend to circulate about aerobic exercise and fat burning.

MYTH #1: You must work out for at least 20 minutes to burn fat.
MYTH #2: Strenuous exercise does not burn fat.

Both myths are based on the same half-truth, says Mildred Cody, R.D., Ph.D., associate professor of nutrition and dietetics at Georgia State University in Atlanta. Our bodies burn a combination of carbohydrate and fat for energy. (That's true.) For the first 20 minutes of exercise, our bodies burn mostly carbohydrate. (That's true.) After 20 minutes, they start burning fat. (That's true.) During mild exercise, our bodies prefer to burn fat and conserve carbohydrate. During vigorous exercise, our bodies prefer to burn carbohydrate and conserve fat. (That's true, too.) So where's the myth?

The myth is the belief that burning fat causes more weight loss than burning carbohydrate, says Dr. Cody. To lose weight, you need to burn *calories*. It doesn't matter whether the calories come from carbohydrate or fat. Our bodies must eventually replace whatever calories we burn during exercise. And that replacement usually comes from stored fat, she says.

Vigorous exercise, however, does tend to build muscle faster than moderate exercise. So a program of mild to moderate exercise will result in faster weight loss in the beginning, while a vigorous program will result in more weight loss down the road when the increased muscle speeds up the metabolism.

abandon. At that time, experts thought that exercise had to be more regimented and strenuous to produce results. But today, experts say that even mild to moderate physical activity can lead to substantial health benefits. Plus, moderate exercise causes fewer injuries than vigorous exercise and is much more pleasant for many people, he says. The new recommendations are not meant to replace the old guidelines but to complement them. The idea is not to stop running or going to the gym if you are already active, the idea is that activity is good for your health at whatever level—so get out there and get moving.

Move slowly to lose quickly. Exercising at a lower intensity seems to take off inches faster than exercising at a higher intensity, when you burn the same number of calories. When researchers studied women who exercised vigorously for a shorter time versus women who exercised mildly but for a longer time, they found that after 12 weeks on the program, the mild exercisers lost 1.2 inches from the waist while the vigorous exercises only lost a fraction of an inch. Both groups lost the same amount of fat, says Mildred Cody, R.D., Ph.D., associate professor of nutrition and dietetics at Georgia State University in Atlanta. But the vigorous exercisers gained more muscle. And that may be why they weighed more on the scale and lost fewer inches, she says.

Though more muscle probably means greater weight loss in the long run, Dr. Cody prescribes moderate exercise at first. "I would start someone out at a lower intensity and a longer period of time because I think that helps you to change behaviors," she says. "A lot of people go into this wanting to look better, and they are going to see these inches lost as being a pretty good indicator of what they are doing." Also, you have more chance losing weight with mild exercise because you are more likely to do it. Mild exercise is usually more enjoyable for beginners or people who have been sedentary, she says.

Be picky. Before you begin your aerobic program, put some effort into selecting your aerobic activity. What's best? "Whatever you can stick with is going to work," says Peggy Norwood, an exercise physiologist, president of Avalon Fitness, and former fitness director of the Duke University Diet and Fitness Center, both in Durham, North Carolina.

Choose something that you enjoy, says Dr. Wilkinson. It doesn't matter if you in-line skate, ski, run, or play hopscotch. And you want to make sure to pick something that you can do for at least 30 minutes, three to five times a week. (For more advice on how to choose your aerobic activity, see chapter 18.)

Start with 5 minutes. Don't worry about exercising for the entire recommended 30 minutes, especially if you are really out of shape. Start with a time that's comfortable, like 5 minutes. Then gradually increase the amount of time up to 30 minutes. That way, you can avoid injuries, aches, pains, and other setbacks, says Norwood.

Weighted Workouts Work Wonders

Resistance training builds muscle much the same way that life builds wisdom. In life, we start out innocent. Then various things stun us— friends gossip about us, our neighborhood associations hike their fees,

Any Time Is the Right Time

What's the best time to work out?

- Some people will tell you to work out in the afternoon so that your body will have had time to warm up. You can exercise more easily than in the morning when your body is naturally sluggish.

- Some people will tell you to exercise in the morning during hot weather because the air temperature is cooler then. Your body won't have to work as hard to stay cool, so you can work out harder.

- Some people will tell you to avoid evening exercise because it will rev up your body, making it difficult for you to get to sleep.

- Some people will tell you to exercise early in the morning to avoid air pollution peaks. Then you will avoid ozone and carbon monoxide levels high enough to affect your lung functioning, causing shallow breathing.

- Some people will tell you to exercise in the morning to rev up your metabolism and burn more calories during the day.

- Some people will tell you to exercise a couple of hours before dinner to reduce your appetite.

"You can find a good reason to exercise at any time of the day," says Susan W. Butterworth, Ph.D., director of wellness services for the occupational health program at Oregon Health Sciences University in Portland. "The best time to exercise is the time that fits into your schedule the best." So, whatever time is most convenient is really the best time because it increases your chances of maintaining your exercise habit, she says.

So, if you enjoy getting up $\frac{1}{2}$ hour earlier than usual, sliding an aerobics video into your VCR, exercising, and then showering and going to work—then mornings are your best time to exercise. If you find you have a spare $\frac{1}{2}$ hour between the time you get home from work and the time you need to cook dinner—then the late afternoon is your best time. If you feel most energetic during your lunch hour—then noon is your best time, says Dr. Butterworth.

The best time is *your* time.

our husbands forget our anniversaries. But eventually, we get used to such happenings, and they don't stun us anymore.

Muscle building is much the same. First, we lift a moderate weight seven or eight times—what's called a set—until we can't lift it anymore. Our muscle gives up under the pressure.

But overwhelm that muscle enough times, and it gets used to the activity by building protein and expanding muscle fibers. The muscle rises to the occasion—and eventually, the weight doesn't feel heavy anymore.

On the Fat-to-Firm Program, you can expect to build an average of about 2 pounds of muscle every eight weeks for the first four months of the program. Then muscle building will slow. Eventually, your hormones will prevent you from building more muscle. But you can maintain what you have throughout life by continuing the resistance program, according to Dr. Westcott.

In one very large study, women lost 3½ pounds of fat for every 2 pounds of muscle that they built. Though that's only a 1½-pound difference on the scale, the change will show up more dramatically on your body. Muscle is more compact than fat. So even if every pound of fat was replaced with a pound of muscle—that is, you lost no weight on the scale—you would still shrink in body size. In the Fat-to-Firm Program, you can expect to lose about an inch around your waist every month, according to Dr. Westcott.

Other than helping us to burn more calories and making us look better, resistance training is an integral part of the Fat-to-Firm Program for yet another reason. Just like it stuns muscles into growing, resistance training also stresses bones, making them stronger, especially the joints. That will protect you from injury in the aerobic part of the program. "There's nothing like a knee or ankle injury to ruin your weight-loss program," says Dr. McMurray. "This type of injury really sabotages weight loss: You can't walk, jog, or even be active at work and around the house. So you can actually end up gaining weight."

Easier Than You Might Think

Though a faster metabolic rate, a slimmer figure, and a stronger skeleton should sound appealing, you might wrongly shy away from weight training because you don't see yourself as the weightlifting type. Maybe you don't know your pecs from your glutes. Or you don't know your dumbbells from your barbells, your squats from your dead lifts, your sets from your reps, or your free weights from your Nautilus.

To tell the truth, maybe you never cared to know any of those things. Plus, you have no intention of resembling a female version of Arnold Schwarzenegger.

Sorry. None of those are good reasons to avoid weight training, also known as resistance training. First of all, you don't need to know the names of your muscles to understand the Fat-to-Firm weight-training program. You simply need to focus on your chest, back, shoulders, stomach, arms, legs, and buttocks. Second, you don't need to know the names of various types of equipment or the names of the various weightlifting poses. The illustrated exercises in chapters 19 and 20 show you how to proceed.

Also, with the Fat-to-Firm Program, you don't need to step foot in a gym (unless you want to). The weight workouts can be done at home, in private. And finally, with the Fat-to-Firm weight-training program, you will never, ever, in a million years come close to resembling Arnold Schwarzenegger. To build that kind of muscle, you need a hormone called testosterone. And women don't have the hormone in large enough amounts, unless they take synthetic steroids.

"Women aren't genetically equipped to build massive muscles, so it won't happen unless they take steroids," says Dr. McMurray. "A woman who combines resistance training with aerobic exercise is going to end up looking firmer and nicely toned. She won't get bulky or muscle-bound."

As you proceed, keep these general guidelines in mind.

Do one set. In the past, most of the advice about weight training was targeted to men who wanted to build huge amounts of muscle. It wasn't uncommon for trainers to recommend lifting a weight eight to 15 times, taking a rest, doing it again, taking a rest, and doing it again. Under such a program weight training lasted for hours.

Experts, however, have begun to study the effects of weight training on women who want to firm up but don't want to build huge muscles. And they found women as well as men only need to do one set—about eight to 15 repetitions all at the same time—to make considerable progress.

Don't worry about time. About 10 different exercises are needed to work the entire body: the arms, shoulders, back, stomach, chest, legs, and buttocks. The Fat-to-Firm weight-training program should take about 20 minutes a day, three days a week. You can add the weight routine to your 30 minutes of aerobic exercise, or lift on the days you don't do aerobics.

Think "Action" All Day, Every Day

Dish washing. Playing twister. Tossing a Frisbee. Bread kneading.

You might not think of cleaning your house, playing games with your children, and baking as exercise, but they all burn more calories than sitting in your recliner. They help create an active lifestyle. And that is crucial for controlling weight.

"We're seeing more overweight people today than at any time in history. Yet we are not eating any more than people did in the 1950s," says Dr. Girandola. "The problem is, we rarely walk anywhere. Most of our leisure activities involve staring at a screen, and we have every conceivable labor-saving device to minimize our activity at home and at work."

Slowly eliminating our dependence on labor-saving devices is one of the easiest ways to live a more active life, says Dr. Girandola.

Here are some things to consider doing without.

- Electric can openers
- Electric car windows
- Elevators
- Escalators
- Power steering
- Riding lawn mowers

This doesn't mean that you have to go back to life in the 1800s and start churning your own butter, says Dr. Girandola. Rather, you need to consciously start making your life more active.

"Women who clean house for a living tend to be relatively healthy because housecleaning is hard work," says Dr. Thomas. "It certainly is not what most people would consider exercise. But activity is critically important."

Dr. Thomas recommends making the following changes to become more active.

- Make it a habit to always park a little farther away from a building entrance instead of waiting for a prime space to open up.

Don't Believe the Scale

Women seem to have a co-dependent relationship with the scale. We trust our scales enough to actually stand on the mechanical device much more than necessary. Then we spend the rest of the time finding ways to not believe what the scale told us.

Over the years, we have developed plenty of ways to argue with our scales.

The "it's broken" excuse: "I wonder where the warranty for this thing is? There's no way I weigh that much."

The rounding down method: "The scale says 143 pounds. I really weigh 140."

The natural fluctuation excuse: "I must be bloated."

The accessory excuse: "My watch (shoes, hair tie, underwear) must weigh at least 3 pounds."

The wet hair excuse: "I just took a shower. I'm still soaking wet. So I weigh more."

Well, get ready for one of the best excuses yet for ignoring the scale. When it comes to going from fat to firm, the scale is probably the least accurate measure of your progress. "Women who are exercising may not lose that much weight on the scale. But that doesn't mean that they aren't making significant progress. They will find that their clothes are looser fitting because they have replaced fat with muscle," says Katherine T. Thomas, Ph.D., assistant professor of exercise science and physical education at Arizona State University in Tempe.

Muscle weighs more than fat. But it's more compact. So an exact exchange of a pound of muscle for a pound of fat will obviously make no change in your actual weight, but it will make you

- Take the stairs.
- Take walking breaks at work.
- Whenever possible, take your bike, in-line skates, or your own two feet instead of your car.

Try to fit in a total of 30 minutes of activity most days of the week, says Elizabeth Howze, Sc.D., associate director for health promotion in the division of nutrition and physical activity in the National Center for

look slimmer, says Wayne Westcott, Ph.D., strength-training consultant in Quincy, Massachusetts, for the national YMCA.

When it comes to health, experts are moving away from focusing on how much you weigh and toward how fat you are. Fatness is measured by the percentage of fat you have to lean body mass (muscle, bones, organs, and so forth). By such standards, someone who weighs 120 pounds but with 35 percent fat could actually be considered fat. And the same woman at the same height who weighs 140 and has only 15 to 18 percent fat could be considered lean, says Peggy Norwood, an exercise physiologist, president of Avalon Fitness, and former fitness director of the Duke University Diet and Fitness Center, both in Durham, North Carolina.

"Some women are not overweight. But they look out-of-shape and frail because they have potbellies. They are round-shouldered. Rather than lose weight, they need to get more fit. They need to exercise," says Alan Weismantel, a physical therapist for Health South in Hanover, Pennsylvania.

You can determine your fat status by getting your body composition tested. Women should try to keep their percentage of fat below 30 percent, says Dr. Thomas. You can get your body composition measured at most health clubs, doctors offices, and university sports-medicine departments.

Or you can use a tape measure. As you progress through the Fat-to-Firm Program, you will replace every $3\frac{1}{2}$ pounds of fat with every 2 pounds of muscle you gain. So for every $1\frac{1}{2}$-pound loss on the scale, you should lose about an inch in your waist measurement simply because the muscle is more compact, says Dr. Westcott.

Chronic Disease Prevention and Health Promotion at the Centers for Disease Control and Prevention in Atlanta. For instance, climb stairs for 5 minutes, walk around the supermarket for 15, and vacuum for 10. On the days when you do ½ hour straight of an activity like aerobic dance, continue to look for opportunities to get more activity during that day. Remember, the more you do, the greater the benefit, she says.

Eventually, leading an active life will become second nature. You won't have to make an effort to do it. But at first, you'll need to do some planning, says Susan W. Butterworth, Ph.D., director of wellness services for the occupational health program at Oregon Health Sciences University in Portland. She suggests sitting down with a family member, friend, neighbor, or co-worker and making a long list of fun things that you can do that don't involve your couch or bed. "The activity can be educational or social. It doesn't have to be a formal exercise session," she says. For instance, your list might include the following:

- Taking your family or a friend to botanical garden or arboretum
- Going to the zoo
- Tossing around a Frisbee with your children, a friend, or your pet
- Playing catch with your dog
- Going shopping

The list can involve home life, work life, or social life. Once you have your list completed, plan at least one activity a week, says Dr. Butterworth.

Though the number of calories you burn will depend on how intensely you do your activity and for how long, you can expect to burn 150 calories a day or about 750 more a week by adding in ½ hour of aerobic activity on most days, according to Dr Howze. (To find more ways to increase your day-to-day activity, see chapter 22.)

Chapter 17

Walking: A Giant Step toward Slimness

Easy, convenient, low-cost, and injury-free, walking is the one exercise that women can stick with.

It was time. Roseanne Welsh Strull had decided that this was the day she would go for her first walk. So she got her 272-pound frame off her living-room chair, went to the front door, opened it, stepped onto her driveway, ambled down to her mailbox, turned around, ambled back up the driveway, entered the house, closed the door, and returned to her living-room chair.

"There," she told herself. "I did it. Now all I have to do is do it again tomorrow."

Today, Roseanne weighs 135 pounds. Walking to the mailbox poses no struggle. Neither does aerobics class, a bicycle ride, a round of badminton, or a night on the dance floor. In fact, Roseanne has been so successful at losing weight that—as a personal trainer and lifestyle counselor in Beaverton, Oregon, the author of *Thinner Winners,* and now eight years at her goal—she teaches other women how to use exercise to do the same.

Though she has branched out since her early exercise days, Roseanne chose walking as her first exercise because it was the only aerobic activity that she knew how to do. And all she needed to get herself started was a good pair of shoes. Once she started, walking never let her down.

Why Walk?

Roseanne started walking for the same reasons that so many other women choose it as their aerobic activity, reasons that make walking an integral part of the Fat-to-Firm Program.

Walking is popular. Call it peer pressure. Walking is the most popular aerobic activity among women who exercise, according to surveys.

Walking sticks. Studies show that four out of five women who walk for exercise keep walking. In contrast, half of the women who try other types of exercise, like swimming, stair climbing, or running, call it quits during the first few months.

Walking is gentle. Many overweight women simply cannot do activities such as jogging or aerobic dance because their joints cannot handle the pounding. But most overweight women can walk, says William Joel Wilkinson, M.D., medical director of the division of epidemiology and clinical applications at the Cooper Institute for Aerobics Research in Dallas.

While the number of calories you burn depends on your weight, muscle mass, and metabolism, a 130-pound woman will burn approximately 70 calories per 15 minutes of walking (about 1 mile), roughly the same as the number of calories burned during 15 minutes of low-impact aerobics.

Walking is an easy fit. Walking is one of the easiest activities to fit into a busy day, says John M. Jakicic, Ph.D., research assistant professor in psychiatry at the University of Pittsburgh. When you split it up into short increments, walking can be squeezed into your day before breakfast or during lunch and coffee breaks at work. You don't have to take the time to change clothes or shower. And you can do it anytime, anywhere. It's as easy as circling your backyard—or your living-room coffee table.

Walking is a bargain. The only thing you need to buy is a good pair of shoes.

Not Just Any Shoe Will Do

Chances are, you have a closetful of shoes—pumps, flats, boots, and sandals for every outfit and occasion. Maybe you even have a pair of ballet slippers or bowling shoes from years gone by. But unless you already own a good pair of walking shoes, you're going to have to do some shopping.

If you walk a mile in a bad pair of shoes, your body isn't going to like you very much, says Howard J. Dananberg, D.P.M., medical director of the Walking Clinic in Bedford, New Hampshire. So a good pair of walking shoes is an essential element of the Fat-to-Firm walking program.

Here's what experts recommend.

Be prepared to spend. Heavier women need shoes with extra support, which tend to be more expensive, says Suki Munsell, Ph.D., director of the Dynamic Health and Fitness Institute in Corte Madera, California. And be prepared to replace your shoes about every three months. For one thing, your feet will shrink as you lose weight. But the heavier you are, the more weight you put on the shoe, wearing it out faster.

Get properly fitted. Start by going to a respected athletic-shoe store where a skilled salesperson can size up your feet, answer questions, and help you select and try on shoes, says Dr. Munsell. Then, to save money on replacement pairs, you can go to a discount store and buy the same shoe for less money.

Look for a firm heel. The heel counter at the back of the shoe should be firm, while the forefoot of the shoe at the ball of the foot should be flexible, says Dr. Dananberg.

Get the right padding. You do want a cushioned shoe to absorb shock and add stability. But you don't want it to be so padded that you can't sense where your shoe stops and the ground begins. You want to be able to feel changes in the surface under your feet so that your body can adjust to changes in the terrain. For instance, if you step onto a stick but can't feel it, you are more likely to trip. "Normal reflexes allow us to absorb impact during walking and tell us when there's a problem, says Dr. Dananberg. "If you don't feel that impact, by the time you know there's a problem, it's often too late."

How Far, How Fast, How Soon?

Convinced? Don't head out the door just yet. In order to make walking an integral part of the Fat-to-Firm Program, take this crash course on the how-tos of walking—how fast, how far, how long to walk. Learn where to walk. And find out ways to ensure comfort, especially if your joints are not as limber as they used to be. And of course, discover how to burn the most calories and lose unwanted weight.

Here's how to get started on your Fat-to-Firm walking program.

Test your endurance. For many women who follow the Fat-to-Firm Program, walking starts out just like Roseanne's first day. If the mailbox is as far as you can go, then that's your first workout. And don't beat yourself up over it. That's as far as a lot of overweight women can go, says Peggy Norwood, an exercise physiologist, president of Avalon Fitness, and former fitness director of the Duke University Diet and Fitness Center, both in Durham, North Carolina.

If simply walking to your mailbox is a challenge, then slowly build up your endurance. "I ask my overweight women how far they can go before they get out of breath or their joints start to hurt. Then we work with that. If it's 5 minutes, then they walk around the house for 5 minutes. Then later on when they have recovered, they do it again," says Norwood.

Take mini-walks. As Dr. Jakicic points out, short walking sessions can make exercise more convenient so that you're more likely to do it. Multiple sessions also allow you to slowly build up your endurance without hurting yourself, say experts.

Increase your time by 10 percent each week. If you start by walking for 10 minutes a day for the first week, then walk 11 minutes a day the following week, says Suki Munsell, Ph.D., director of the Dynamic Health and Fitness Institute in Corte Madera, California. That should allow you to eventually work up to at least 30 minutes a day, the ultimate goal of the Fat-to-Firm walking program.

Aim for long, slow distance. Concentrate more on the amount of time that you walk rather than how fast you walk, says Dr. Munsell. "Kind of underdo it each time, so you don't hurt yourself or exhaust yourself. Don't create a reason to stop doing it."

Make it pleasant. At this point you're probably thinking, "Yeah, but if I go faster, I can burn more calories in less time." That's true. But that's not what the Fat-to-Firm Program recommends. You want to walk at an intensity that doesn't make you exceptionally tired, says Dr. Wilkinson.

You don't want to make your walk so hard that eventually it becomes too unpleasant for you to keep doing it. "If you want to stay with it, it needs to be as pleasant as possible," says Mildred Cody, R.D., Ph.D., associate professor of nutrition and dietetics at Georgia State University in Atlanta.

Talk to yourself. Walk at a slow enough pace that you can talk about what happened on *Seinfeld* last night but not so slowly that you can whistle the *Andy Griffith Show* theme. "We know that people who can reach a level where they can walk a mile in 15 to 20 minutes are getting many of the health benefits they need from that exercise," Dr. Wilkinson says. "They just need to get out and be moving. If they are doing that, then they will be burning calories while improving their health and fitness level."

Walk the Fat-to-Firm Walk

You probably learned how to walk somewhere around your first birthday. So it probably seems silly to read pointers on how to walk. But the pointers are important. It's not uncommon for beginning walkers to use bad form. And if your walking form is bad, you'll feel it, says Howard J. Dananberg, D.P.M., medical director of the Walking Clinic in Bedford, New Hampshire. And if you're overweight, you'll feel it in the knees, he says. That kind of pain can sidetrack any walking program.

By looking for oddities, you can pinpoint bad form before the pain sets in, says Dr. Dananberg. If one bra strap repeatedly falls down your shoulder, for instance, that's a sign that you are carrying one shoulder higher than the other, he says.

Before setting off onto your first walk, try to keep the following pointers in mind.

Stand tall. You want to hold your body in the posture Mom always nagged you to hold as you grew up. To learn how to walk more erect, stretch your arms toward the sky, says Dr. Munsell. Once you lower them, exhale, keep your shoulders relaxed and head in the same place.

Strive for equal footing. Nobody's body is perfectly aligned. Still, you want to avoid moving differently on one side of your body than the other, says Dr. Dananberg. So watch for one foot that turns out while the other stays straight or one shoulder that is higher than the other, he says.

20 Surprising Places to Walk

Walking the same route again and again is like eating leftover spaghetti night after night. It's easy to pop in the microwave. But eventually, even the laziest cook will opt for another dish. Finding new places to walk isn't that hard, though.

Whether you live on the rocky Maine coast or in downtown San Diego (or somewhere in between), you can always find a great walking trail nearby by writing to the American Volkssport Association at 1001 Pat Booker Road, Suite 101, Universal City, TX 78148-4147.

The association will let you know about walks in your area or an area that you plan to visit, says Sandra Ward, director of public affairs for the American Volkssport Association.

Here are some examples to get you started.

Mansion tours
Historic districts of cities
Orchards
Vineyards
Botanical gardens
Lakefronts
Waterfronts
Boardwalks
Biking trails
Canal towpaths
River gorges
Wildlife refuges
Zoos
College campuses
School playgrounds and tracks (during off-hours or
    vacation periods)
Golf courses (perimeters only, where permitted)
Downtown pedestrian malls
Large shopping malls
Convention centers
Cranberry bogs

Also be on the lookout for unequal stride lengths and arm swings, says Dr. Munsell.

Admittedly, it's hard to watch yourself walk. So Dr. Dananberg suggests having a friend observe you to see if you look fairly symmetrical.

Hold your head erect. Keeping your head aligned with your shoulders—neither tilted forward or arched back—will help your neck support your head, says Dr. Munsell. If you lead with your chin, you'll probably end up with neck pain, she says.

Don't lead with your hips. Some people walk with their hips in the lead as if someone had just stuck a cane around their necks and yanked their upper bodies backward. Walking that way strains the lower back, says Dr. Munsell. So try to keep your hips aligned with your shoulders, not jutting forward.

Don't model a waddle. If you're overweight, your thighs might rub together when you walk. And that might cause chafing. Inadvertently, you might waddle by bowing your legs. Instead, Dr. Munsell suggests swiveling. It's like doing the twist. Stand tall and concentrate on moving your hips instead of pushing your legs far apart.

Fat-to-Firm Treadmill Tips

Your fat cells and muscle tissue don't know whether you are walking outside or inside on a treadmill. So theoretically, walking on a treadmill should burn the same number of calories as walking on other surfaces, says Ed Burke, Ph.D., associate professor of biology at the University of Colorado in Colorado Springs and editor of *The Complete Home Fitness Handbook.*

In reality, however, most people burn more calories on a treadmill than walking elsewhere, says Dr. Burke. Because treadmills force you to walk at an even clip, many walkers tend to walk slightly faster when indoors, thus burning more calories than when outside. "Treadmills keep the pace consistent. You can't let up. There's no stopping to smell the flowers. From a calorie standpoint that's good because it makes the work more consistent," he says.

Treadmills also offer other advantages.

- There are no sticks to trip over.

- There are no worries about walking too far away from home and not being able to make it back.

Plan a Walking Vacation

Walking vacations are great ways to visit interesting places you've read about—and get some exercise. Below we have listed the walks that get top billing year after year in a contest held by the American Volkssport Association. (For more information and directions for any of these walks, contact the association at 1001 Pat Booker Road, Suite 101, Universal City, TX 78148-4147.)

West Point, New York: Starting at the Hotel Thayer Gift Shop on Route 218, the walk winds along the West Point Military Academy campus, takes you past historic monuments, and offers great views of the Hudson River. The trail ranked number one two years in a row.

South Portland, Maine: Starting at the Shop 'n Save on Cottage Road, the route winds along local sidewalks, pathways, and beaches, allowing you to see many of the areas famed lighthouses and offering a beautiful view of the capes.

San Antonio, Texas: Starting at the Four Points Sheraton on Lexington Avenue, this trail goes along the Riverwalk through the city's King William District, the Hemisfair Park, and the historic Alamo.

Devils Tower, Wyoming: The trail starts at the Devils Tower trading post and takes you through and around Devils Tower, the first landmark in the United States to be declared a national monument.

Niagara Falls, New York: Starting at the Schoellkopf Geolog-

- Because of their cushioned rollers, some treadmills absorb about 40 percent of the jarring that you would get by walking on a road, making them joint-friendly.

- Because you use a treadmill indoors, you don't have to worry about the weather messing up your walking plans.

- And most important, many treadmills have a device to monitor your heart rate while you walk, making sure that you don't over-stress your heart early in the program, says Dr. Munsell.

No wonder sales of home treadmills are booming. But treadmills are not without a downside. There is really no comparison to walking outside, where you can take in the sights and be at one with nature. "It's healthier

ical Museum on Robert Moses Parkway North, the trail offers a great view of the falls from Prospect Point and Goat Island.

Guernsey, Wyoming: Starting at the Bunkhouse Motel on Highway 26, the walk runs along a section of the famous Oregon Trail, where ruts left behind by early settlers are still visible.

Washington, D.C.: Starting at the Columbia Plaza Pharmacy on 23rd Street, this popular walk takes you along city streets and through historic monument sections. You'll get to see the Lincoln Memorial, the Washington Monument, the Capitol Building, the White House, and Vietnam Memorial.

Alexandria, Virginia: Starting at King Henry Corner Deli on King Street, the walk goes through the historic Old Town of Alexandria, on city sidewalks, and through parks along the Potomac River. The town dates back to the seventeenth and eighteenth centuries.

Virginia City, Montana: Starting at Stonehouse Inn Bed and Breakfast on West Wallace Street, the trail quickly becomes challenging, with mountain terrain at an elevation of 6,000 feet.

Silver Falls State Park, Oregon: Of all the states, Oregon ranks as the most popular place to walk because it is so scenic. And among one of the better walks is Silver Falls State Park, which will take you past nine waterfalls, including one that's 150 feet high. The walk starts at Roth's IGA on North First Street.

to be outside," explains Hy Levasseur, an exercise physiologist and director of health education and fitness at the U.S. Department of Transportation in Washington, D.C. "Statistics suggest that depression is much more prevalent among people who have to stay inside because of the weather."

But that's not a big enough reason to forgo treadmills. "I think people need treadmills to ensure convenience," says Dr. Burke. "If it's rainy or cold or windy or wet, they don't have an excuse not to do it."

To use a treadmill as part of your walking program, follow these tips.

Use a shock absorber. Just about every treadmill manufacturer carries a line of joint-friendly treadmills, says Dr. Burke. Those treadmills are designed to absorb more shock. And they are also more expensive

(continued on page 244)

Stretch First

To avoid strain, stretching is a part of the Fat-to-Firm walking program, says Howard J. Dananberg, D.P.M., medical director of the Walking Clinic in Bedford, New Hampshire. He suggests doing the following stretches before and after every walking session.

Calf Stretch

A

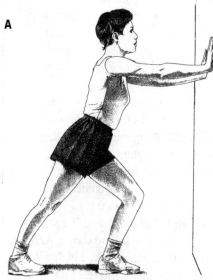

A. Face a wall, standing about 2 to 3 feet away from it. Place your right foot about 2 feet behind your left foot and bend your left knee, keeping your right leg straight. Both heels should be on the ground. Lean into the wall using your hands to press against it, keeping your back straight. Hold for about 25 seconds.

B

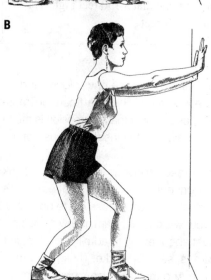

B. To stretch the lower calf, remain in the same position and bend the back knee, keeping the heel to the ground. Hold for about 25 seconds. When a muscle is particularly tight, the stretch should be held for 90 seconds, at which time considerable relaxation should be felt. An additional gentle stretch can then be given. Repeat on other side.

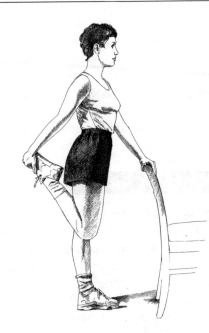

Thigh Stretch

Use your left hand to balance yourself by placing it on the back of a chair or against a wall. Bend your right leg, grasping your right foot with your right hand. Pull your foot toward your buttocks, keeping your leg and foot directly behind you. Your knees should be kept together. Hold for 25 seconds. When a muscle is particularly tight, the stretch should be held for 90 seconds, at which time considerable relaxation should be felt. An additional gentle stretch can then be given. Then switch legs.

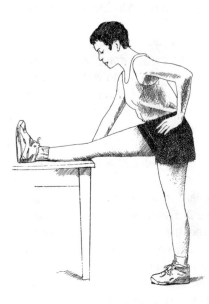

Hamstring Stretch

Place the back of your lower right leg on a table that is waist high or at a comfortable height that enables you to keep your right leg straight. Your standing leg should be slightly bent with your foot pointed forward in a walking position. Then slowly bend forward toward your right leg. Hold for 25 seconds, feeling the stretch in the back of your leg. When a muscle is particularly tight, the stretch should be held for 90 seconds, at which time considerable relaxation should be felt. An additional gentle stretch can then be given. Repeat with your other leg.

than other models. But it's worth it for the overweight woman who has joint problems, he says.

Get used to it. Some people have Jetson phobia during their first walk on a treadmill, says Dr. Burke. They picture the cartoon character George Jetson crying out, "Jane, stop this crazy thing," as he gets sucked underneath the conveyer belt. It will probably take a few times walking on a treadmill to get used to the belt moving under your feet. So start off on a slow speed until you feel comfortable, he says.

Comfort Cues

When Donna J. Kinoshita, 48, of Lafayette, Colorado, first started walking, she would routinely think to herself, "One block. Two blocks. Three blocks. There's the utility pole. Time to turn around. Three blocks to go. Two blocks. I can see the trailer from here." Each day she walked the same three blocks. Each day she counted them down as she went. And each day she become more and more bored.

Then Donna realized that if she simply wore a wristwatch, walked anywhere she wanted, and then headed back after a given amount of time, she could stop counting blocks and begin to take in the scenery instead.

"If you're just counting blocks as you walk and not looking at the flowers and the trees and the sky, something's wrong," says Donna.

Avoiding boredom is only one reason not to walk the same way every day. Avoiding injury is another, says Dr. Dananberg. For instance, when your walk takes you along the same crested road over and over again, your legs compensate by taking unequal steps. One leg bends more than the other because the ground isn't as far away. And many times your entire body will tilt to the side. All of those things can cause pain over time, he says.

Even if you walk an evenly flat surface each day—such as at the mall—it can create problems, says Dr. Dananberg. Again, the problem is lack of symmetry. Most women's feet are not exactly the same size. Neither are our hands. Or our legs. That's normal, but potentially problematic. "When you walk on a flat surface every day, your body adjusts by leaning to the left or to the right," he says.

To avoid problems, experts offer these tips.

Change terrain. Opt for trails where the ground offers a variety of stepping surfaces—dirt, gravel, sand, pavement, and so forth. Also, switching routes will help, says Dr. Munsell.

Consider pool walking. For people with joint problems, simply walking on treadmills and trails and switching routes may not be enough to avoid injury. But there are options. One is pool walking, says Dr. Munsell. And if you are really overweight, pool walking might be a better place to start than on land, she says. The water cushions the body and eliminates stressful impact on the joints. "If you are more than 60 pounds overweight, then you should balance any walking you do on land with equal time in the pool," she says.

Grab a staff. Another way to avoid joint pain is to use walking poles (such as hiking sticks), says Dr. Munsell. The poles help elongate the spine, distributing your body weight more evenly and putting less stress on your knees, ankles, and hips. As a bonus, the poles also involve working your upper body, increasing the number of calories you burn, she adds.

Crank Up Your Effort

At first, concentrate on making walking a regular part of your life, says Norwood. Once you can walk comfortably for at least ½ hour a day, use these strategies to increase the number of calories you burn with each walk.

Pump those arms. The more you swing your arms, the more calories you burn. "If you can activate both the upper and lower body, you are going to use up more oxygen—and burn more calories," says Hermann J. Engels, Ph.D., professor of exercise science at Wayne State University in Detroit.

Step up the terrain. Some surfaces are easier to walk on than others. And the easier it is to move, the fewer calories you burn. So if you want to increase the amount of calories you burn, increase the incline on the treadmill or scout around for surfaces that are somewhat difficult to walk on, such as sand, says Dr. Engels. Walking on a soft sand beach can burn almost twice as many calories as a walking on a paved road. Basically, the softer the surface you walk on, the more effort you have to put into each step, making you burn more calories.

Speed up. Another way to increase intensity is to pick up the pace for short periods of time, suggests Norwood. Start by walking faster than

Walking Enthusiasts Share Their Secrets

Plenty of women start exercise programs. That's the easy part. But sticking with it is another matter. That's why we asked exercise experts and long-time walkers for their advice on how to stay with the Fat-to-Firm walking program. Here's what they said.

Don't park out front. When Donna J. Kinoshita, 48, of Lafayette, Colorado, kept forgetting to walk, she finally decided to park her car a few blocks away from home. That way she had to walk. As she got in better shape, the car got farther and farther away from home, until finally she got rid of it and opted to walk everywhere. That was June of 1992. Donna is fortunate enough to live in a town where many grocery stores, restaurants, and businesses are within walking distance. Also, if necessary, she can opt for public transportation. When Donna is running late, she takes the bus. "I haven't had a car since 1992 and I love it," she says.

Bet on it. Find a walking partner, then make a wager. "In the beginning chip in more than you can afford to lose—$50 or $100. Put that into a pot and any time that you miss one of your walking appointments, the other person takes $10 out of the pot," says Suki Munsell, Ph.D., director of the Dynamic Health and Fitness Institute in Corte Madera, California.

Count things. When walking in a mall, make a game out of it. Memorize the order of the stores. Learn what's hot and what's not by scouting out window-front items in music and clothing stores. If you are walking with a group, organize a treasure hunt where one person scouts out some storefront items that other walkers must try to spot, suggests Thomas Cabot, president of the National Organization of Mall Walkers in Hermann, Missouri.

Get a dog. Marilyn Knight, 42, of Lewisburg, Kentucky, was never a dog person. But when she began her walking program to lose weight, she knew she would need some extra help. So she went to the pound and bought a golden retriever. Now when she's feeling kind of blah and thinking about skipping the routine, she sees Dusty staring intently out the front door, signaling that it's time for a walk. The

usual for 5 minutes of your walk or treadmill session. A week or two later, try to pick up the pace for 8 minutes. Keep increasing the amount of time you are walking faster until you can keep up the higher pace for ½ hour.

dog's look of yearning prompts Marilyn to get the leash, and they head outside together.

Take commercial breaks. There's about 10 minutes of commercials for every hour of television programming. So if you find yourself glued to *Roseanne* reruns when you should be out walking, at least make a habit of doing circles around your coffee table during the commercials, says Peggy Norwood, an exercise physiologist, president of Avalon Fitness, and former fitness director of the Duke University Diet and Fitness Center, both in Durham, North Carolina. In the course of a night's TV viewing, you could spend quite a bit of time walking.

Do errands on foot. One rule Norwood asks women to follow is the convenience-store rule. Find a convenience store that is within walking distance. Then when you need one item—say, you ran out of milk—don't drive. And don't borrow it from your next-door neighbor. Instead, walk to the convenience store to get what you need.

Become a walking encyclopedia. Fill your life with walking. Read about it. Talk to friends about it. Buy instructional walking tapes. Join walking organizations and groups. Make it so much a part of your life that you couldn't possibly think of quitting, says Dr. Munsell, who holds workshops on walking nationwide.

Stick on some 'phones. When walking on the treadmill became tedious for Kathy O'Connor, 54, of Peekskill, New York, she bought a tape player that fits into a carrying case attached to her belt. Then she popped in some tapes she hadn't listened to in a while and was amazed at the difference. "It almost makes you overexert yourself. You really can get lost in the music," says Kathy. She suggests trying books on tape as well.

Just remember not to blast your eardrums. To safeguard your hearing, make sure you can still hear someone talk in a normal conversation-level voice while the music is playing, says Kathleen Hutchinson, Ph.D., an audiologist and assistant professor in communications at Miami University in Oxford, Ohio.

Skip the hand weights. Theoretically, using hand or ankle weights should increase the amount of calories you burn because you have to work harder for each step and arm swing. At least that's what

Problem Solved

Solitude Works for Her

For Mindy Kane, 38, of Houston, walking was her secret to losing 50 pounds.

What she did: "Being overweight, I didn't feel comfortable or coordinated starting a fitness program involving classes," she says. "But I liked walking because it was just me, walking at my pace. Pretty soon, I was challenging myself to walk faster and longer."

Why it works: Slow and steady does win the race when it comes to fitness, says Larry T. Wier, Ed.D., director of the health-related fitness program at the NASA Johnson Space Center in Houston. Begin any new program at a comfortable pace, with an activity you enjoy. "It may take some getting used to, but after a short time, you'll love it," he says. "The important thing is to build a habit for a lifetime."

ppens in laboratory studies, says Dr. Engels. But when he gave lkers some weights and asked them to walk, he found that the people wore hand weights didn't swing their arms as much as they did when weren't holding hand weights. The compensation actually negated ncrease in calorie burn that would have resulted from using the ts, he said.

Doctors caution against walking with weights strapped to your wri r ankles because weights can cause pain in the lower leg or arm and increase blood pressure to high levels. It's safer to wear weight on th so. Problem is, carrying weight there won't up your calorie burn much ause it is so close to your center of gravity, says Dr. Engels. The hu body is designed to most efficiently carry weight along its center avity such as the head, shoulders, chest, and back. That's why som omen in African cultures can carry such heavy loads on their heads, he ys.

Chapter 18

More Fat-to-Firm Aerobic Options

When it comes to aerobic exercise, "easy does it" is the key to weight loss, firming, and better health. Here's how to pick the best easy exercise for you.

Forget about those get-thin-quick exercise videos where a perky, leotard-clad woman makes you jump up and down dozens of times while she yells, "Can you feel the burn? Work it! Work it!"

Forget about the television sitcom character wrapped in bulky sweat clothes who half runs and half limps here, there, and everywhere, all in the name of weight loss. Forget about all the ouch, all the strain, all the sweat, and all the pain that come to mind when you hear the word *aerobics.*

Aerobics is not synonymous with anguish.

"No, it doesn't have to hurt," says Peggy Norwood, an exercise physiologist, president of Avalon Fitness, and former fitness director of the Duke University Diet and Fitness Center, both in Durham, North Carolina.

Easy Does It

If it doesn't mean anguish, what does aerobics mean? Technically, aerobic exercise is any type of repeated physical movement that makes

Start Slow

Expert after expert says that the secret to losing weight and keeping it off is to start slowly with an exercise routine you like and stick with it. That's also the advice of woman after woman who succeeded at permanent weight loss. Here's how three women lost weight—and kept it off once and for all.

Donna Gettings, 42, of Williamsburg, Virginia: "When I realized that I couldn't walk my 278-pound body across a soccer field to watch my daughter's game, I knew I had to start exercising. I had swam competitively as a child. So I began swimming 10 laps a day, five days a week. After a month I bumped it up to 15. After another month, 20. Then, 50 lengths—which is a little less than ¾ mile. Then one day I made a mile. Then I made a mile again. It took a long time to get to a mile—a long time. And I lost 111 pounds getting there."

Regina Pascucci, 37, of West Trenton, New Jersey: "When I started losing weight in 1993, I was so out of shape that I could barely take a mile walk with my husband along the Delaware River near our house. I started exercising to a beginner's step-aerobics tape every other day. Then I worked up to three days on, one day off. I started with no step at all. Then my husband bought me a step. Eventually, the tape was too easy. So I got a more advanced tape. Then I added 4 inches to the step; then 6. By April 1994 I had lost 35 pounds, exchanging my size 18 clothes for size 10s. And I could walk along the trail with my husband and not get tired."

Donna J. Kinoshita, 48, of Lafayette, Colorado: "On my first walk, I had to stop to catch my breath. I just remember thinking, 'I'm 42 years old. I just walked 4½ blocks. I can't be this out of breath. If I don't get in shape, I'm not going to be able to get out of my chair by the time I'm 50.' At first, I did six blocks every other day. Then I began walking every day. I started adding distance. I began walking to the store instead of driving my car. I walked 15 minutes here, 10 minutes there, 20 minutes here. Eventually, I walked so much that I just got rid of my car—I didn't need it anymore, and it was too much of a headache, so I simplified my life. Then I walked about 10 miles a day, four days a week, and 5 miles a day, three days a week."

you breathe more than usual and improves the strength of your heart and lungs. But what qualifies as aerobic exercise has changed over the years. In the past, exercise experts thought we should work out for 20 to 60 minutes, at least three times a week, at a moderate-to-vigorous rate. For maximum health and weight loss, they recommended exercise that involved a lot of sweating, huffing, and puffing.

But today's exercise experts have refocused their recommendations. Now, they say we only need to exercise at a light-to-moderate pace for 30 to 60 minutes, three times a week, to be healthier and to lose weight. What's moderate? It's taking 15 to 20 minutes to walk 1 mile, compared to a vigorous pace of 10 to 12 minutes, which requires fast walking or jogging, says William Joel Wilkinson, M.D., medical director of the division of epidemiology and clinical applications at the Cooper Institute for Aerobics Research in Dallas. Leisurely cycling, swimming, and canoeing are examples of other moderate-intensity activities.

"People don't need to be exercising so intensely that they are breathing hard and sweating and having to push themselves to keep up that pace," says Dr. Wilkinson. "Exercise should be comfortable. It should feel as though they are pushing themselves a little bit more than normal. They should breathe slightly harder or faster. But exercise shouldn't feel hard."

Why did exercise experts change their tune? They came face-to-face with this reality: People who exercise at a light-to-moderate pace are likely to stick with their exercise programs. People who exercise intensely are likely to quit. "Imagine a woman who wants to lose weight who has never exercised before," says Dr. Wilkinson. "All of a sudden, she starts exercising intensely—and all of a sudden, she feels more tired than usual. That woman is not going to continue to exercise. That's why we stress light-to-moderate activity—because it helps people maintain their exercise programs."

Exercise for Life

Okay, so you don't have to be a triathlete to firm your body and stay healthy. You want to find an easy, enjoyable kind of aerobic exercise—or even a couple kinds—that you're likely to do today, next week, next month, next year...and the rest of your life. "Pick what you think you might stick with," says Dr. Wilkinson. "I don't really think there's one best exercise. It's the long-term commitment that's important. It doesn't matter if it's

Set a Goal, Break a Record

People who get into the *Guinness Book of Records* do some amazing things. But you can be just as amazing.

Did you know that if you...

...skied the NordicTrack at a moderate pace for an hour, five days a week, it would take you seven weeks to surpass Sisko Kainulaisen's women's Guinness record for the longest 24-hour cross-country skiing run. Actually, you would beat her by 26 miles. In 1985 she covered 205.05 miles during a 24-hour nonstop skiing adventure.

...ran 3 miles a day, five days a week, in 39 weeks you could beat Hilary Walker's 1991 ultra-run. She ran the 590-mile length of Friendship Highway from Tibet to Nepal in 14 days.

...rode an exercise bike at a moderate speed for an hour, five days a week, for one year, you could surpass Bill Narasnek's Guinness record by 149 miles. In 1991, he cycled the distance of Canada from Vancouver, British Columbia, to Halifax, Nova Scotia, traveling 3,751 miles.

walking, swimming, or riding a stationary bike. It just needs to be something that you can do for the long term."

Finding an exercise you enjoy is the first step. But there are other criteria to think about. Is it affordable, or is it too expensive? Is it convenient, or is it a hassle? Is it comfortable, or does it cause discomfort and pain?

To help you pick the right exercise, we asked top exercise and weight-loss experts to comment on the pros and cons of 10 different types of aerobic exercise. First, they discuss exercises that are "just right" for women who haven't exercised for a while, who have at least 20 pounds to lose, and who may have joint or back pain. Next, they evaluate some higher-intensity exercises, like running, that are possible choices for women who are already somewhat fit and who have few medical problems.

One final clarification before you begin reading: The experts have evaluated cost and convenience as either "low," "medium," or "high." To do that, they compared the exercises to walking (lowest cost, highest convenience) and downhill skiing (highest cost, lowest convenience).

Water Aerobics

Calories burned: up to 155 calories in 15 minutes
Convenience: medium
Cost: medium

If you think there's no exercise that's right for you, then water aerobics may be your best bet. The gentle support of the water almost guarantees that you'll have no discomfort or injuries, according to Luye Lui, personal trainer, certified aquatics instructor, and director of Luye Aquafit in New York City. And water aerobics accomplishes three goals of exercise in one session: It burns calories, builds strength (because of the resistance of the water), and increases flexibility (because of water's natural fluid support).

Some women learn to do water aerobics from a book or a video, Generally, though, you need some instruction. And either way, you need a pool, which could be one problem. Another is that you have to be seen in a swimsuit, not a happy idea for some women. Luye Lui suggests wearing a T-shirt over your suit if you feel self-conscious.

Or take a cue from Donna Gettings, 42, of Williamsburg, Virginia, who used swimming to lose 111 pounds. "At first, I was concerned about the perceptions of others who would see me in my size 24 bathing suit that was way too tight," she says. "My thoughts vacillated between being seen as someone foolish or someone determined. I chose to be seen as someone determined—and swam."

Here are some other hints to follow if you choose water aerobics.

Talk to the instructor. If you have a medical problem, like back pain, or you're afraid of water or you don't know how to swim, tell the instructor. Nonswimmers can stand in the front of the class where the instructor can see them better. And exercises can be modified for orthopedic problems, says Luye Lui.

And ask about the class. Look for a class where the teacher allows you to work out at your own pace. That's one of the pluses of water aerobics, says Luye Lui: You shouldn't have to move at the same speed as your neighbor.

Swimming

Calories burned: up to 200 calories in 15 minutes
Convenience: medium
Cost: medium

Like water aerobics, swimming is also kind to your joints. But improper form might put some strain on your lower back, says Luye Lui.

You may have heard some say that swimming won't really help women lose weight. Evidently, one scientific study, which has never been duplicated, found that women who swam didn't lose weight. To test that finding, Laurie Grubbs, Ph.D., associate professor of nursing at Florida State University in Tallahassee, measured the fat-burning levels of women who swam and women who walked. Her conclusion? Both groups burned the same amount of fat.

"I'm not really sure why the women in that one study did not lose weight," says Dr. Grubbs. "They might not have been swimming continuous laps. It might be that people who swim eat more than people who do other types of exercise." She says that out-of-water exercises like jogging and biking increase your body's inner temperature, which tends to squelch your appetite. Swimming doesn't make you hot, so it may not reduce your appetite the way other exercises do. In fact, she says, it might have the opposite effect: If the water is cold, your body may crave extra calories to keep warm.

So, to make swimming optimal for weight loss, Dr. Grubbs suggests that you swim in a heated pool that's at least 80°F and be sure to swim continuous laps. Here are some other hints to help you make swimming a part of your Fat-to-Firm Program.

Vary your strokes. "A lot of people jump in the pool and do 30, 40, or 50 laps of the crawl stroke over and over and over at the same pace," says Luye Lui. To keep swimming fun, she suggests alternating between backstroke, sidestroke, breaststroke, and freestyle. Luye Lui also says to do some laps at a pace that's fast, some moderate, and others slow.

Isolate a muscle group. Increase the intensity a notch by isolating muscle groups. Use a kickboard to isolate your leg muscles. Or isolate your arms by hugging a flotation device between your legs—the device prevents you from kicking, forcing you to use your arms to move your body through the pool. Or, says Luye Lui, try running in place in waist- or chest-high water or treading water in the deep end.

Bicycling

Calories burned: up to 119 calories in 15 minutes
Convenience: high
Cost: high

Biking is a great aerobic activity for overweight women because it involves little or no bouncing—your legs spin in a circle, with little impact on your joints.

Fat-to-Firm Exercise Advice for New Moms

Yawn.

That's the telltale sign of a new mom. The recent arrival of a new baby means that she's getting up over and over again every night. She's tired.

Besides getting some shut-eye, that new mom may also want to get rid of her extra pounds. But hours of exercise aren't going to do it. In fact, too much exercise might actually hinder the weight-loss efforts of new moms—because it can cause even more fatigue.

In a scientific study of women who had recently given birth and were breast-feeding, those who exercised for 45 minutes, five days a week, didn't lose any more weight than the group that didn't exercise. But in another study, a group of postpartum women who worked out aerobically for ½ hour to 1 hour only three times a week did lose weight.

What's going on? Diane Habash, Ph.D., nutrition research manager in the General Clinic Research Center at Ohio State University in Columbus, who lead the second study, concurs with the authors of the first study. "Unfortunately, because the women had just had babies, they didn't get much sleep. They had to get up several times throughout the night. And exercising five times a week just wore them out. They went home, sat down, overate, and didn't do anything for the rest of the day," she says. "Exercising three times a week for a postpartum women is probably more realistic than five times a week."

Biking is also incredibly convenient. You can ride for pure exercise, or you can ride with your husband or children, commute to work, or bike to the store. If you use a stationary bike, you can read or watch television while you pedal.

But biking does involve fairly expensive equipment. You'll need to buy either an outdoor or indoor bike, or a gym membership.

Biking also has some physical drawbacks. Some outdoor bikes require the rider to hunch over, which can be hard on the back, says Hy Levasseur, an exercise physiologist and director of health education and fitness for the U.S. Department of Transportation in Washington, D.C. That's especially a problem for women who are extremely overweight,

Why Mix-and-Match Exercise Is Best

Joan goes jogging for the 15th day in a row.

Her body sneers: "Not again. That's it. I'm not standing for this treatment anymore!" Joan's body puts its foot down. And suddenly, Joan gets a wicked pain in her calf.

She can't exercise for the next two weeks.

Joan is fictional, but her problem a fact of life, experts say. Whenever you do the same movement over and over again, you increase the chance of developing what doctors call an overuse injury. Every sport has them. Runners get shinsplints. Tennis players get tennis elbow.

But these injuries are easy to avoid—by cross-training, or participating in more than one exercise. "Cross-training decreases the chance of getting hurt," says William Joel Wilkinson, M.D., medical director of the division of epidemiology and clinical applications at the Cooper Institute for Aerobics Research in Dallas. It also gives you other exercise options if you do get injured. If you develop shinsplints from running, for example, you can stop running but keep up other activities that don't stress the shins, like swimming. Cross-training also helps you mentally, he says, by preventing the boredom that can come from doing the same exercise every day.

In order to cross-train, Dr. Wilkinson suggests alternating between at least three activities. Try to alternate between activities, such as aerobic dancing or running, that put pressure on the joints, and activities, such as swimming and cycling, that don't.

he says, and he suggests those women buy a recumbent bicycle, which allows them to lean back while riding.

If biking is your choice on the Fat-to-Firm Program, here are some hints to get started.

Sit and spin. When riding a stationary bike, don't set the resistance so high that you can barely pedal. "A lot of people don't spin their legs around enough, and that's where the aerobic workout comes from," says Nancy C. Karabaic, a certified personal trainer in Wheaton, Maryland. If you're a beginner, aim to ride at 80 revolutions per minute. Once you get in shape, shoot for 90 to 100 revolutions per minute, she says.

Protect your knees. When adjusting the seat on a stationary or outdoor bicycle, make sure that there is a slight bend in your knees. If your legs are too straight, you will hurt your knees. If your knees are too bent, you won't be able to power the bike as well, says Karabaic.

Dancing

Calories burned: up to 150 calories in 15 minutes
Convenience: high
Cost: low

Three times a week, Kathy O'Connor, 54, of Peekskill, New York, drives to the gym and uses the treadmill and the stair-climbing machine for 30 minutes. She knows it's good for her, but sometimes she has to force herself to go.

But on Monday nights, motivating herself to exercise is never a problem—because that's when she and her husband take an Irish folk dancing class.

Dancing? As exercise?

You bet—it qualifies as light-to-moderate activity, and it's lots of fun, too. Any kind of dancing is aerobic: square, rock 'n' roll, disco, belly, salsa, and ballroom. Just pick your favorite music and start moving. It requires no equipment besides a radio or a tape or CD player. And there are no rules to follow. As long as you're moving, you're exercising, says Levasseur, who suggests that you start with 10-minute sessions and work up to 30 minutes or more.

At-Home Aerobic Dancing

Calories burned: up to 125 calories in 15 minutes
Convenience: high
Cost: low

Regina Pascucci, 37, of West Trenton, New Jersey, is a morning person. Good thing. When she started her step aerobics, she had to leave for work by 6:30 A.M., which meant—because the morning was the only time she could exercise—that she had to get up at 4:45 A.M. to work out. Gyms weren't open at that hour. And it was too dark to exercise outside.

So she turned on the VCR, stuck in a step-aerobics tape, and exercised for 30 to 45 minutes. "How I was motivated to exercise at that hour of the day, I don't know," she says. "But step-aerobics exercise tapes are what did it for me. I went down from a size 18 to a size 10 and lost 35 pounds."

▶

As a term, *aerobic dance* covers many different forms: from "low-impact" moves, in which there's no bouncing, to "step," which involves (no surprise) using a low, benchlike step, to "weighted workouts," which use rapid movements and light hand weights, to...well, to whatever a creative aerobics teacher can invent. But no matter what the form, aerobic dance can burn a lot of calories—from 300 to 500 an hour.

Aerobic exercise tapes work for so many women because they are incredibly convenient, says personal trainer Roseanne Welsh Strull, 48, of Beaverton, Oregon, who lost 137 pounds and co-authored the book *Thinner Winners* to help other women do the same. "You can use aerobics tapes in your own home. You can use them at midnight or 6:00 A.M. You can use them with earphones so that the family doesn't hear you. And you can dress any way you want."

Of course, you can do just about anything you want at home—which might also include not working out when you don't feel like it. "At-home workouts are always in danger of becoming nonworkouts," says Diane Habash, Ph.D., nutrition research manager in the General Clinic Research Center at Ohio State University in Columbus. To cure a case of the at-home exercise blahs, find tapes you really enjoy.

Roseanne suggests trading tapes with friends or checking them out of the library. Also, the company Collage Video will send you a free guide to home exercise videos that offers detailed descriptions of tapes, For a catalog write to Collage Video, 5390 Main Street, N.E., Minneapolis, MN 55421-1128.

One last caution from Roseanne: Those just starting to exercise should look for low-impact-aerobics tapes for beginners.

Aerobic Dance Classes (including step or slide classes)

Calories burned: up to 125 calories in 15 minutes
Convenience: medium
Cost: medium

Dr. Habash asked one group of new mothers to do stretching, toning, abdominal exercises, and aerobics classes with an instructor and another group of new mothers to do stretching, toning, and abdominal exercises at home with a videotape, but not to include aerobics. Well, home might be where the heart is, but there wasn't too much exercise going on. "Most of the women who exercised at home ended up doing nothing," she says. "Once in a while, they would really work on their sit-ups. Then all of a sudden, they just quit."

Exercising in an aerobics class—which incinerates approximately the same 500 calories an hour as working out to an at-home aerobics tape—is a wonderful way to have a literal "exercise routine." Classes also score high for sociability and inspiration, since you're spending a lot of class time and locker-room time with other women who want to be healthy and firm.

The problem with aerobics classes is that you have to keep up with the instructor. Every woman has a war story of the aerobics teacher from Planet Perky who wouldn't stop until everyone had to be wheeled out on a gurney. Such classes are especially tough on beginners, who are perpetually one move behind, still doing the "grapevine" when the rest of the class has moved on to the "pony."

Luye Lui, who is also a certified aerobics instructor, suggests starting with a low-impact class designed for beginners. And if you find that coordinating your arm movements and leg movements is too difficult (a common frustration for beginners), she says to just do the footwork until you get used to the movements.

Don't worry about choosing the type of aerobics—step, slide board, or the traditional variety. They all work. Just make sure to start with low-impact—that means no bouncing—until the pounds come off, says Luye Lui. Otherwise, the pressure of your body weight can hurt your ankles, knees, or hips.

Cross-Country Skiing

Calories burned: up to 150 calories in 15 minutes
Convenience: medium
Cost: high

Cross-country skiing—whether in the snow or on a machine—was once thought of by exercise scientists as the king of aerobics, burning more calories per hour than any other exercise. Sorry, indoor cross-country machine, but treadmills and stair-climbers come out ahead.

Researchers at the Medical College of Wisconsin and the V.A. Medical Center, both in Milwaukee, taught people how to use a treadmill, a stair-climbing machine, a cross-country ski machine, a stationary bike, and a rowing machine. Then they measured the calories burned at a given perceived effort on all those simulated machines. The winners? Jogging on the treadmill with 705 calories per hour and stair climbing, with 627 calories per hour. Simulated cross-country skiing burned 597. These results were gotten at an intensity that felt "somewhat hard," according to the researchers.

Now, that doesn't mean that you shouldn't take up simulated cross-country skiing. It's a great workout for the upper and lower body and easier on your joints than running, but you shouldn't expect it to be the best calorie-crusher. You also shouldn't expect to master the machine on the first day, since it requires coordinating arm and leg movements.

"Start with your legs and get used to that motion—then add the arms. Take it slow. Don't go on the machine and expect to be an expert right away," says Mike Smith, spokesperson for NordicTrack, one of the leading manufacturers of cross-country ski machines. Stick with it, and you'll eventually get the hang of it, he adds.

Rowing

Calories burned: up to 150 calories in 15 minutes
Convenience: medium
Cost: high

In the Wisconsin study of various exercise machines, scientists found that rowing machines burned about 600 calories an hour at a perceived effort described as somewhat hard. They also work your entire body and don't jar your joints.

The key to using a rowing machine is to put your back into the motion, says Karabaic. She says to start with your knees bent and your arms forward. Then push back with your legs as you keep your arms and back straight. Once your legs are extended, lean back from the hips and pull your arms to your chest. Then sit up, push your arms forward, and bend your knees to the starting position. This instruction is guaranteed to trigger your past-life memories as a galley slave, she says, so be prepared.

Jogging

Calories burned: up to 149 calories in 15 minutes
Convenience: high
Cost: low

"If you asked me what was the best single thing that you could do for yourself to help you trim down and lose weight, it would be jogging, provided your hips, knees, and ankles can handle the stress of jogging," says Levasseur.

Jogging uses the muscles of your whole body: your legs to push off and your arms and trunk for balance. Using all that muscle translates into burning a lot of calories, about 600 an hour. Which gets to the reason that jogging isn't it ranked *numero uno* in the Fat-to-Firm Program. In a word: pain. Because jogging puts so much pressure on your joints, you literally run the risk of injury to your ankles, knees, and hips. Almost every expert consulted said that people who are overweight should not run.

Is there any way to avoid injury? Yes, says Alberto Salazar—world-class marathon runner and coach to fellow running champion (and injury-prone) Mary Decker Slaney. Here's the (slow) steps he advises for beginning runners.

1. Start by alternating between 1 minute of walking and 1 minute of running for up to 10 minutes. Do that for two weeks.
2. Proceed to 2 minutes of running for every 1 minute of walking and increase your total time to 15 minutes.
3. Gradually build up to a nonstop 20-minute jog followed by a 10-minute walk.
4. Then try for a full ½-hour jog.
5. Stay at a ½ hour for a few months—even if it feels easy, says Salazar. That will give your joints a chance to get used to jogging.

Stair Climbing

Calories burned: up to 150 calories in 15 minutes

Convenience: medium

Cost: low to high

Who ever thought that climbing stairs would be the "in" thing to do? Enter the stair-climbing machine—and a whole new way to exercise. It's a great workout for a woman's buttocks, thighs, hips, and calves. And because it doesn't involve bouncing, it's easy on the joints.

Some experts, however, think that stair climbing may be too much of a good thing because it's so effective in building buttock, hip, and thigh muscles—precisely the places where most women want to lose inches. "It will make your thighs and hips firmer, but they might not get smaller," says Levasseur. To stair-step to slimness, he suggests stair-stepping at low intensities.

Another way to avoid bulky hips is to make stair stepping only one part of the Fat-to-Firm exercise mix, says Karabaic. That way, you will avoid overworking those large leg muscles that you are trying to shrink.

When using a stair-climbing machine, think form not speed, says Cedric Bryant, Ph.D., director of sports medicine for StairMaster, L.P. in Kirkland, Washington. Many people set the machine on the fastest motion, thinking they're burning maximum calories. But at that intensity most people compensate for the super-fast speed by leaning on the console, tightly gripping the handrails, and locking their arms—all of which cut calorie burning by 20 to 25 percent, no matter what the readout on the machine says.

To use the machine correctly, set it at an intensity that allows you to stand up straight and only loosely grip the handrails for balance.

Here are some other pointers from Dr. Bryant.

Step up. Instead of pushing down on the pedals, try to step up. The pedals are designed to lower at a controlled rate. It's the stepping-up motion that prevents the pedals from sinking to the floor and provides the workout, he says.

Find your sweet spot. The bigger the step you take, the more calories you will burn. But Dr. Bryant cautions against going for the highest step possible. You want to find the exact stepping motion that is right for you, your "sweet spot." While it might be comfortable for the person next to you to step up 9 inches, you might only be comfortable with 5, and that's fine.

In fact, Dr. Bryant's final words about stair-climbing machines apply to all the aerobic exercises discussed in this chapter: "The real trick with any type of exercise routine aimed at weight control is that you want to find your comfort zone. That way, you are going to be able to do the exercise longer and more consistently, which will allow you to maintain your body weight or lose weight."

Chapter 19

Strength Training: Boost Your Metabolism in an Hour a Week

**Here's the best way to firm
your body, lose weight faster, slow aging,
and look great in clothes.**

Joyce Stoner's 44-year-old body was beginning to reveal its age. Joyce meticulously watched what she ate, yet unwanted pounds slowly attached themselves to her hips. She regularly sweat to step aerobics, yet found flab on her thighs and a pouch on her tummy.

Joyce knew that she couldn't stop the aging clock, but she wanted to at least slow it down. So she hired a personal trainer to take her through a weightlifting and aerobics routine two days a week.

Six months later, Joyce looked in the mirror and liked what she saw. It was as if she had traded in her old body for a new model.

"People had always told me that I had great legs, but I didn't see it," says Joyce, an administrative assistant from New Carrolton, Maryland. "Now, I'm noticing that I have great legs. My buttocks are firm. And I just love my arms. Before, I wouldn't wear a tank top. Now, I wear sleeveless clothes without hesitation. And my breasts—they seemed small before. After strength training, they look bigger."

"My husband has never said that I needed to lose weight," adds Joyce. "But he's noticed the changes."

They're Firm and Feminine

The biggest obstacles that stand between a woman and a weightlifting program are fear and not knowing how to begin. Fear of building too much muscle. Fear of walking into a gym where so many already-muscular people hang out. Well, listen to these women. They'll tell you how they overcame those fears—and incorporated weight lifting into their weight-loss efforts.

Shiela Ward, 38, of Washington, D.C.: "I'm broad-shouldered, and I wanted to make sure that weight lifting didn't make me excessively broad-shouldered like a man. My trainer assured me that would not happen. So I took her word for it. And I haven't gotten more broad-shouldered. Weight lifting helped me whittle down the size of my body so that I could fit into a wedding dress that a friend gave me. I feel like I'm tightening my body up. And I no longer feel self-conscious when my husband sees me walking around in the nude."

Julie Nava, 49, of San Marino, California: "In a year and a half, I went from a size 0 to a size 14. One day I really got a good look at myself and noticed I had three chins. I couldn't fit into my size 14s. And I couldn't hide the weight anymore. So I began eating differently, and I hired a personal trainer to help me weight-lift and exercise aerobically five days a week.

"At first, I was worried. I had never been in a gym before. I thought everyone would have a perfect body and then there would be fat little me. But I was inspired by Oprah Winfrey's success and by the threat of some health problems.

Why Strength Training Works

As you age, your metabolism slows. So, like Joyce, you start putting on pounds even though you're not eating more food. In some cases, you may even eat less food—and still gain weight. That slower metabolism is caused, in part, by an age-related loss of muscle. Well, strength training (or weight lifting, as it is also called) reverses that process. It builds muscle and speeds metabolism, says Wayne Westcott, Ph.D., strength-

"When I started, I could only do 15 seconds on the treadmill and barely pedal the bike. My trainer probably thought I wouldn't last a day or two. Now I can bike and run for an hour. I can leg-press 200 pounds. My body fat has gone down from 36 percent to 18 percent. My waist has shrunk from 31 to 25 inches. At 4 feet, 11 inches tall, I weigh 97 pounds."

Crystal Thompson, 37, of Fort Washington, Maryland: "I started to use weights, but I didn't want to walk around with arms that looked like Arnold Schwarzenegger's. When I first started lifting weights, I noticed that my arms looked swollen. I thought they looked fatter, not defined. I considered quitting. But my trainer told me to be patient. So I kept with it. And two months later, my arms were defined. Now, I shop for shirts that will show off my arms."

Joyce Stoner, 44, of New Carrolton, Maryland: "I thought that I didn't need to lift weights, that I just needed to tone up and lose a couple pounds. So when a friend of mine asked me to start a weight program with her, I thought I was going to bulk up like a competitive bodybuilder. I didn't want to look like one of those muscle people. But after talking with a trainer, I realized there's more to weight lifting than building big muscles.

"After lifting weights for six months, I'm really pleased with what I'm seeing. I've toned up a lot. I don't mind wearing sleeveless clothes. I think I look good for a change. It has built my confidence. I feel better about myself on the job, at home, everywhere."

training consultant in Quincy, Massachusetts, for the national YMCA. The result is that you burn more calories—even when you're sleeping. And you lose weight, or don't gain any extra.

That's why strength training is such a crucial ingredient of the Fat-to-Firm exercise equation—it helps speed up the metabolism. Sure, there are other ways to burn calories: lifestyle changes like walking up the stairs instead of taking the elevator or doing aerobic exercise. But only strength training builds the kind of muscle that's needed to give your sluggish metabolism a...well, a swift, firming kick in its sagging posterior.

What makes strength training such a powerful muscle builder? And why doesn't aerobic exercise do the same?

In aerobic exercise, the muscle is building predominantly endurance, not strength. When you walk or bike, you are increasing the capacity of your body to deliver more blood to the muscle so that it can work longer without being fatigued, says Morris B. Mellion, M.D., clinical associate professor at the University of Nebraska Medical Center and team physician for men's and women's sports at the University of Nebraska, both in Omaha. But in strength training, the cells of your muscles actually grow. When you ask a muscle to handle more weight than normal and then rest the muscle to let it recover, the muscle cells thicken. The muscle is bigger, firmer.

Building muscle also sculpts the body. A pound of muscle is smaller, firmer, and more shapely than a pound of fat. So as you replace fat with muscle, your body will take on a firmer shape. Try this: Press your finger against the top of your forearm. Your forearm is primarily muscle, so it probably feels pretty hard. Now press your finger against your abdomen, which tends to collect fat. Chances are, your abdomen gives considerably. While fat jiggles, muscle stays in place. And while fat hangs limply, muscle hugs the body, giving you a distinct shape.

Besides making you look better, strength training also makes you stronger. As you progress from fat to firm, you'll find groceries easier to carry, stairs easier to climb, and boxes easier to lift.

Body Sculpting for Women

If you asked a guy why he lifts weights, he would probably tell you that he wants to get bigger. He would say that he wants a chest like a bull, shoulders like a tank, and biceps like bowling balls.

Know any women who want to look like that?

"Women's strength-training goals are very different than men's goals," says Mia Finnegan, a Fitness America Pageant National Champion and Miss Olympia Fitness, who with her husband operates a training service called Tru Fitness in Pasadena, California. "The man wants a big, thick chest; a woman wants a shapely breast line. A man wants huge biceps and triceps; a woman wants toned arms. Women want to shrink their lower bodies—shrink their hips, butt, and thighs. Most men don't even care about their legs. They just care about their upper bodies."

Weight lifting can make a guy larger. And the image of the super-muscled male weight lifter can make women shy away from the weight room. Not to worry, though. Only in the rarest of cases do women have the natural ability to build huge amounts of muscle, says Dr. Westcott.

Take Finnegan, for example. At 5 foot, 4 inches, she weighs 125 pounds. At around 15 percent body fat, her arms are sculpted and toned. Her buttocks never jiggle. Her abdomen is enviably firm. But she's feminine and petite. If you saw her walking down the street, you would never suspect that she's a fitness champion who's featured regularly in muscle magazines.

When women tell Finnegan they worry that weight lifting will make them big, she asks, "Do you think I'm big?" "No," the women tell her. They say they want to look just like her. So Finnegan puts them on an exercise program that includes weight lifting.

"Nobody ever says, 'I want to get big. I want to look like one of those women in the bodybuilding magazines.' Women want to be tight, toned, and small," says Finnegan. "Women think that those overly muscular women in the magazines are natural. But those women often have breast implants and have drug-enhanced physiques. Few natural woman can gain muscle like that."

So, you won't have biceps like Arnold—or Arnoldette. But you will have firmer muscles and a faster metabolism. Before you begin, however, you need some guidelines for lifting correctly.

Give yourself enough room. Women who begin to lift weights don't give themselves enough elbow room, says Nancy C. Karabaic, a certified personal trainer in Wheaton, Maryland. We tend to keep our arms at our sides and our legs close together to appear ladylike. To train properly, you need to spread out and take up as much room as you need to be comfortable, she says.

Pay particular attention when doing squats and upright-rowing motions, says Karabaic. To do a squat correctly, you have to stick your butt out, which at first makes many women self-conscious, she says. And upright rowing involves bringing your elbows out to the sides, as if you were trying to jab someone next to you. To do rowing motions correctly, you need to get used to bending your elbows out to the sides.

Start right, start light. Ultimately, your goal for each strength-training exercise will be to lift a weight light enough that you can lift it at least eight times and heavy enough that you can't possibly lift it more than 15 times, says Tereasa Flunker, an exercise physiologist at ReQuest Physical Therapy in Gainesville, Florida, who won the Miss Gainesville title in 1988. But for the first couple of weeks of your weightlifting program, use weights that are slightly lighter than the description above so that you can make sure you use proper form. If you start out with weights that are too heavy, you'll tend to cheat. That is, you'll throw your back into the motion, do repetitions too quickly, or rely on momentum. So in the beginning, concern yourself more with lifting the weights correctly than with lifting heavy weights.

Add more weight. Once you're able to do between eight to 15 repetitions of an exercise comfortably, then you should move up in weight for that exercise, says Karabaic. Some women will feel comfortable doing eight, and some will need to wait until they do 15 before adding more weight. In the beginning of your program, you should expect to move up in weight every month to two months. After six months to a year, however, your muscles won't grow as quickly, so you'll advance in weight more slowly, every three to six months.

Visualize the exercise. To lift weights correctly, you need to feel your muscles move. Yet some women who are overweight or uncomfortable with their bodies for any reason tend to be out of touch with what it takes to move their bodies, says Kathy Mangan, a certified lifestyle and weight-management consultant and a certified personal trainer at the Women's Club, an all-women's health and fitness facility in Missoula, Montana. So at first, weight lifting may feel foreign.

Visualization can help overcome that awkwardness and help you lift correctly, says Mangan. Before you actually start the strength-training exercises on the pages that follow, picture yourself doing the motions depicted in the illustrations. In particular, think about what parts of your body you will use to do the motion correctly and how that might feel.

Don't lock your joints. When doing any exercise, make sure that you don't lock your elbows or knees. If you do, you'll end up putting weight on the joint instead of on the muscle, possibly causing elbow or knee pain, says Karabaic.

Straighten your wrists. Though you don't want to lock your elbows or knees, you do want to keep your wrists straight, says Karabaic. Otherwise, you may end up with wrist or forearm pain.

Breathe. Don't forget to breathe when lifting weights. Breathe out while lifting the weight and in while lowering it, says Karabaic. Don't hold your breath.

Ladies, Choose Your Weapon

The Fat-to-Firm Program uses quite a variety of strength-training exercises to both sculpt and strengthen muscle. You can do a complete routine in about 20 minutes, and it should be repeated three times a week.

Weight machines. Most often found at fitness centers, weight machines employ weights and pulleys, or other forms of resistance, to work specific muscle groups in specific ways. They offer a controlled workout, taking you through a safe range of motion with constant resistance throughout the entire motion.

Since you don't have to worry about dropping a heavy weight on your head or neck, weight machines are somewhat safer than *free weights*—dumbbells and barbells. But many machines are designed for the average male body. So unless you're 5-foot-7 or taller, you may find yourself constantly trying to adjust the machine and still never quite feeling comfortable. Don't blame your technique or know-how. Most likely, the machine does not fit you properly. So, for short women, machines may not be the best option, says Karabaic.

Resistance bands. Sold in many sporting goods stores and medical supply stores, stretchy, oversize rubber bands are an inexpensive way to begin a strength-training program. To work your arms, legs, and various other muscle groups, you simply stretch the oversize rubber bands in various directions. Commercial brand-name resistance bands are sold in sets, with different amounts of tension in each band. So as one resistance band becomes too easy, you can progress to a more-difficult-to-stretch band.

Resistance bands are convenient: They're easy to store, and you can even take them with you on vacation. But the bands can be unwieldy. As you pull on the band in a circular motion, such as when doing a biceps curl, you'll feel more tension at some points than others, making the movement feel jerky. Also, you need to do more repetitions with resistance bands than you would with using dumbbells or a barbell to get the same workout, says Karabaic.

Dumbbells and barbells. Free weights might be your best bet. Dumbbells and barbells are nothing more than hand-held rods with varying amounts of weight at each end, offering many of the same benefits as weight machines. Dumbbells come in pairs, one for each hand. A barbell is longer—you lift it with both hands.

You can get a good workout using dumbbells alone. They're fairly

How Dumbbells Got Their Name

Dumbbells aren't shaped like bells. And they're no dumber than a chin-up bar. So why do we call this handheld weight a dumbbell?

For the answer, we need to go back in time to the year 1711, when the word *dumbbell* was coined. At that time, churches lacked the technology to stick a cassette tape into a tape player attached to an amplifier and press "play" to blast what sounds like a real bell from church steeples. Bell ringing was a job. A hard, demanding job. A job only a strong person could do.

Problem was, if you needed to ring the church bells just once a week, you didn't ring them often enough to get in shape for the job. And to get in shape, bell ringers couldn't run up to the church tower and ring the bells whenever they wanted to—townspeople would never know whether the bell tolled for thee or whether the bell ringer was just getting a workout. So during the week, bell ringers began to exercise using a handheld weight that looked much like the apparatus used to swing a church bell, but without a bell. Because no sound came from the bell-like apparatus, the ringers referred to it as a dumbbell.

inexpensive and convenient for home use (in between workouts, you can store them under a bed).

Getting Set

For the Fat-to-Firm strength-training workout, you'll need various sizes of dumbbells and some sort of a bench. Experts offers these tips for getting equipped.

Buy varying sets of weights. Because different muscles will be stronger than others, you'll need more than one pair of dumbbells. Buy sets of 3-, 5-, and 10-pound dumbbells. Later, as you become stronger, you'll probably need heavier dumbbells. But most beginners don't need anything heavier than 10 pounds, Flunker says. If, however, you find 10 pounds is too light, don't hesitate to get heavier weights, she says.

Shop secondhand. You can save money on dumbbells by going to a secondhand sporting goods store, such as Play It Again Sports; by scouting garage sales; or by offering to buy lighter weights from body-builders who have moved on to heavier levels, says Flunker.

Go for comfort. Unlike treadmills, stair-climbers, and other exercise machines, buying free weights doesn't require a lot of research or comparison shopping. Dumbbells haven't evolved much since the day of their invention, says Mike May, spokesman for the National Sporting Goods Manufacturers Association in North Palm Beach, Florida.

Your main objective is to find dumbbells that are comfortable to hold, says Mangan. Dumbbells vary in length and width. You'll probably feel more comfortable with shorter dumbbells. The longer the dumbbell, the more unwieldy, she says.

You also want a comfortable bench. Some are wider than others. When at the store, lie on the bench to make sure it is wide enough to support your body, says Mangan. You don't want your shoulders or sides to hang over the edge to the point that you feel as though you'll fall off. Also, some benches are taller than others. Make sure that your feet can comfortably touch the floor when you are lying down, she says.

Make do with water jugs. If you aren't ready to purchase dumbbells, you can use plastic gallon milk jugs filled with water, says Molly Foley, an exercise physiologist and director of ReQuest Physical Therapy. A 1-gallon milk jug filled with water weighs about 8½ pounds. How much water you use depends on how much weight you intend to lift. Experiment to determine how much water is right for you. You'll probably have to add water or dump some out as you go from one exercise to the next, she says.

Improvise a bench. For beginners, a piano bench, padded picnic-table bench, or other rectangular-shaped object can suffice as a strength-training bench, says Foley. Make sure that your bench allows you to lower your elbows below body level, in order to do bench presses and similar exercises, she says. Lying on the bed or the floor won't work.

Slip on the gloves. You can get through your routine without them, but you'll feel more comfortable with a pair of weightlifting gloves. Gloves help you grip the weight securely and prevent calluses.

The Fat-to-Firm Workout

For allover body toning, follow the Fat-to-Firm workout, suggested by Michael Pollock, Ph.D., exercise physiologist and professor of medicine and exercise science at the University of Florida, with help from Gainesville exercise physiologists Tereasa Flunker and Molly Foley. The routines that comprise this workout target the chest, shoulders, neck, back, arms, legs, and buttocks, in that order. (For exercises that target the abdomen, see chapter 21. To focus more specifically on other trouble spots—thighs, hips, buttocks, and triceps—see chapter 20.)

When doing the program, follow these guidelines.

Go in order. Do the exercises in the order that they are listed. The exercises are arranged so that you can work the larger muscles in your chest and back before you work the smaller muscles in your arms. The smaller arm muscles assist the large chest and back muscles during exercises such as the bench press and upright row. If you worked the smaller muscles first, you would be too tired to complete the chest and back exercises, says Flunker.

Try to fail. Muscles get stronger more quickly if you work them to failure. That means you have worked your muscle to the point where you can't do a single additional repetition without resting. You want to lift a heavy enough weight so that between eight to 15 repetitions you have no option but to give up, says Dr. Pollock. Muscle failure makes stronger muscles. As you progress and are comfortable doing between eight and 15 repetitions, you can do another set or add more weight if using barbells, he adds.

Take breaks. After each exercise, rest for up to 2 minutes before moving on to the next exercise. Rest breaks give your muscles a chance to recuperate and prepare for further effort. When you first begin to work out, you may need to rest for the full 2 minutes before you feel able to do the next exercise. As time progresses, however, you will probably be able to shorten your rest time, says Foley.

Use good posture. Good posture will help you protect your joints and spine from strain, says Flunker. Before each movement check to make sure that you have good posture. Stand with your feet about shoulder-width apart and your knees slightly bent. Let your arms relax at your sides. Lift your breastbone by pulling your shoulders back and down. Roll your pelvis so that your lower back is straight instead of curved inward. Then assume that pose whether you're vertical (standing) or horizontal (lying on a bench), she says. When bending over, keep your back and chest straight by bending from the hips.

Take every other day off. Ideally, you should try to do the routine three days a week with at least one day of rest in between workouts. The rest will give your muscles a chance to recuperate, explains Dr. Pollock.

Give the gym a try. Though the following workout involves dumbbells, you can do similar moves on machines at a gym. For each exercise, you'll find the name of the machine you can use at the gym that works the same muscles as that exercise.

Dumbbell Bench Press

Muscles toned
The chest (pectoralis major) muscle around the breast builds up. The flabby back of the upper arms (triceps) gets hard. The shoulders (anterior deltoids) take on more shape.

What to do
A. Lie flat on a bench with your knees bent and feet flat on the bench. (If you have trouble keeping your balance, you can put both feet flat on the floor.) Hold a dumbbell in each hand, palms forward, with your arms held at a 90-degree angle from your chest—that is, arms straight up, as pictured.

B. Lower the dumbbells to your chest. Try not to let them wobble as you lower them as far as you can. Then return to the starting position and repeat.

In the gym
Use the chest press machine.

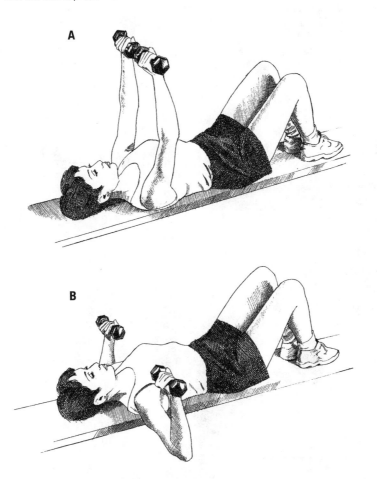

A

B

Dumbbell Flies

Muscles toned
The chest (pectoralis major) builds up, helping to accentuate the breasts. The shoulders (anterior deltoids) take on more shape.

What to do
A. Lie on a bench with your knees bent and feet on the bench. Hold the dumbbells above your chest, with your palms facing each other and elbows slightly bent.

B. Lower the weights as you move them out to the side of your body in a wide arc as far as you can. Keep your palms facing each other and elbows slightly bent to reduce stress on the shoulders. Once you have reached the maximum stretch, arc the weights back to the starting position, as if you were giving someone a huge bear hug. Then repeat.

In the gym
Use the arm-cross/butterfly machine.

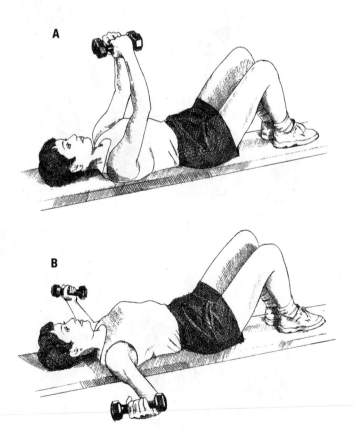

A

B

Dumbbell Press

Muscles toned
The shoulders (deltoids) take on shape, the neck (trapezius) builds up slightly, and the back of the upper arms (triceps) gets firm.

What to do
A. Sit on a bench with your back straight. Hold dumbbells in both hands. Bend your elbows to hold the dumbbells even at shoulder level, to the sides of the shoulders. Your palms should face forward.

B. Press the dumbbells overhead. Make sure to keep the weights above your shoulders, elbows slightly bent. Then return to the starting position and repeat.

In the gym
Use the overhead press machine.

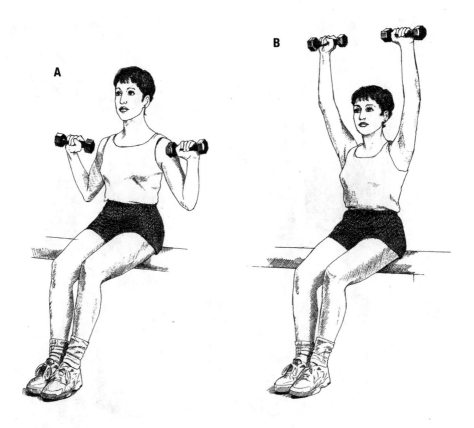

Upright Row

Muscles toned
The shoulders (deltoids) and the neck (trapezius) build up slightly and take on shape.

What to do
A. From a standing position, hold dumbbells in both hands with your knuckles facing forward. The dumbbells should be in front of your body below waist level. Your arms should hang downward, with your elbows straight.

B. Bend and raise your elbows to pull the dumbbells toward the ceiling. Try to keep the weights as close to your body as possible. Once you have the weight to armpit level, return to the starting position and then repeat.

In the gym
Use the lateral raise machine.

A

B

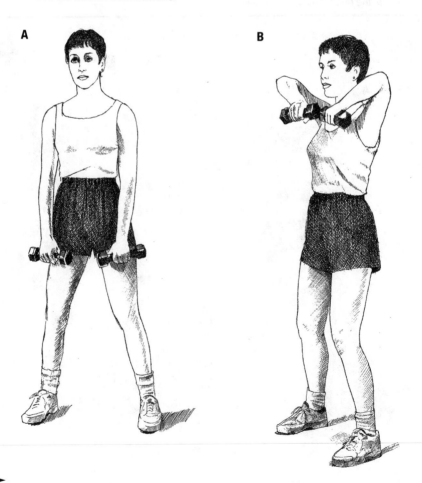

Bent Row

Muscles toned
The back muscles (latissimus dorsi, rhomboids) create a triangle from your shoulders to your waist, tapering your torso.

What to do
A. Kneel on one end of a padded weight bench with your left knee, keeping your right leg slightly bent. Support yourself with your left arm and hold a dumbbell with your right hand. Keep your back slightly arched.

B. Lift the dumbbell until your right elbow is a few inches higher than your back, as shown. Remember to keep your back slightly arched and your support leg straight. Return the dumbbell to the starting position and then repeat. After you complete your repetitions, repeat on the opposite side.

In the gym
Use the seated rowing machine.

A

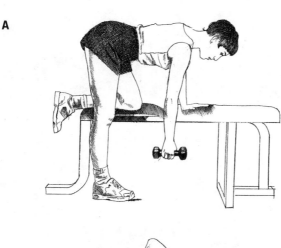

B

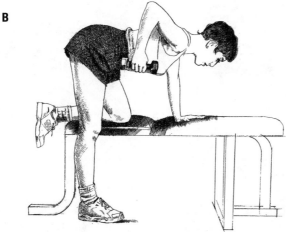

Back Extension

Muscles toned
The lower back (erector spinae) and buttocks (gluteals) firm up, further toning your torso, waistline, and hips.

What to do
A. Roll up two towels so they are each about 2 inches thick. Lie on your stomach and place one towel under your abdomen and the other under your forehead. Extend both your arms above your head.

B. Tighten your buttocks as you raise one extended arm and the opposite leg. Your arm should be straight, with your fingers pointing. Your toes should be pointed. Hold for 5 to 10 seconds and then repeat on the other side.

In the gym
Use the Roman chair or hyperextension machine.

A

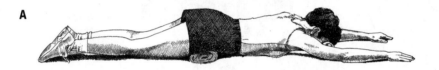

B

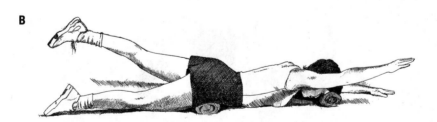

Standing Dumbbell Curl

Muscles toned

The upper front of the arms (biceps) take on shape and are less apt to jiggle when you move.

What to do

A. Stand with your knees slightly bent and your feet shoulder-width apart. With your back straight and head up, hold dumbbells in both hands, with your arms resting at your sides and your palms facing your outer thighs.

B. Rotate one arm so the palm is facing forward.

C. Curl that arm, bringing the forearm toward your biceps, with your palm facing up. Lower the weight, twist the arm back to the starting position, and repeat on other side. Continue switching sides until you have completed your repetitions. If you prefer, you can also do both sides simultaneously.

In the gym

Use the biceps curl machine.

A   B   C

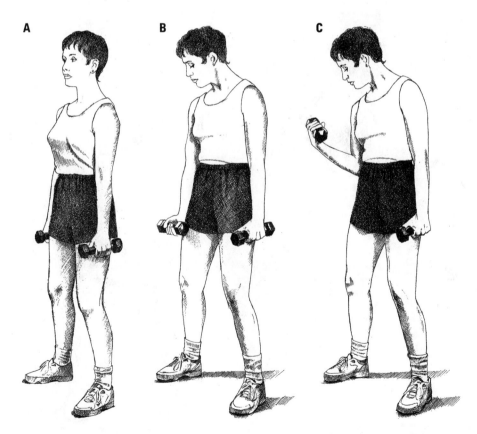

Seated Curl

Muscles toned
The upper front of the arms (biceps) take on shape, improving how you look in sleeveless tops.

What to do
A. Sit on the edge of a bench. Put your feet on the floor, about 2 feet apart. Hold a dumbbell in one hand with your palm facing up. Bend slightly forward and place the hand not holding the dumbbell on the knee on the same side. Then rest the elbow of the hand holding the dumbbell on the thigh, slightly above the knee on that side with the arm hanging down.

B. Curl the dumbbell toward your shoulder, making a semicircle while keeping your elbow on the thigh. Then lower the weight. After you complete your repetitions, repeat on the opposite side.

In the gym
Use the biceps curl machine.

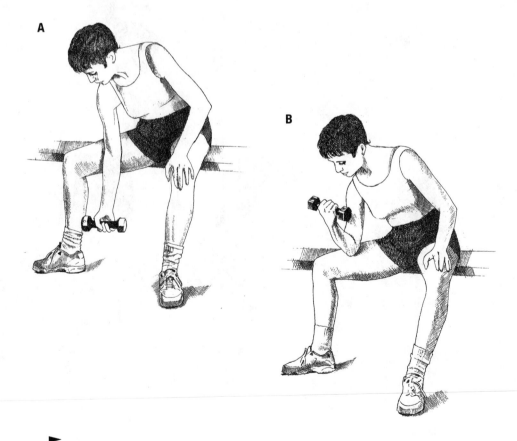

A

B

French Press

Muscles toned

Firms up flab on the upper back of the arms (triceps) so that your arms don't jiggle.

What to do

A. Hold a dumbbell just behind the top of your head with both hands. Cup your palms and thumbs around the handle of one end of the dumbbell, elbows extended. Stand straight with your feet shoulder-width apart or sit on the edge of a bench.

B. While keeping your upper arms close to your head, lower the weight behind your head in a semicircular motion until your forearms almost touch your biceps. Return to the starting position, then repeat.

In the gym

Use the triceps extension machine.

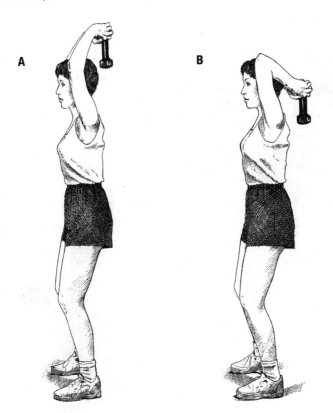

A   B

Dumbbell Kickback

Muscles toned
Firms the flab on the upper back of the arms (triceps), eliminating jiggliness.

What to do
A. Stand with your knees slightly bent, with one foot in front of the other at a comfortable distance. Place one hand on the bench or on your front knee for balance. Keep your upper torso parallel to the bench. Take the dumbbell in the other hand. Bend that arm and raise your elbow close to your side to shoulder height. Make sure your arm is at a 90-degree angle with your palm facing your side.

B. Your elbow should remain in place as you complete the movement. Press the weight back until your forearm is parallel to the floor. Do not raise it above your body. Hold for a count of two and then slowly return to the starting position. After you complete your repetitions, repeat on the opposite side.

In the gym
Use the triceps extension machine.

A

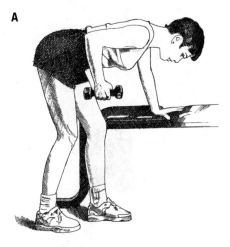

B

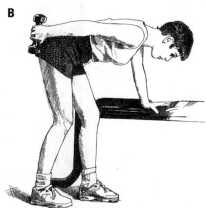

Dumbbell Squat

Muscles toned

Tightens, firms, and adds shape to the front thighs (quadriceps) and buttocks (gluteals), giving your legs a sleeker, firmer appearance.

What to do

A. Stand with a dumbbell in each hand. Raise the dumbbells to the outside of your shoulders with your palms facing forward, as shown.

B. Keeping your head and back in a straight line, bend forward slightly as you bend your knees and lower yourself as if you were going to sit into a chair. Keep your head and neck in a straight line. Lower yourself into a squat as far as you comfortably can but only until your thighs are almost parallel to the floor, as shown. Then raise yourself to the starting position and repeat.

In the gym

Use the leg press machine.

A

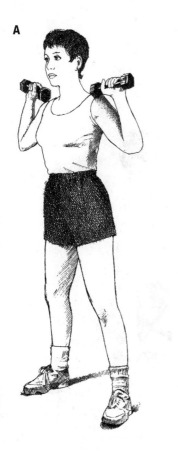

B

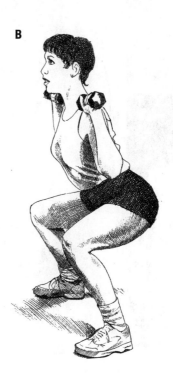

Dumbbell Lunge

Muscles toned

Firms, tightens, and adds shape to the buttocks (gluteus medius, gluteus maximus) and the front thighs (quadriceps).

What to do

A. Hold a dumbbell in each hand, with your arms at your sides and your palms facing in.

B. While keeping your head up and back straight, take a large step forward until your thigh is almost parallel to the floor. Bend your front knee while bringing the trailing knee almost to the floor, as shown. Push yourself back to the starting position and then repeat with the other leg.

In the gym

Use a leg press machine that works one leg at a time.

A

B

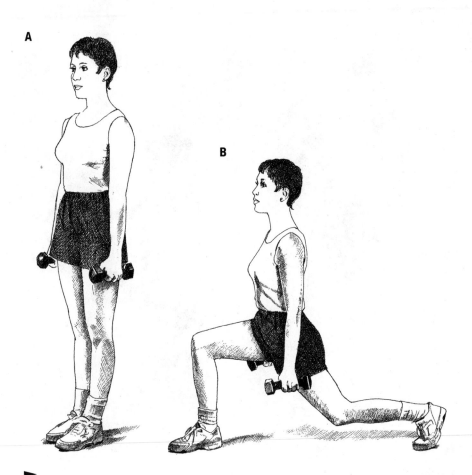

Standing Calf Raise

Muscles toned

Firms, tightens, and adds shape to the calves (gastrocnemius, soleus).

What to do

A. Stand with your toes and balls of feet on a step with your heels extended off the step.

B. Lower your heels as far as you can toward the floor or toward the step below while keeping your knees slightly bent, as shown.

C. Then raise up on your toes as far as possible. Repeat.

In the gym

Use the standing or seated calf-raise machine.

A

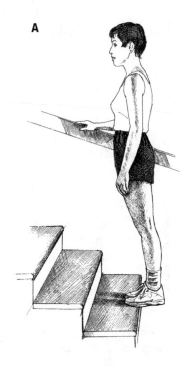

B

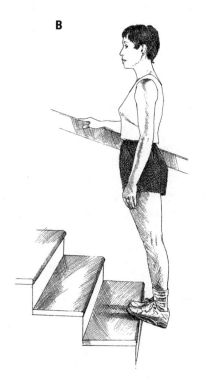

C

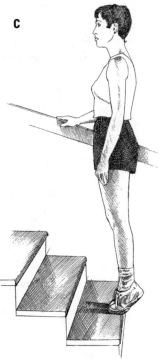

High Weights, Low Reps? Or the Reverse?

One piece of misinformation might confuse your early weightlifting efforts. Women who work out might tell you that doing a lot of repetitions at a low weight will prevent you from getting big.

They are partially correct. High repetitions at a low weight will build up muscle endurance instead of muscle strength, which means your muscles won't grow as much. Problem is, you are defeating the purpose of your entire weightlifting program if you chose the high repetition workout. You want your muscles to grow in strength and size to boost the number of calories you burn a day. You are better off doing fewer repetitions with more weight, building more muscle, and burning more calories to burn off more fat, says Wayne Westcott, Ph.D., strength-training consultant in Quincy, Massachusetts, for the national YMCA.

Staying Limber

Many weightlifting exercises tend to shorten the muscles, which makes you less flexible, says Flunker. Regular stretching will elongate those muscles, reduce any soreness, lower your injury risk, and give you a greater range of motion. Try to do the following stretches before and after each weightlifting session, in the order given, and do each one three times, holding each stretch about 10 to 20 seconds, she says.

Shoulder circles. Starting with your shoulders relaxed, slowly rotate them backward until you feel loose. Then change directions, rotating them forward.

Shoulder blade squeeze. Stand with your hands clasped behind your back. Lower your shoulder blades by pulling your clasped hands down and lifting your breastbone. Then raise your clasped hands toward the ceiling as high as you can. Your body may bend forward. Hold for about 20 seconds and then relax.

Chest stretch. Stand in a doorway with one foot a few inches in front of the other for balance. Extend your arms to the side, placing your hands, palms flat, against each wall along the doorway. Lean forward so that you can feel the stretch. Hold for about 20 seconds. Then vary the stretch by moving your hands higher and lower on the walls.

Back flex. Lie on your back. Using your arms, pull one knee to your chest. Hold for 20 seconds, then release. Repeat on the other side.

Back stretch. Get down on the floor on your hands and knees like a baby beginning to crawl. Your lower legs and thighs should form a 90-degree angle at your knees. Your back should be straight and your arms extended straight down directly under your shoulders. Lower your buttocks toward your heels. (Don't let your hands move out of position). You will look like a cat stretching. Feel the stretch through your spine. Hold for 20 seconds.

Hip flexor stretch. Get down on one knee, like someone making a marriage proposal. Keep both knees at 90-degree angles. Then, perform a pelvic tilt: Keeping your chest upright, lean forward, until you feel a stretch in the leg that has the knee on the floor. Most people cannot bend past their bent knee while maintaining a pelvic tilt. Hold for 20 seconds and then repeat on the other side.

Hamstring stretch. Lie on your back with your left knee bent and your foot on the floor, the right leg extended straight up at a 90-degree angle to the floor. Flex your right foot. Use your hands to pull the extended leg toward your chest. Hold for 20 seconds. Repeat with the right leg bent and the left leg lifted.

Thigh stretch. While standing, put your left hand on a wall for balance. Use the right hand to reach behind you and grab the ankle of your right leg so your foot comes as close as possible to touching your buttocks. Do not lean forward or allow your back to arch. Hold for 20 seconds. Repeat on the other side.

Calf stretch. With one leg in front of the other, about a walking-distance apart, push against a wall as if you were trying to push it down. Keep the calf you are stretching straight and its knee straight while the other knee is bent and lunging forward in front of you. Keep your heels on the floor and body straight so that you feel the stretch through the calf of your rear leg. Hold for 20 seconds. Repeat on the other side.

Forward neck stretch. Sit or stand with good posture. Bring your chin as close as you can to your chest. Hold for 20 seconds.

Side neck stretch. Sit or stand with good posture. While keeping your face forward, tip one ear toward the shoulder on the same side. Hold for 20 seconds. Repeat on the other side.

Side stretch. Hold your arms straight overhead and clasp both hands together. Lean to one side without leaning forward or backward. Hold for 20 seconds. Repeat on the other side.

Chapter 20

Taming Your Trouble Spots

You probably can't look like a supermodel, say the experts, but you can look like the best possible version of yourself.

Thunder thighs. Hippo hips. Blubber butt.

Such mean, nasty words we call our bodies. We use that kind of exaggerated and critical language to describe thighs that spread out and greet one another every time we sit down. Or hips that prevent us from yanking those old Jordache jeans up to our waists. Or rear ends that overflow the boundaries set by the swimsuit industry. Four body parts take the brunt of our criticism: thighs, hips, butts, and upper arms (the kind that swing like pendulums as you hang laundry out to dry).

We use that kind of language because we want to look like the women who are the exception, not the rule, in body shapes. Women who seem to have no fat whatsoever on their hips, thighs, buttocks, or upper arms.

But there's an easy explanation why we're not those women, why most of us are a little heftier in certain spots: Our genes designed us that way. From the day Dad's X chromosome hooked up with Mom's, many of us were genetically destined to collect fat below the waist, above the knees, and under the arms.

Fat, According to Plan

How do genes do their dirty work? They produce hormones and enzymes that influence the distribution of the fat, says Claude Bouchard, Ph.D., professor of exercise physiology at Laval University in Ste. Foy, Quebec. He cites these examples: Women who have more active cell enzymes that promote fat storage—partly a genetic trait—tend to have large thighs, hips, and buttocks. Women with higher amounts of female hormones like estrogen and progesterone—again, partly a genetic trait—tend to have larger lower bodies. And, to make it really obvious, women with large thighs usually have mothers and grandmothers with large thighs.

When we exercise and eat low-fat food, the weight also seems to leave in a predetermined manner—and not one that we might choose. Chest fat tends to go first, making our breasts smaller. At about the same time, we lose abdominal fat. (Well, at least *that's* good.) But the fat on our legs, hips, and buttocks acts like a bunch of stubborn tenants who ignore eviction notices and must be dragged away kicking and screaming as the wrecking ball demolishes the apartment.

There is a sunny side, however, to this seemingly bad cosmic joke, in which our genetically given body shape looks something like a pear. Being shaped like a pear is healthy, although too much fat overall is not. Being shaped like an apple—with most of your weight around your tummy—is unhealthy. That's why when women begin to resemble apples, they develop the same health risks as their potbellied menfolk: diabetes, high blood cholesterol, and heart disease.

Realistic Resizing

Whatever your genetic destiny, the Fat-to-Firm exercise program can help you improve the appearance of your hips, thighs, buttocks, and upper arms. For firming success, however, you need to set realistic, attainable goals, says Keli Roberts, certified fitness trainer in Hollywood, California, author of *Fitness Hollywood,* and maker of numerous exercise videos.

Women commonly make two mistakes when it comes to setting firming goals, she says. First, we compare ourselves to an ideal woman, whether she is Demi Moore, Cindy Crawford, or a composite of a bunch of famous women's body parts. And we somehow expect exercise to

▶

make us look just like our ideal woman—not only slimming down and toning up our trouble spots but also miraculously lengthening our bodies or changing our bone structure.

Exercise, however, can only do so much. For instance, celebrities like Tina Turner, supermodel Vendela Kirsebom, and Melanie Griffith have long, lean legs. The length enhances the leanness. If your legs are shorter, you may be able to get them just as toned, but they will never be longer, says Greg Isaacs, corporate fitness director for Warner Brothers in Los Angeles, author of *The Ultimate Lean Routine,* and fitness trainer to both Griffith and Kirsebom.

So instead of fantasizing about looking like a fashion model or a celebrity, suggests Roberts, imagine looking like an improved version of yourself.

Our second mistake, says Roberts, is that we try to tone specific body parts rather than our entire body. For instance, some women who want to tone their legs will do leg lifts as their only form of exercise. Although they feel a bit stronger, they get poor toning results. To get real results, you need an aerobic workout to burn fat and strength training to build metabolism-boosting muscle, says Michael Pollock, Ph.D., professor of medicine and exercise science at the University of Florida in Gainesville. So the Fat-to-Firm exercises for taming trouble spots are designed to be used in conjunction with aerobic exercise and other overall toning exercises.

Besides the fact that it works, this whole-body approach has another advantage: It helps us avoid injury. Working only one set of muscles—like our legs—creates an imbalanced body in which some muscles are much stronger than others. The stronger muscles then take on more work than the weaker muscles can handle, which can injure the weaker muscles, says Dr. Pollock.

Firming Your Trouble Spots

The Fat-to-Firm exercise plan that follows was created by Dr. Pollock and by Molly Foley, an exercise physiologist and director of ReQuest Physical Therapy in Gainesville, Florida; and Tereasa Flunker, an exercise physiologist also at ReQuest Physical Therapy. These exercises firm the thighs, hips, buttocks, and upper arms, in that order. For best results, follow these guidelines.

Don't get total-body amnesia. Don't focus on one figure flaw and neglect the rest of your body. Combine your trouble-spot workout with the total-body strength-training program that is outlined in chapter 19 and do some form of aerobic exercise, recommends Dr. Pollock. To firm up your thighs, hips, and buttocks, for example, start with the squats and/or lunges that are described on pages 283 and 284. Then do the thigh, hip, and leg exercises that are shown on pages 292 through 300, in the order given.

To firm your upper arms, begin with the French press and dumbbell kickbacks described on pages 281 and 282. Then do the upper arm exercises shown on pages 301 through 302 and 305 through 306.

Choose what you like. You don't necessarily need to do all of the Fat-to-Firm exercises to sculpt shapely legs and arms. Start with the first two exercises, which are leg lifts. To customize your program, you can mix and match your program according to which exercises you like. For instance, the fourth leg lift and both pelvic tilts will all work the buttocks. The first and second leg raises both work the inner thigh. And the triceps extension and bench dip both work the upper back of the arms. Out of those groups, pick out the exercises that you most enjoy, suggests Flunker.

Add some weight. You can do the exercises without added weight. As you progress, however, you may want to incorporate added resistance by using dumbbells or cuff weights. The extra weight will add intensity to the exercise and give you better results with fewer repetitions, according to Dr. Pollock. How much weight you add depends on your comfort and fitness level. He suggests increasing the weights by 2 to 3 pounds.

Tips on using added weight, such as ankle weights, accompanies various exercises. Look for ankle weights in sporting goods stores. Cuffed ankle weights, with a pouch to insert various weights, are economical. Instead of buying additional weights as you progress, you can insert more weight as you get stronger. And once using one fully loaded cuffed weight gets easy, you can use two on one leg instead of buying a heavier set, says Flunker.

Count your reps. For each exercise, do one to three sets of eight to 15 for best results, says Flunker. Hold the muscles being worked for a count of two and relax for a count of four.

Breathe. Be sure to exhale as you contract your muscle and inhale as you relax them, says Dr. Pollock.

Leg Lift #1

Muscles toned
Tightens and shapes the front thighs (quadriceps).

What to do
A. Sit on a sturdy table, bench, or chair. Place your palms against the chair, bench, or table for support. You can lean on your hands for balance, but try not to grip the edges.

B. Straighten one leg while keeping your foot flexed, as shown. Rest the other leg on the floor or on a stool, depending on the height of your platform. Hold this position for a count of two, then lower your leg. Do one set of repetitions with one leg, then repeat with the other leg.

For added resistance, you can do this exercise using light ankle weights. Begin with 1 pound. When you can easily do three sets, increase the weight.

In the gym
Use the leg extension machine.

A

B

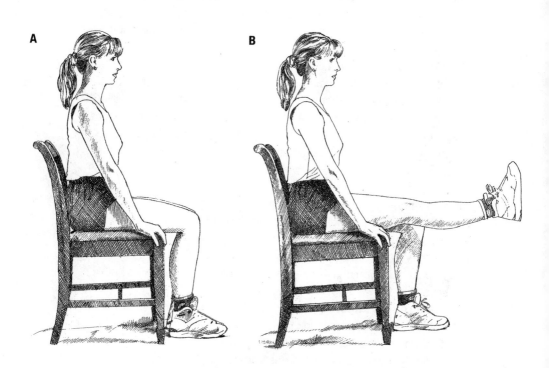

Leg Lift #2

Muscles toned
Firms and shapes the back thighs (hamstrings).

What to do
A. Stand while resting your hands on a table for balance.

B. Slowly bend one knee, bringing your heel toward your buttocks, stopping when you get to a 90-degree angle. Hold for a count of two and then slowly lower the leg. Do one set of reps with one leg, then repeat with the other leg.

For added resistance, do this exercise using light ankle weights. Begin with 1 pound. Once you can easily do three complete sets, increase the weight.

In the gym
Use the leg curl machine.

A   B

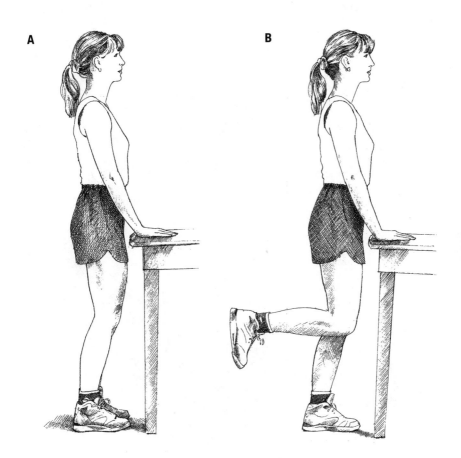

Leg Lift #3

Muscles toned
Tightens and shapes the front thighs (quadriceps).

What to do

A. Lie on your back with one knee straight and the other knee bent.

B. Keeping your leg completely straight, raise it to a 45-degree angle. Hold for a count of two. Then lower and repeat. Do one set with one leg, then repeat with the other leg.

For added resistance, you can do this exercise using light ankle weights. Start with 1 pound. When you can easily do three complete sets, increase the weight.

In the gym
Use the leg extension machine.

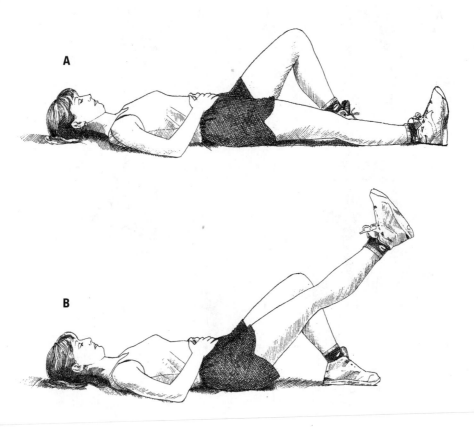

A

B

Leg Lift #4

Muscles toned

Firms up the back thighs (hamstrings), the buttocks (gluteals), and lower back (erector spinae).

What to do

A. Lie on your abdomen with a pillow under your hips, as shown.

B. Raise one leg off the floor as high as you can without arching your back. Hold for a count of two and then release and repeat. Do one set with one leg, then repeat with the other leg.

For added resistance, you can do this exercise using ankle weights. Begin with 1 pound. When you can easily do three complete sets, increase the weight.

In the gym

Use the lower back machine.

A

B

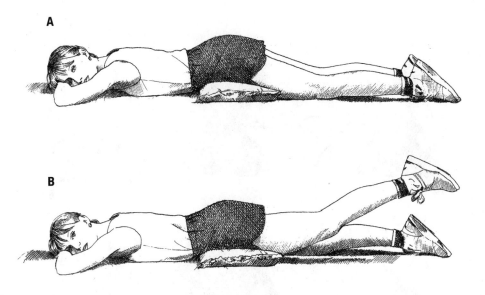

Pelvic Tilt #1

Muscles toned
Tightens and shapes the buttocks (gluteals) and the abdominals.

What to do
A. Lie on your back with both legs bent and your feet flat on the floor. Contract your abdominals and press the small of your back down to the floor.

B. Raise your torso off the floor as high as you can while tightening your buttocks and keeping your buttocks, back, and shoulders aligned. Hold for 5 to 10 seconds and then repeat.

In the gym
Use the lower back machine.

A

B

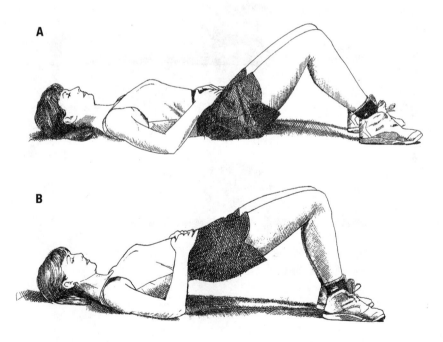

Pelvic Tilt #2

Muscles toned
Tightens and shapes the abdominals and buttocks (gluteals).

What to do
A. Lie on your back with both legs bent and your feet flat on the floor. Contract your abdominals and press the small of your back down to the floor. Raise your torso off the floor as high as you can while tightening your buttocks and keeping your buttocks, back, and shoulders aligned.

B. Extend your right leg out while contracting your left thigh muscles. Keep your pelvis, outstretched leg, and back in a straight line. Hold for 5 to 10 seconds. Return your right leg to the starting position. Alternate right and left legs for 5 to 10 extensions per leg. Rest between leg extensions, when necessary.

In the gym
Use the lower back machine.

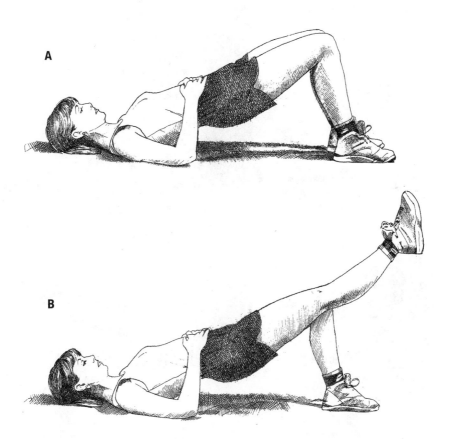

A

B

Leg Raise #1

Muscles toned
Firms up the flab on the inner thighs (adductors).

What to do
A. Lie on one side, supporting your head with the hand of the bent arm that rests on the floor. Bend the upper leg so that your foot is in front of the knee of the leg that rests on the floor.

B. Raise the leg that rests on the floor toward the ceiling. Hold for a count of two. Release and repeat. Do one set with one leg, then repeat with the other leg.

For added resistance, you can do this exercise using an ankle weight on the leg that rests on the floor. Begin with 1 pound. When you can easily do three complete sets, increase the weight.

In the gym
Use the hip adduction machine.

A

B

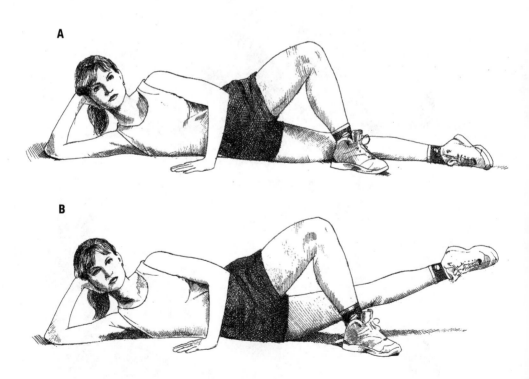

Leg Raise #2

Muscles toned

Firms up the flab on the inner thighs (adductors).

What to do

A. Lie on your back with your legs raised and straddled, heels resting against a wall, as shown.

B. Pull your legs together as you slide your heels against the wall. Straddle and repeat.

For added resistance, you can do this exercise using ankle weights. Begin with 1 pound. When you can easily do three complete sets, increase the weight.

In the gym

Use the hip adduction machine.

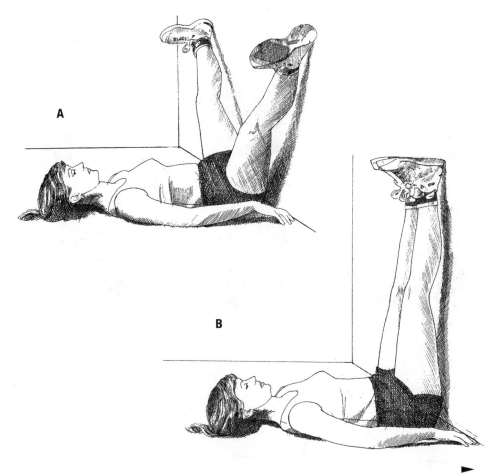

A

B

Leg Raise #3

Muscles toned
Shapes and firms the outer thighs (abductors).

What to do
A. Lie on your side. Bend your lower leg slightly, as shown.

B. Raise your top leg with a flexed foot straight up as high as you can. Keep the extended leg aligned with your hip, and your hips aligned vertically. Don't let the top hip lean forward. Hold for a count of two. Repeat. Do one set with one leg, then repeat with the other leg.

For added resistance, you can do this exercise using an ankle weight on the top leg. Begin with 1 pound. When you can easily do three complete sets, increase the weight.

In the gym
Use the hip abduction machine.

A

B

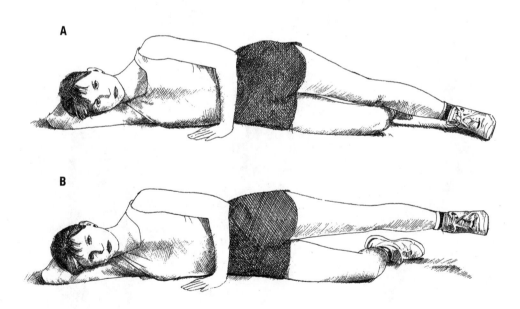

Triceps Extension

Muscles toned
Firms up the flabby back of the upper arms (triceps). Improves ability to extend your arm, to push yourself up out of a chair or off the floor.

What to do
A. Hold a lightweight dumbbell in one hand. Lie on your back with your arm straightened up toward the ceiling, as shown. Use your other hand to support your biceps just below your elbow with your fingertips facing the outside and your thumb inside.

B. Bend your arm back toward your ear, with your elbow pointing toward the ceiling, letting the dumbbell touch your ear or the floor. Hold for a count of two. Return to the starting position and repeat. After you complete your repetitions, repeat with the other arm.

In the gym
Use the triceps extension machine.

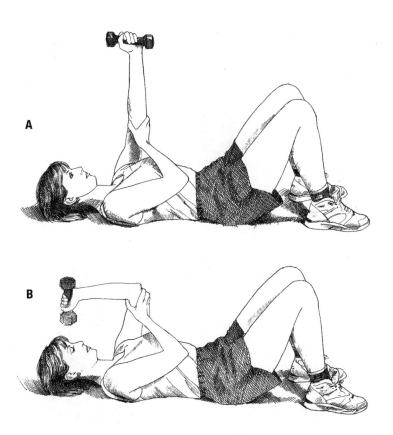

A

B

Bench Dip

Muscles toned
Firms the flabby back of upper arms (triceps).

What to do
A. Sit on the edge of a chair. Place your hands next to your buttocks with your fingers pointing forward. Extend your legs so your heels are resting on the floor and your legs are straight.

B. Slowly lower yourself off the chair, allowing your feet to slide and bringing your buttocks toward the floor. Try to keep your elbows straight back and not pointing out toward the sides. Once your upper arms are parallel with the floor, slowly push yourself back up. Repeat.

In the gym
Use the triceps extension machine.

A

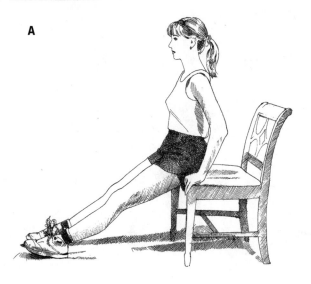

B

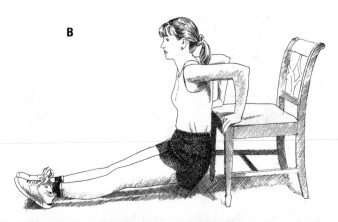

Move to Lose

You can also work your thighs, hips, and buttocks while performing other activities that are already a part of your aerobic program or daily activities, says Isaacs. Cycling, stair climbing, walking, and running all work the legs and buttocks. To work your lower body during some of your daily activities, try some of the following strategies.

Stroke it. If you choose swimming as your aerobic option, try squeezing your buttocks muscles as you do the breaststroke kick. Or, while wearing a pair of flippers and using a kickboard, concentrate on using your buttocks muscles to butterfly-kick you through the pool, suggests Isaacs.

Sprint for it. If you are in good enough shape to run, try sprinting for short distances for a great leg and butt workout. If you are out of shape, just walking uphill will give you a good workout, says Dr. Pollock.

Walk it. When walking or when climbing stairs, be conscious of what muscles you are using. Make an effort to squeeze your butt cheeks when doing such activities, says Isaacs.

Just squeeze it. When standing in line at the bank or when caught in a traffic jam, squeeze your butt cheeks together, suggests Mia Finnegan, a Fitness America Pageant National Champion and Miss Olympia Fitness, who with her husband operates a training service called Tru Fitness in Pasadena, California.

Hike at home. To work your thighs a little bit harder on stairs, take the stairs two steps at a time. To avoid losing your balance or tripping, hold on to the railing.

Dip at the sink. When standing at the kitchen sink or bathroom vanity, grasp the lip of the sink and do 5 to 10 squats. Your goal is to lower yourself until your backside is almost parallel with your knees. If you're unaccustomed to this maneuver, start gradually. You may be able to lower yourself only a few inches at first. You'll feel the effort in your quadriceps, the large muscles that run up the front of your thighs.

Extend and flex. When you're watching television, sit on the floor with your legs extended in front of you, resting your weight on your hands. Roll a bath towel or blanket under your knees. Hold the soles of your feet perpendicular to the floor, squeeze each thigh 10 times, and hold for a count of 10.

Volunteer to mow the lawn. If you don't customarily cut the grass and you have a push mower, you can also firm your thighs by pushing a lawn mower every week.

A Natural Breast Lift

After two childbirths, after breastfeeding, after more than three decades of gravity, Crystal Thompson, 37, of Fort Washington, Maryland, told her husband that she was saving money for a breast lift.

But instead of a consulting a surgeon, Crystal hired a personal trainer. She began lifting weights. And six months later she didn't need a breast lift after all. "Now, my husband looks at me and says I don't need to have the breast lift done—and I agree," she says.

A magic weight program for saggy breasts? Hardly. Crystal's personal trainer put her on an abbreviated total-body workout program, focusing on two exercises—the bench press and dumbbell flies. These exercises work the muscles supporting the breasts, not the breasts themselves, which are primarily fat and glands. Working the surrounding pectoralis muscles can help lift up the breast tissue, which is especially important for full-breasted women like Crystal.

But chest exercises can also help women with smaller bosoms improve the appearance of their breasts. When you diet to lose weight, the breasts lose fatty tissue, so they grow smaller. By building up the surrounding pectoralis muscles, you create the illusion of cleavage and fullness.

To do bench presses, see page 273. To do dumbbell flies, see page 274. Then try the following two exercises, designed by Michael Pollock, Ph.D., professor of medicine and exercise science at the University of Florida in Gainesville; Molly Foley, an exercise physiologist and director of ReQuest Physical Therapy in Gainesville; and Tereasa Flunker, an exercise physiologist also at ReQuest Physical Therapy.

Push-Up

Muscles toned
Builds up the chest (pectoralis major), helping to accentuate the breasts. The flabby back of the upper arms (triceps) gets hard. The shoulders (anterior deltoid) take on more shape.

What to do
A. Lie face down on the floor with your elbows bent and hands next to your chest.

B. Straighten your arms as you push your upper body up, as shown. Keep your knees on the floor and your back straight. Lower, then repeat.

In the gym
Use the chest press machine.

A

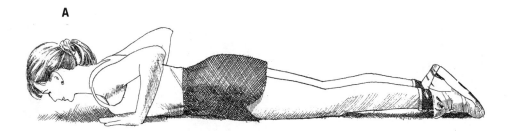

B

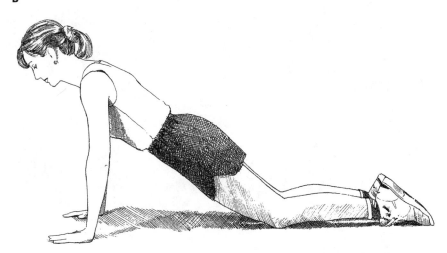

Dumbbell Raise

Muscles toned
Builds up the largest muscle in the chest (pectoralis major), helping to accentuate the breasts. The flabby back of the upper arms (triceps) gets hard. The shoulders (anterior deltoid) take on more shape.

What to do
A. If you have an adjustable bench, raise the back up to about a 75-degree angle. Or sit on a carpeted step and lean back until the step above supports your back. Hold a dumbbell in each hand, with your palms facing forward at shoulder height, as shown. Use weight light enough so that you can do a set of eight but heavy enough so that you can't squeeze out much more than 15.

B. Without arching your back, lift both dumbbells straight up, trying to keep them directly above your collarbones. Lower, then repeat.

In the gym
Use the bench press or chest press machine.

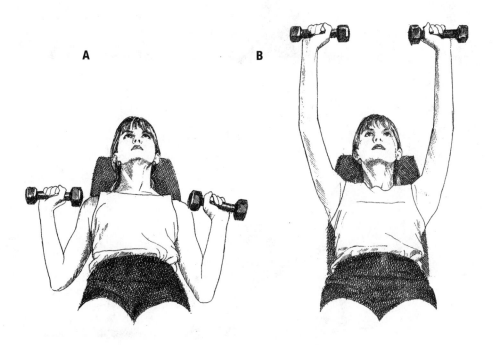

A   B

Chapter 21

You *Can* Flatten Your Tummy

For many women, a toned abdomen is the Holy Grail of body shaping. All the sit-ups in the world won't help. Here's what will.

Donna Michaels never used to worry about her abdomen.

The former bodybuilder from Miami expects to look in the mirror and see well-defined muscles etched into her midsection. But as she approaches her fifties, Michaels now sometimes looks down at her abdomen and notices a belly that she never thought she would have. Unlike apple-shaped women, who collect fat around their midsections, Michaels had always carried her weight on her hips and thighs—a classic pear shape. Until now, that is.

"Now that I'm older, my abdomen is betraying me," she says.

As a certified personal trainer, fitness director, and author of *Underneath It All: Either You Live It or You Diet,* Michaels knows what she needs to do: With every year, she'll have to work smarter (not harder) to keep her tummy flat. That's because she is nearing menopause, one of the most common belly bloaters.

"It's not impossible to control abdominal fat at my age. But it is a little more difficult," says Michaels. "I have to stay on top of it. I can't let abdominal exercise slide."

The Two Enemies of a Tight Tummy

Menopause can have a dramatic effect on the shape of a woman's body. Women who have fought off hip fat for most of their lives hit menopause and find a new foe, tummy fat.

Just when some of us get used to our pear shape, menopause turns us into apples. Researchers are not entirely sure why. But the drop in the female sex hormones that coincides with menopause may have something to do with the change in fat patterning, says Claude Bouchard, Ph.D., professor of exercise physiology at Laval University in Ste. Foy, Quebec.

Menopause isn't the only life event that bulges our bellies. Pregnancy also creates problems. As the baby grows inside the womb, the surrounding abdominal muscles stretch. And stretch. And stretch. Let's put a microscope on that problem.

Muscles consist of proteins that are woven together in the shape of a ladder. When the muscle is overstretched, the proteins that form the sides of the ladder move away from the proteins that form the steps. Imagine how a real ladder like that would be; well, a ladder of stretched-out protein is just as flimsy, says Diane Habash, Ph.D., nutrition research manager in the General Clinic Research Center at Ohio State University in Columbus.

And the protein loses not only its strength but also its elasticity, its rubber-band-like ability to expand and contract. A rickety ladder, a worn-out rubber band—not a pretty picture of your abdominal muscles after pregnancy. But, unfortunately, a true one. And it can get worse. You can have another baby. Or a cesarean section, which also weakens abdominal muscles by slicing them apart. And the result of all that abdominal stress is that those muscles have trouble performing even the most basic duty: holding your internal organs in place.

That's news that's hard to stomach. But it can be old news: "Abdominal exercises can get your abdomen as strong as before," says Dr. Habash.

The Three Areas You Can't Neglect

When you exercise your abdominal muscles, you make them tighter. The tighter they are, the more they hold in your stomach and other internal organs so that they don't protrude. "It's like putting on a tighter belt," explains Rudolph Leibel, M.D., associate professor at the laboratory of human behavior and metabolism at Rockefeller University in New York City.

But all the abdominal exercises in the world won't help you reduce a potbelly unless you combine them with fat-burning aerobic exercise and a calorie-zapping total-body strength-training program, according to Michael Pollock, Ph.D., professor of medicine and exercise science at the University of Florida in Gainesville. That's because a big middle is caused not only by sagging organs but also by the fat that surrounds them. Abdominal work will shape up your midsection as you're whittling away your fat.

And when it comes to the abdominal work in the Fat-to-Firm Program, *quality* counts more than *quantity.* To get a flat tummy, experts say you need to work three different areas: the upper rectus abdominis, the lower abdominals, and the obliques.

Plenty of women work the upper rectus abdominis, the portion of this muscle that runs from the belly button to the rib cage, says Mia Finnegan, a Fitness America Pageant National Champion and Miss Olympia Fitness, who with her husband operates a training service called Tru Fitness in Pasadena, California. But fewer women work the obliques, the muscles that travel diagonally along the sides of the torso. And even fewer women work the lower abdominal muscle that lies below the belly button. Yet the lower abdominal area is where most women notice a bulge, she notes.

How do you work those areas? Traditional crunches do little to work your obliques or the lower abdomen, which is why you may have failed at flattening your tummy even if you did as many as 200 sit-ups a day. To work your obliques, you need to modify a traditional crunch by adding a twist, or try other twisting movements. To work your lower abdominals, you can tilt your pelvis while raising and lowering your legs, according to Finnegan.

If you have back problems, consult your doctor before doing these. If you have back pain or discomfort while doing these, stop immediately and consult your doctor, advises Dr. Pollock.

Your Personal Belly-Busting Routine

The following program of abdominal exercises addresses all three areas. It was developed for the Fat-to-Firm Program by Dr. Pollock; Molly

(continued on page 312) ▶

Problem Solved

No More Abominable Abdominals

When it comes to New Year's resolutions, doing crunches is probably one of the most commonly ignored goals. Sure, come January 2 we get up and do a set of 40 before work. Maybe we do another set the next day. And if we're lucky, the next. Then we might only have time for 10. Then we tell ourselves that we'll do them at night. But by the time we remember, we're lying in bed, drifting off to dreamland. No crunches today.

Why do we hate crunches so much? Two problems, say trainers: boredom and neck pain. To combat both, here's what they suggest.

Stretch first. Before doing crunches, stretch your neck muscles by doing a few slow neck rolls, suggests Nancy C. Karabaic, a certified personal trainer in Wheaton, Maryland.

Lower your back. The correct crunch position involves keeping your back flat on the floor. Sounds easy. But few women do it correctly, says Diane Habash, Ph.D., nutrition research manager in the General Clinic Research Center at Ohio State University in Columbus who also studied exercise science. When you lie on the floor with your legs bent—the classic starting position for both crunches and the pelvic tilt—your lower back may arch slightly. Be sure to press your lower back to the floor so that there is no space between your back and the floor, she says. (In fact, holding this position for a few seconds provides a great lower abdominal workout even without lifting the head and shoulders.)

Women can start out just doing the pelvic tilt (shown on page 320) without a crunch until they get used to the position, says Dr. Habash. Also, once you add the crunch, continue to do the pelvic tilts alone a few times before crunching, she says.

Prop yourself. To support your lower back, rest your bent legs on a bench or chair, suggests Dr. Habash. Propping your legs up will encourage your lower back to drop to the floor into the pelvic tilt position.

Use your abs. Sounds like common sense. But many women do crunches by using their arms to jerk their heads off the floor. Instead, concentrate on contracting your abdominal muscles. You shouldn't use your arms, except for balance. As you contract your abdomen, your head will rise, says Karabaic.

Put your finger on it. To help concentrate on using your abdomen and not other body parts such as your arms and neck, occasionally rest a finger near your belly button when doing crunches. Make sure you feel that area contract, says Dr. Habash.

Star-gaze. As you crunch, pretend you are searching for the Big Dipper, says Donna Michaels, a certified personal trainer, fitness director, former bodybuilder from Miami, and author of *Underneath It All: Either You Live It or You Diet.* In other words, look up. Point your chin toward the ceiling instead of bringing it into your chest, she says.

Forget about height. Concentrate more on form than on lifting yourself as high as you can go. Initially, you may only have the strength to bring your shoulders an inch or two away from the floor. That's fine—you're still working your abs. If you bring your shoulders up higher but have to cheat to do it, you may end up straining your neck or back, says Michaels.

Slow down. Crunches are not a race. In fact, you'll get more benefit from doing them slowly and accurately than from doing them quickly and sloppily, says Dr. Habash. Quick, jerky movements are often what causes that pain in the neck.

Pause. After each crunch, pause before the next. That will give you a chance to check your form, preventing you from jerking your head first, says Karabaic.

Practice. Because many women hate doing abdominal work, they do it sporadically. Then they never really get the hang of it, and it always seems difficult. "You have to learn how to do ab work. And that means you have to practice," says Karabaic.

Don't count. One reason many women hate crunches is that they're boring. One way to combat boredom is to not count. Instead, crunch until your muscle fatigues and you just can't do another one. This signals that you have worked your abs enough to make them stronger, so it's more effective than counting, says Michaels.

Mix it up. To further prevent boredom, trainers suggest doing different kinds of crunches to add variety. So do one type of crunch one day, and another the next. Or do a few of one type, and a few of another within one set, says Michaels.

Foley, an exercise physiologist and director of ReQuest Physical Therapy in Gainesville, Florida; and Tereasa Flunker, an exercise physiologist also at ReQuest Physical Therapy. The program offers plenty of options, but make sure to follow the following guidelines.

Work the whole abdomen. Make sure to do at least one of each type of abdominal exercise—upper abdominals, obliques, and lower abdominals—to ensure that you work your entire abdomen. If you only focus on your upper or lower abdominals, you won't achieve your goal, says Dr. Pollock.

Go in sets. Because your body weight does not provide enough resistance to sufficiently fatigue your abdominal muscles, you'll probably need to do multiple sets. Start with one set of eight to 15 repetitions. When you're ready and feel comfortable doing so, move up to two or three sets of each exercise, says Dr. Pollock.

Contract slowly. To get the most benefit out of crunches, contract for a count of two and release for a count of four, says Dr. Pollock. Or, where indicated, hold the pose for as long as possible.

Do them either first or last. Crunches should be done along with the total-body exercises that make up the rest of the Fat-to-Firm Program. It doesn't really matter whether you do your abdominal work before or after your strength-training routine, just as long as you do it. If you find that you tend to avoid abdominal work, then doing the exercises before your strength training is probably better, according to Flunker. After a workout you'll be more tired and more inclined to skip your crunches, she says.

The Rectus Abdominis: Working the Upper Abs

Probably the most familiar part of your abdomen, the upper portion of the rectus abdominis runs along the front of your belly, going from your rib cage to your belly button. Working this area of your abdomen involves doing one of the most hated exercises, crunches. You simply can't avoid them. But take solace. You only need to do crunches to work this section of your abdomen. You don't have to do crunches to work the sides of your abdomen or the lower part of your abdomen below your belly button.

You can opt to do crunches in any of the ways illustrated here. All three variations will have the same effect on your abdominal muscles. The difference is personal preference. Pick the type of crunch that is most comfortable to you, says Flunker.

Crunch #1 for Upper Abs

A. Lie on your back with your knees bent, your feet flat on the floor, and your arms to your sides.

B. Extend your arms, reaching forward, and curl up toward your knees, as you pull your shoulders and head off the floor enough to touch your fingertips to your knees. Hold for 5 to 10 seconds. Then lower yourself and repeat. Keep your chin away from your chest as if holding a tennis ball under your chin.

A

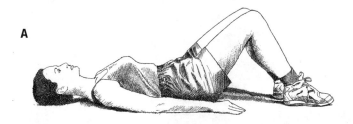

B

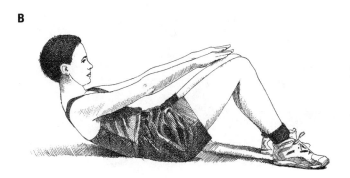

Crunch #2 for Upper Abs

A. Lie on your back with your knees bent and feet flat on the floor. Cross your arms on your chest.

B. Contract your abdomen as you curl up and raise your head and shoulders off the floor about halfway toward your knees. Keep your neck straight and chin pointing up, as shown.

A

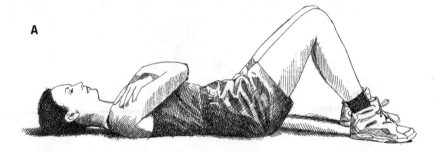

B

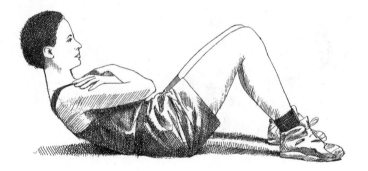

Crunch #3 for Upper Abs

A. Lie on your back with your knees bent and your feet flat on the floor. Put your hands behind your head. Your fingers should not touch. Instead, they should support your head just behind your ears. Your elbows should remain aligned with your fingers, out to the side, as shown.

B. Without yanking your head up with your hands, use your abdominals to lift your upper body. You should not be able to see your elbows in your peripheral vision. Hold for a few seconds. Then lower yourself and repeat. Be sure not to pull your neck forward.

A

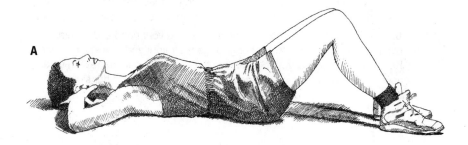

B

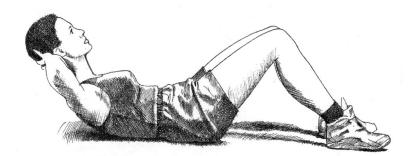

The Obliques: Creating a Natural Girdle

Strong oblique muscles act like a girdle along the sides of your body, cinching in your waist. Obliques also help stabilize the trunk during twisting movements like snow shoveling. The following exercises are all good workouts for the obliques. Pick the exercise that you find most comfortable.

Crunch #1 for Obliques

A. Lie on your back with your knees bent and your feet flat on the floor. Place your hands on your abdomen and rest your elbows on the floor by your sides.

B. Reach toward the ceiling with one arm, raising your head and shoulder blade off the floor, as shown. Keep your neck straight and look at the ceiling. Keep the other side of your body flat on the floor with your arm resting across your abdomen. Hold for a few seconds, then repeat on the other side.

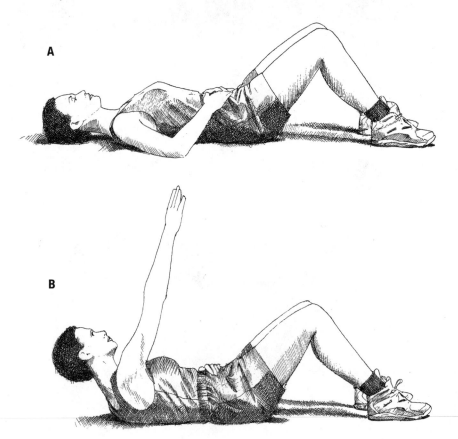

A

B

Crunch #2 for Obliques

A. Lie on your back with your knees bent and feet flat on the floor. Put your hands behind the lower part of your skull for support. Your fingers should not touch. Do not yank your head forward. Make sure to keep your elbows out to the side, as shown.

B. Curl upward about halfway toward your knee as you bring one elbow toward the opposite knee, as shown. Again, make sure to keep your elbows parallel with your ears. Also, don't pull yourself up with your hands. Hold for a few seconds, then lower yourself and repeat on the other side.

A

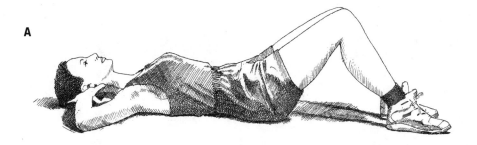

B

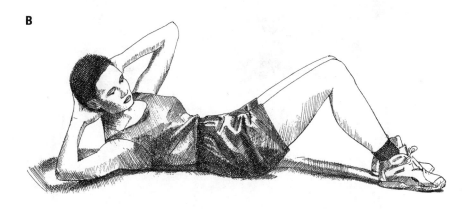

Crunch #3 for Obliques

A. Lie on your back with your knees bent, feet flat on the floor, and arms resting at your sides, as shown.

B. With your arms extended, reach toward one of your knees, curling your head and shoulders off the floor, as shown. Hold for a few seconds. Lower yourself. Then repeat on the other side.

A

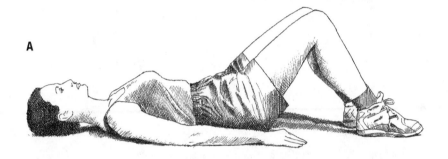

B

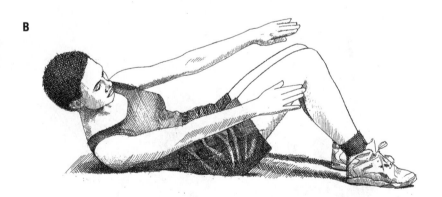

Beyond Crunches: The Stress-Diet Connection

Crunches are not the only answer to eliminating a potbelly. Sometimes other factors are at work. Claude Bouchard, Ph.D., professor of exercise physiology at Laval University in Ste. Foy, Quebec, has studied big bellies for years. And he says that there are two common problems that seem to contribute to abdominal fat: your diet and the way you respond to stress. Here is what you need to do to eliminate those problems.

Go low-fat. A high-fat diet seems to make people store fat in the abdomen, says Dr. Bouchard. Try to keep your fat intake to below 30 percent of your daily calorie intake. On an 1,800-calorie-a-day diet, that's 600 or fewer calories from fat, about the amount in 5 tablespoons of oil, butter, or hidden fats in baked goods and milk.

Calm down. When we respond negatively to stress, our bodies start producing a hormone called cortisol. Besides wreaking havoc on our arteries, stomach linings, and intestinal linings, this hormone also somehow coaxes the body into storing more fat in our abdomens. "Stress in general is not bad. You need stress to keep you alive," says Dr. Bouchard. "But when you have stress and you cannot cope, your cortisol levels are elevated." He has found that people who have elevated cortisol also tend to have more abdominal fat.

The Lower Abdominals: Your Greatest Challenge

Because we use them so rarely, the lower abdominals are usually the weakest area of our bodies. The lower abdominals also are the muscles that get stretched out so severely during pregnancy. Because they are so weak, beginners can probably get a good workout by simply drawing in the muscles and holding for a few seconds, says Flunker. A strong lower abdomen will not only help flatten your tummy, it will also help with posture and protect your lower back, she says.

The lower abdominal exercises for the Fat-to-Firm Program appear in order of increasing difficulty. Start with the first exercise—the pelvic tilt—which does not involve lifting your hips off the floor. Then progress at your own pace. All of the other exercises use the pelvic tilt in combination with other motions, says Dr. Pollock.

Crunch #1 for Lower Abs

A. Lie on your back with your knees bent and your feet flat on the floor. Cross your arms over your chest, as shown.

B. Squeeze your buttocks, tighten your abdomen, and push your lower back into the floor. Hold for 10 to 20 seconds, without holding your breath. Relax and release, then repeat.

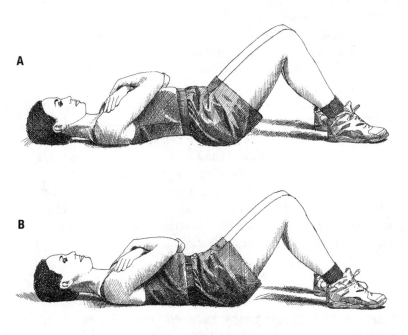

A

B

Crunch #2 for Lower Abs

A. Lie on your back with your legs straight, as shown. Press your lower back into the floor.

B. Raise one leg, bending at the knee, and raise your head and shoulder. Use the opposite arm to push against the thigh of the raised leg, as shown. The leg should resist the pushing motion of the hand. Hold for 10 to 20 seconds, and then repeat on the opposite side.

A

B

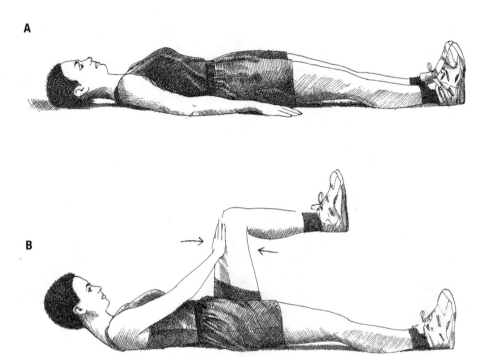

Crunch #3 for Lower Abs

A. Lie on your back with your legs straight and your back flat against the floor, as shown. Then bend both knees and put your feet flat on floor.

B. Raise both knees off the floor and toward your chest.

C. Slowly straighten one leg so that the knee is about 4 to 6 inches off the floor, keeping the other knee bent and your back flat. Don't allow the heel of either leg to touch the floor. Repeat on other side.

A

B

C

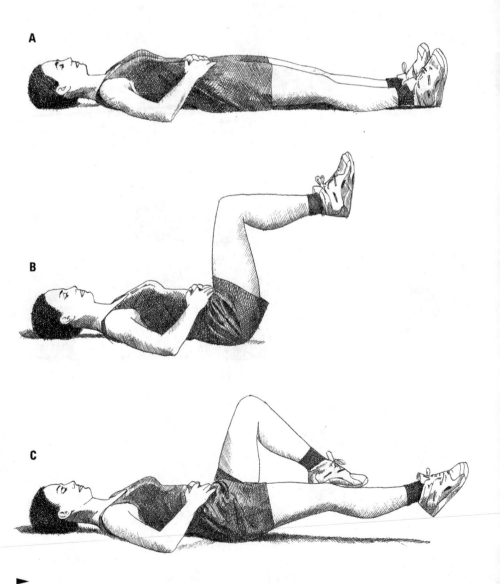

Crunch #4 for Lower Abs

A. Lie on your back with your knees bent. Reach your arms above your head and hold onto a stable object such as a heavy desk or bed frame.

B. Squeeze your abdomen as you raise your torso up, as shown. Keep your knees bent as in the starting position. Be sure to bring your knees toward the ceiling and not toward your chest. Hold for 10 to 20 seconds, without holding your breath. Lower, then repeat.

A

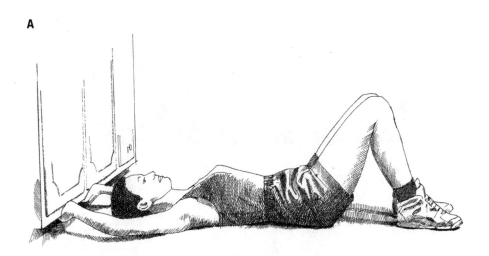

B

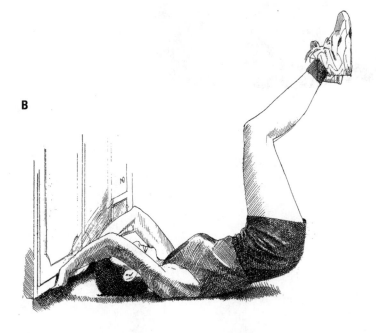

Crunch #5 for Lower Abs

A. Lie on your back with your knees bent and arms crossed over your chest, as shown.

B. While keeping your back flat and your knees bent, lift both legs off the floor so that your thighs are nearly perpendicular to the floor and your calves are almost parallel to the floor. Your feet should be flexed. Hold for 10 to 20 seconds, without holding your breath. Slowly lower your legs, then repeat.

A

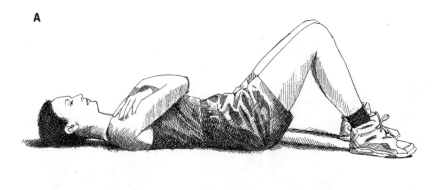

B

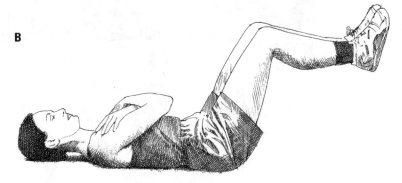

Crunch #6 for Lower Abs

A. Lie on your back with your legs straight in the air and your toes pointed, as shown. Your knees should be straight. Put your arms above your head and hold on to a stable object such as the bottom of a desk or couch.

B. Squeeze your abdomen as you raise your feet, hips, and pelvis toward the ceiling. Hold for 10 to 20 seconds, without holding your breath. Lower, then repeat.

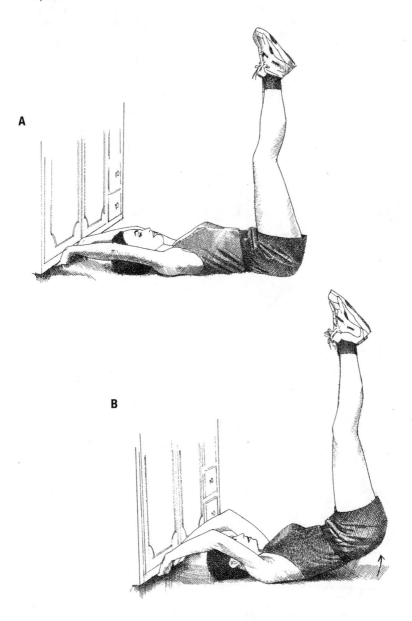

A

B

Crunch #7 for Lower Abs

A. Lie on your back with your knees bent and arms close to your sides, as shown. Tightening your buttocks and abdomen, hold your back in place against the floor, and relax your neck and shoulders.

B. Lift your arms and feet off the floor, as shown. Your legs should be bent, with your knees aligned with your buttocks, at a 90-degree angle to the floor. Your arms should be elevated off the floor with your hands at the level of your mid-thigh. Slowly extend one arm overhead as you extend and straighten the leg on the same side. Then switch, and repeat. This can be difficult. If you have pain, stop immediately. If you have a back problem, consult a doctor before doing this exercise.

A

B

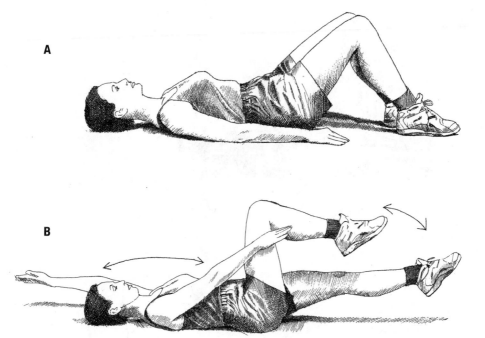

Chapter 22

50 Easy Ways to Burn 150 Calories

You don't have to go to the gym to burn calories. Here's how to exercise without exercising.

Welcome to the land where garage doors open at the push of a button, where bread is kneaded and baked by machines, where conveyor belts transport you through airports, where automatic-teller machines let you bank without ever leaving your car, where most of the lawn mowers have seats, and where walking to work, to school, or to the store seems as quaint as taking a carriage.

Welcome to the land where sitting is the national hobby. Where intentionally burning an extra calorie seems almost as shocking as arson.

Welcome to the land of...weight gain.

"People are getting more obese," says Mildred Cody, R.D., Ph.D., associate professor of nutrition and dietetics at Georgia State University in Atlanta. "All of these labor-saving devices are making people more sedentary. We're not walking as much as we used to. We're not taking the stairs. All of those things really add up."

When Dr. Cody says "add up," she's not talking about a dozen unburned calories a day. According to a study from the United Kingdom, people in that country are burning about *800 calories less per day* than

Problem Solved

Exercising in Tight Quarters

Say you are flying out of New York City tomorrow for Paris. You'll be stuck on a plane for hours. Then you'll get on the metro, then in a taxi.

Sounds like lot of time sitting, burning the average 1 to 2 calories a minute, doesn't it?

Well, you may be stuck in a seat. But that doesn't mean that you can't exercise. You can work almost every major muscle group in your body without getting out of your seat by doing isometrics, says Robert Lavetta, a fitness trainer in Palm Desert, California, who works with Lorenzo Lamas and owns Healthy Lifestyles, a nutrition, fitness, and stress-reduction counseling service. Isometrics involves pushing against static resistance. For a total-body isometric workout that you can do in an airplane, on a bus, or in a subway, here's what Lavetta often recommends to his busy celebrity clients.

1. Put your hands together as if you were going to clap. Your elbows should be out, parallel to the floor. Your fingers should be facing away from your sternum. The heels of your hands and backs of your wrists should rest against your chest. Squeeze your hands together while breathing out. Hold until you finish exhaling and then release. You should feel as though you just worked your chest.

2. Put your hands together as if you were in a praying position. Your fingers should be pointed up and your elbows out, parallel to the

---

they did in 1970, mostly because of automation and labor-saving devices. Those of us in the United States are probably burning even fewer calories, since we outpace the United Kingdom in car ownership, television watching, and drive-through restaurants, says the author of the study, WPT James, director of the Rowett Research Institute, a nutrition and biological sciences research center in Aberdeen, Scotland.

Change Your Ideas about Exercise

Why, when so many of us want so desperately to lose weight—or at least stop the yearly addition of another couple of pounds—do we ig-

floor in a straight line with your wrists. Use your right hand to push against your left hand. Keep your left hand stable. Breathe out as you push. Once you have exhaled, stop pushing, take a breath and then do the same movement pushing against your right hand. You should feel as if you worked your shoulders and chest.

3. Put your palms against the top of your outer thighs. Apply firm pressure and exhale as you slide your hands toward your knees. As you return your hands to their original position, relax and inhale. Concentrate on flexing the back of your arms to work the triceps as much as possible.

4. Put both hands underneath your right knee. As you exhale, use your hands to pull your right thigh and knee toward your chest. Your right leg should act as dead weight. Make sure to use your arm muscles and not your leg. You should feel as though you just worked your biceps.

5. Sit with your knees together and place your hands on either side of them. Exhale and push your legs against your hands to work the outer thigh and shoulder muscles. You can easily reverse this exercise to work the inner thigh. Just put your hands between your knees to provide some resistance and squeeze your legs together as you exhale.

nore perhaps the easiest way to stay trim: the calorie-burning power of everyday activities?

A team of government researchers in the United States may have found the answer. When they talked with people who were sporadically active to learn why they were not regularly active, the researchers were surprised to learn those folks simply didn't know that everyday activities burned lots of calories. "For the men and women interviewed, the word *exercise* meant going to the gym or doing some activities that were uncomfortable and made them sweat," says Elizabeth Howze, Sc.D., associate director for health promotion in the division of nutrition and physical activity in the National Center for Chronic Disease Prevention and Health Promotion at the Centers for Disease Control and Prevention in Atlanta.

But when researchers used the words *physical activity* and explained that that included activities like mowing the lawn, vacuuming, raking leaves, and mopping the floor, these same people were much more receptive to the notion of being active for ½ hour on most days of the week, says Dr. Howze.

So, says Dr. Howze, instead of thinking of exercise as pain and sweat, think of it as your body in motion—any kind of motion. Or to put it another way: The more often you move your arms or legs, the more calories you burn. The more you sit or lie still, the fewer calories you burn.

"Consider any activity exercise, whether it is climbing stairs, gardening, or carrying groceries," says Frank Butterfield, a certified fitness trainer in Las Vegas and chairperson of the professional development committee for the American Council on Exercise. "As long as what you are doing is more than what you were doing before, you'll benefit. Sitting up is better than lying down, standing is better than sitting up, walking is better than standing."

The 30-Minute Miracle

As mentioned in other parts of the Fat-to-Firm Program, people are more likely to be successful in reaching and maintaining their optimum weight if they combine a healthy diet with regular physical activity. And not only that, they will feel better and reduce the risk of dying prematurely. You should stay in motion long enough to burn at least an extra 150 calories on most days, says Adele L. Franks, M.D., assistant director for science with the National Center for Chronic Disease Prevention and Health Promotion at the Centers for Disease Control and Prevention and scientific editor for the 1996 Surgeon General's report on physical activity.

Most moderate physical activities—dancing, walking briskly from room to room, and raking leaves—will burn 150 calories in about ½ hour. So instead of counting calories, you can count minutes, aiming for at least 30 minutes of motion a day, says Dr. Howze.

If you can't get it in all at once, consider amassing your 30 minutes in small chunks of time rather than doing it all in one shot, says Dr. Howze. "Research suggests that women who are trying to lose weight by increasing their activity are more likely to do so when they break up their activities. Think about exercise as something that can be done over the course of the day and that does not require extra time. It's sort of like putting money in the bank. You get in 10 minutes here and 5 minutes there, and 10 minutes at another time. Your time adds up."

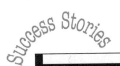

Everyday Activity Can Help Burn Calories

Here are some smart methods women just like you use to put more activity into their days.

Lori Kaminski, 37, of Avonmore, Pennsylvania: She made walking an integral part of every day. At every chance she can find, Lori walks. For instance, she walks to the neighbor's instead of driving, and she parks in the space farthest from the supermarket door instead of the one closest.

Veronica Canfield, 31, of San Antonio: She runs with a skip when answering the phone, going from one room to another, going from the car to the house, crossing the street, and at any other time the opportunity presents itself. When at school, teaching, Veronica walks extra fast down the halls—so fast that other teachers call her the blur. She uses a cordless phone so that she can walk while she talks.

Kathie Chew, 50, of San Jose, California: She offers to deliver and pick up items at work so that she can walk from one place to another in the large Stanford-area hospital where she works as an administrative assistant. Instead of phoning her co-workers, Kathie walks to their desks. During nice weather, she walks the perimeter of her office building at lunchtime.

Lynn Oatman, 46, of Liverpool, New York: She climbs the stairs to her second-floor apartment.

Donna J. Kinoshita, 48, of Lafayette, Colorado: Donna gave up driving a car and walks everywhere, including trips to and from the supermarket. At the same time, she started drinking more water, which she buys at the supermarket and has to carry home. So she burns even more calories.

For instance, during the next few days, clock yourself every time you climb a flight of stairs, walk, clean, garden, or do any other activity that involves putting your body in motion. Then, at the end of the day, add up your active time. You'll probably find yourself looking for ways to add 5 minutes of activity here and there. Suddenly, exercise will seem easy and enjoyable, says Dr. Howze.

How does increasing your activity in small chunks throughout the day fit in with your aerobic exercise program? That depends on you. You have your choice of two methods.

- The lifestyle activity method. You can rely solely on adding moderate activity throughout the day. Depending on the intensity of effort over 30 minutes, at least five days of the week, you could burn the same amount of calories (or more) as you would by walking, jogging, swimming, or cycling for 30 continuous minutes, three days a week, says Dr. Franks.

- The mix-and-match method. You can mix your aerobic workouts with your daily activity. For instance, one or two days a week, work out for 30 minutes by walking, swimming, or cycling. Then, on the other days, amass your 30 minutes of activity by raking leaves, vacuuming, or washing windows, says Dr. Howze.

The best method is the one you'll actually do, says Dr. Howze. Whichever method you choose, just remember that 30 minutes is the minimum. As physical activity becomes a bigger part of your routine, you'll probably want to increase your duration or intensity to become healthier and lose more weight, says Dr. Franks.

"The more you do, the better off you are," says Dr. Franks. "Thirty minutes of moderate activity, five times a week is a guide. You can achieve measurable health benefits by exercising moderately for 30 minutes, five days a week. But you can get an even greater benefit if you increase the time or the intensity."

Take Your Pick

Thirty minutes is only a rough estimate of how much motion you need to burn 150 calories (and then only if you weigh 150 pounds). An activity like snow shoveling, for example, burns calories more quickly than an activity like window washing: 15 minutes of snow shoveling burns the same amount of calories as an hour of window washing.

To ensure that you burn your 150 calories, take your pick from these 50 activities.

- Ironing clothes for 68 minutes
- Shooting pool for 58 minutes

- Canoeing leisurely for 50 minutes
- Cooking for 48 minutes
- Wallpapering for 45 minutes
- Washing and waxing a car for 45 to 60 minutes
- Washing windows or floors for 45 to 60 minutes
- Playing volleyball for 45 minutes
- Ballroom dancing for 43 minutes
- Stocking shelves for 40 minutes
- Playing croquet for 38 minutes
- Cleaning blinds, closets, and shelves for 36 minutes
- Fishing for 36 minutes
- Mopping floors for 36 minutes
- Grocery shopping for 36 minutes
- Walking 1¾ miles at a moderate pace in 35 minutes
- Dusting for 34 minutes
- Vacuuming for 34 minutes
- Playing horseshoes for 33 minutes
- Playing table tennis for 33 minutes
- Gardening for 30 to 45 minutes
- Wheeling yourself in a wheelchair for 30 to 45 minutes
- Shooting baskets for 30 minutes
- Bicycling leisurely 5 miles in 30 minutes
- Dancing fast for 30 minutes
- Doing a country line dance for 30 minutes
- Pushing a stroller 1½ miles in 30 minutes
- Raking leaves for 30 minutes
- Walking briskly 2 miles in 30 minutes
- Mowing the lawn with a power push mower for 29 minutes
- Snowmobiling for 29 minutes
- Golfing on foot (no cart) for 26 minutes
- In-line skating leisurely for 26 minutes
- Stacking firewood for 25 minutes
- Snorkeling for 24 minutes
- Bowling for 23 minutes
- Playing leisurely badminton for 22 minutes

- Playing Frisbee for 22 minutes
- Scrubbing floors for 20 minutes
- Sawing wood by hand for 18 minutes
- Grooming a horse for 17 minutes
- Backpacking with an 11-pound load for 17 minutes
- Riding a motorcycle for 16 minutes
- Forking hay for 16 minutes
- Twirling a baton for 16 minutes
- Bicycling fast 4 miles in 15 minutes
- Shoveling snow for 15 minutes
- Climbing stairs for 15 minutes
- Doing the twist for 13 minutes
- Snowshoeing in soft snow for 13 minutes

The Fidgeting Factor

The average woman will burn 1 to 2 calories a minute while sitting. Veronica Canfield, 31, of San Antonio, however, is not your average woman. As she sits in front of her home computer, she burns more calories than the average sitting woman by shaking her legs, squirming in her seat, tapping her feet, and twirling a pencil between her fingers. She fidgets. By doing so, Veronica burns somewhere between 110 and 620 more calories a day than she would if she sat still, according to one study that measured that calorie-burning potential of fidgeting.

Fidgeting is just one small way to work activity into your inactivity. You have probably already heard about a few other methods, like parking farther away from your destination or opting for stairs instead of elevators and escalators. But those tips just scratch the surface of possible ways to make extra calorie-burning part of your day, experts say. Here are 30 more from weight-loss specialists and fitness trainers.

Become an inefficiency expert. When it comes to going somewhere or getting something done, try to be as inefficient as possible. Chances are, you'll burn more calories, says Vicki Pierson, a certified fitness trainer and weight-management consultant in Chattanooga, Tennessee. For instance, instead of using a big sponge to wipe up a mess, use a smaller one. Instead of using a mop, get down on your hands and knees and scrub that floor. When cleaning windows, get rid of the labor-saving squeegee and use a rag instead. "We are all so busy with our schedules that the last thing we think about is being inefficient," she says. "Ironically, when it comes to our bodies and keeping them healthy, inefficiency in our movements may actually benefit us."

Tote more groceries. Instead of trying to lug every single grocery bag into the house in one trip, make multiple trips by carrying one bag at a time, says Kathy Mangan, a certified lifestyle and weight-management consultant and a certified personal trainer at the Women's Club, an all-women's health and fitness facility in Missoula, Montana.

Clean to be lean. When cleaning the house, use large, exaggerated movements, says Pierson. For instance, when cleaning windows, use big arm circles. And when vacuuming, use long, slow rhythmic movements. Switch arms to work both sides of your body equally.

Boycott the car wash. Instead of taking your car to a drive-through car wash, get out the soap and hose and do it yourself, says Mangan.

Kid around. Instead of popping in a video, play actively with your children or grandchildren. Play catch, jump rope, climb on the monkey bars, push them on a swing, or run foot races, suggests Pierson. "Most anything a child enjoys will give you a good aerobic workout."

Say good morning to your body. Before getting out of bed in the morning, kick down the covers and raise your arms as if you were reaching for the sun. Take a breath and drop your arms forward on the bed toward your legs. Repeat three or four times to get your heart beating slightly faster. Then get out of bed, says Robert Lavetta, a fitness trainer in Palm Desert, California, who owns a nutrition, fitness, and stress-reduction counseling service called Healthy Lifestyles.

Walk a long distance. When answering the phone, scurry to the one that is farthest away from you instead of the one that's closest, says Pierson.

Don't use the parking lot. To work more walking into your day, park ½ mile away from work, suggests Dr. Cody. "I know everybody wants to park their car right next to the door. But parking farther away is such a small behavior change, and it has tremendous, positive results."

Rediscover the stairs. Whenever possible, take the stairs instead of the elevator or escalator, says Mia Finnegan, a Fitness America Pageant National Champion and Miss Olympia Fitness, who with her husband operates a training service called Tru Fitness in Pasadena, California. If you work on the 108th floor and couldn't possibly walk up that many steps, take the first few flights and then ride the elevator, she says.

You can add a few more flights to your workout each day. When walking stairs, walk them as quickly as you can. Or for variety, take two steps at a time, says Pierson.

Leave the cart in the store. When at the supermarket, carry your groceries to the car instead of using a cart, says Pierson.

Lunge for breakfast. As you walk through your kitchen to put toast in the toaster, fix some cereal, or grab some orange juice, do lunges. Every time you reach for something, lunge instead of simply walking over to it. This will give your legs an early-morning workout, says Lavetta.

Take exercise breaks. During breaks at work, walk the stairs or walk around the building instead of reading the paper or visiting the water cooler, says Pierson.

Earn your inactivity. Think of inactivity as something you have to earn, suggests Dr. Cody. For instance, if you enjoy reading, don't allow yourself to read your book until after you've walked.

Take a "longcut." Whenever walking somewhere, take the long route, whether you are on your way to the mailroom or to the corner store, says Pierson.

Hike to the ladies room. Start using a bathroom on a different floor than the one on which you work, or at least one that is farther away from your office, says Mangan.

Make dancing dates. Go out with your partner once or twice a month to a dance club, says Pierson, or take dance lessons.

Curl your drink. Whenever you grab a gallon plastic jug from your refrigerator, make it your habit to do a biceps curl with it a few times before opening it and pouring yourself a drink, says Lavetta.

Go in circles. While at work, get up every so often and walk two circles around your desk, says Finnegan.

Give up sunbathing. When at the beach, stay active by swimming, wave surfing, renting a rowboat or paddleboat, or playing paddleball, says Pierson.

Do the lunch-box lift. If you make your child's lunch, assemble the food and Thermos in the lunch box, close it, and then French-press the box behind your head for a triceps workout, pictured on page 281, suggests Lavetta. After some time, when the lunch box feels too light, try French-pressing a 5-pound bag of potatoes.

Get back to basics. If you have a riding mower, switch to a push mower. If you have a power push mower, switch to a manual, says Pierson.

Be a Ms. Fix-It. Whenever possible, take on home-improvement projects—such as painting and wallpapering—yourself. You will not only get a workout but also save money, says Pierson.

Have a motorized locker room. Designate an area in your car as the "locker room." Keep a pair of sneakers, clean socks, a clean towel, a Frisbee, some tennis rackets, a basketball, or any other items that you think you might use. Then the next time you are out and about with a little extra time, stop at a park and shoot some hoops, take a jog, hit a tennis ball against a wall, or do some other activity, says Pierson.

Be your own squeeze. When driving, standing in line at the deli counter, or waiting at the doctor's office, tighten your butt cheeks, thighs, and abdominals to give your muscles a workout, says Finnegan.

Give yourself a raise. While washing dishes, do toe raises to work your calves, says Tereasa Flunker, an exercise physiologist at ReQuest Physical Therapy in Gainesville, Florida.

Squat, don't bend. When getting clothing out of the dryer, instead of bending over, do a squat to work your leg and butt muscles. Do the same when picking things up from the floor, says Flunker.

Play this game. Take 5 minutes here and there throughout the day and play a game with yourself: You can do anything except sit or lie down, says Peggy Norwood, an exercise physiologist, president of Avalon Fitness, and former fitness director of the Duke University Diet and Fitness Center, both in Durham, North Carolina.

Lose control. When you don't have a remote control, you have to get up and walk to the television to change the channel. You also may watch less television, in general, says Norwood.

Get down. When in the house, put on some of your favorite tunes and dance. Dance while you are doing other activities. Dance while walking from the table to the sink. Dance while picking things up off the floor, says Hy Levasseur, an exercise physiologist and director of health education and fitness at the U.S. Department of Transportation in Washington, D.C.

Do television waist-whittlers. While watching television or doing any other activity that involves sitting, you can still work the muscles along your waist, says Norwood. To do them, place one hand on your opposite knee and lift that leg 6 to 8 inches off the floor. Flex your stomach muscles and you gently apply counterpressure with your hand, allowing your elbow to bend slightly.

Chapter 23

Customizing Your Fat-to-Firm Exercise Program

**Become your own personal trainer.
Design the program that works for you.
There's one right way to exercise: *your* way.**

A dress that makes every woman look beautiful. A job suited to every woman's career. An eye shadow that's right for every woman's eyes. A man every woman can fall in love with.

All these things make the same amount of sense: none. The same goes for an exercise program that's right for every woman who wants to get fit.

"Unfortunately, there is no magic formula," says Vicki Pierson, a certified fitness trainer and weight-management consultant in Chattanooga, Tennessee. "No one exercise works for everybody."

If you want exercise to work for you, if you want to lose weight, firm up, feel great, and enjoy reaching those goals, you must customize your exercise program, say experts. You need to think about your personality—whether you're a morning person or a night owl, a loner or an extrovert. You need to think about your body type—big-boned or small, delicate or hardy. You need to think about your past—what activities you've tried and hated, what you've tried and liked. And, taking all those factors into account, you need to create an exercise program that's right for you. And, finally, you need to remember that if you quit exercising in the past, you were not a failure. No, the workout failed you.

The Fat-to-Firm Program offers a broad range of exercise options—aerobics, everyday activities, strength training, stretching—so that you can design your fitness program to meet your needs. This chapter takes you step-by-step through the design process. So read on—and get ready for fitness that is actually fun.

Make a Plan

You wouldn't go on a trip without a map or build a house without a blueprint. So why would you start something as important as an exercise program without a plan?

Before making any big change—whether you're beginning an exercise program or giving up smoking—you need a game plan, says Elizabeth Howze, Sc.D., associate director for health promotion in the division of nutrition and physical activity in the National Center for Chronic Disease Prevention and Health Promotion at the Centers for Disease Control and Prevention in Atlanta.

And the first step in that plan, says Dr. Howze, is to make a list of problems and how you intend to face them. Your list could include these (and many other) questions.

- What will I do if it rains or snows?
- How can I balance my exercise with my family life?
- What will I do with my children when I exercise?
- What activities can I do with my family so that we can all become more active?
- What will I do during fall and winter when it gets dark early?
- What will I do if I keep forgetting to exercise?

"It's important for anyone who is thinking about becoming active to plan for difficulties rather than just relying on willpower," says Dr. Howze. "People who make changes are more successful if they first plan for how they are going to deal with difficulties."

Your solutions to these problems may be entirely different from someone else's. So brainstorm for the solutions that work best for you, she says.

For Kathie Chew, of San Jose, California, her "problem" was her 6-year-old daughter—what to do with her while she exercised. Kathie knew that she couldn't count on her husband to babysit every time she exercised. So she decided against walking, biking, or in-line skating because she knew her daughter wouldn't be able to keep up. Plus, she couldn't do those activities in bad weather. She decided against a stationary bike because she had tried one at the gym and hated it. So she tried a cross-country ski machine. She didn't have to worry about the weather. She didn't have to worry about her daughter, who played in the house while she worked out. And Kathie lost 35 pounds.

Figure Out What You *Don't* Want to Do

The next step in designing your fitness program is to examine your past and pinpoint your exercise likes and dislikes, says Kathy Mangan, a certified lifestyle and weight-management consultant and a certified personal trainer at the Women's Club, an all-women's health and fitness facility in Missoula, Montana. What a lot of women don't like about exercise is...exercise. "Some women hate exercise," she says. "They don't want to sweat, and they don't want to get hot. Exercise feels foreign to them. It's uncomfortable."

If you're in this category, don't feel as though you've failed before you've started. Mangan and other experts say that there are ways to design an exercise program that even a confirmed exercise-hater will love. Here's how.

Don't try anything new. A crucial element of an exercise-hater's program is familiarity, says Mangan. You want to try exercises that you already know how to do. Most often, walking will be part of the plan, she says. But think about all the aerobic activities you have tried. Ask yourself, "Which was comfortable?"

Avoid post-traumatic gym syndrome. Many women have bad memories of that dreaded day in gym glass when...you were forced to run a mile in under 10 minutes...you were the last girl to get picked for softball...Freddy Kurtz threw a dodgeball into your face while everyone else giggled...you desperately tried to climb the rope but only progressed 1 inch.

If you know from experience that a particular exercise isn't for you, if running, for instance, seemed like torture or team sports embarrassed you, cross it off as one of your aerobic options, at least at the beginning,

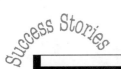

How She Did It

Here's how one women customized her exercise program to fit her personal needs.

Lynn Oatman, 46, of Liverpool, New York: "I joined a commercial gym where the staff there suggested that I begin with 5 minutes each on the treadmill, rowing machine, and StairMaster. After about a week, I incorporated a weight program in with my aerobic exercise. I worked out three times a week, gradually increasing my aerobic time. After a while, however, I found that I dreaded my workouts. I was bored. So I added more variety. Now, on Mondays I do 15 minutes on the leg curl and leg extension machines, 10 minutes on the treadmill, and 10 minutes on the rowing machine as well as weights. On Tuesdays, I do 10 minutes on the ski machine, 15 minutes on the arm machines, 10 minutes on the treadmill, and then my abdominal workout and leg lifts. On Fridays I do 20 minutes on the leg machines, 5 minutes on the ski machine, and 5 minutes on the cross-aerobic machine and weights. In one year, I lost 30 pounds."

says Mangan. You can always try it again later as you gain experience and confidence.

Be patient. While your list of hated exercises may fill a page, don't despair. Experts interviewed for this book say that they've never met a woman who couldn't find at least one activity she enjoyed. You will find an exercise you like—though you may need to experiment to find out what it is.

Make it a chore. Well, make it part of your chores. If you don't like the idea of a formal bout of exercise, try a new approach. Make your daily activities your exercise, says Dr. Howze. Be aware of the amount of time you walk up the stairs, wash your car, vacuum—anything active that you do during the day. And then make sure that you do those types of activities for a total of at least 30 minutes a day. That type of "exercise" can be just as effective at providing health benefits as 30 minutes of walking, swimming, or other aerobic activities, she says. (For more on using everyday activity as exercise, see chapter 22.)

Don't push yourself. "If you go to a gym and it seems as though they are pushing you too hard, they are," says Robert Lavetta, a fitness trainer in Palm Desert, California, and owner of Healthy Lifestyles, a nu-

Baby on Board

Choosing an exercise program for when you're pregnant requires a special set of guidelines. First, of course, consult your obstetrician. Then, follow this advice from Douglass Hall, M.D., of Ocala, Florida, who founded Pregnagym, a group of gyms throughout the country that help women to prepare their bodies for pregnancy and labor.

Stay off your back. Abdominal exercises help you get in shape for the pushing and bearing down during labor. And keeping your abdomen in shape during pregnancy will speed up the time it takes to trim your tummy after your delivery. But, after the fifth month of pregnancy, you shouldn't do any abdominal work that involves lying on your back—your larger uterus could compress the main blood vessel that runs from your trunk to your heart. (That compression can cause a pregnant woman to pass out when she lies on her back.)

Instead, Dr. Hall suggests doing the following two abdominal exercises.

For the oblique abdominal muscles, which run along the sides of your body, sit on a stool and place a broomstick or long barbell behind your neck and across your shoulders. Use your hands to hold the bar as your twist from one side to the other, keeping your lap and face pointed forward.

For the rest of your abdomen, stand with your back 3 inches away from a wall, with your feet shoulder-width apart and your knees slightly bent. Contract your abdominal muscles as you push your back into the wall. Hold the muscles tight for 4 seconds, then release and repeat. (Or use a Nautilus or Cybex abdominal machine at the gym that allows you to do a crunch while sitting up.)

Stay off your feet. After the fifth month of pregnancy, you should avoid any upright aerobic activity. Standing activities such as jogging and floor aerobics will pull your pelvis forward, which will lengthen and weaken your abdominal and hamstring muscles, causing lower back pain. Instead, try aerobic activities such as swimming, cycling, or other sitting exercise options like upright rowing

trition, fitness, and stress-reduction counseling service. "Exercise should produce positive physical and emotional fitness."

One way to make sure that you don't overdo is to breathe through your nose while exercising, says John Douillard, D.C., a chiropractor and

machines designed to pull your arms toward you while pushing your legs forward. The best known of these is the HealthRider.

Stretch and strengthen. As your uterus and breasts grow, some muscles will get weaker, others will get tighter. Larger breasts can pull your shoulders forward, tightening your chest, shoulders, and some back muscles. And as your uterus grows, your lower back muscles, quadriceps, and inner thigh muscles will also tighten. So you want to pay special attention to those areas when stretching.

- For your chest, put your palms on the edges of a door frame and lean your body forward.
- For the shoulders, pull your right arm across your chest. Use your left hand to push your right arm closer to your chest while pulling it to the left. Then repeat on the other side.
- For the lower back, sit on the floor with your legs forward and knees bent slightly. Try to lower your chest so that you hug your legs while rounding your back.
- For the quadriceps, stand facing a wall with one hand on the wall for support. Bend the leg opposite that hand back toward your buttocks. Hold the front of that foot with your free hand and, while keeping your thighs aligned, try to make your foot touch your buttocks. Repeat on the other side.
- For your inner thighs, sit on the floor with the bottom of your feet touching, in the chicken-wing position. Try to push your knees to the floor.

At the same time, your trapezius muscles in your neck and shoulders get weakened. You can strengthen that area by using a rowing machine or by doing a rowing motion with weights, like the upright row on page 276. Your hamstring muscles will also weaken. Target your hamstrings with the leg lift pictured on page 293 or by using a Nautilus machine that allows you to do leg curls while lying on your side.

certified fitness trainer, who is president of the Life Spa Clinic in Boulder, Colorado, and author of *Body, Mind, and Sport*. At first, he says, you may find it a little bit hard to breathe. But after a few weeks you should be able to breathe effortlessly through your nose. This type of breathing guarantees that you will exercise in a relaxed state. "Once you lose the feeling of calm and comfort, you are doing too much," he says. "If you drive yourself to exhaustion, you will not like your workouts, you will not do them for a long time, and when you stop, the fat will come back."

But to reap the full health and weight-loss benefits of exercise, Dr. Douillard says that you should push your pace slightly—your intensity should be right at the level where you feel as though you might have to breathe through your mouth.

Gung-Ho or Ho-Hum: Determine Your Motivational Profile

Mangan divides women exercisers into two motivational types. The "gung-ho" type is full of energy and optimism; she can't wait to get started and see results. The "ho-hum" type thinks she has seen it all before; she'll try exercise (again) but doesn't have much faith that it will make a difference in her life. Mangan says you need to customize your approach to your type.

Gung-ho seeks balance. The gung-ho exerciser tends to pick a high-impact exercise like running—and then runs herself into the ground. Mangan says to balance high-impact exercises with joint-gentle activities like bicycling and swimming. For example, if you want to exercise five days a week—typical of a gung-ho—run two of them and swim three of them, she says.

The ho-hum needs challenge. The ho-hum person needs to find fun, new ways to challenge herself, says Mangan. But first, pick an activity you don't mind doing, like walking. Then do something a little different: Walk up a big hill. Walk faster for a block. And try to do a more difficult activity once a week, like stair climbing or working out on a cross-country skiing machine. "Take what you are comfortable doing, and do a little more," says Frank Butterfield, a certified fitness trainer in Las Vegas and chairperson of the professional development committee for the American Council on Exercise.

Match Your Exercise to Your Body Type

The ancient medical science of India—Ayurveda—categorizes all human beings into three body types: vata, pitta, and kapha. Dr. Douillard believes that discovering your type—and then picking the right exercise for your body type—is crucial for an enjoyable exercise program. To determine your body type, fill out the worksheet on page 346 designed by Dr. Douillard.

Vata. If you circled column one most often, you are the hypermetabolic vata body type. You have a small-boned, naturally lean physique. You are fast, but have little endurance. You will excel in exercise activities that require brief bursts of speed and agility such as racquetball, sprinting, aerobics, and dance. But to protect your delicate joints, you should balance those activities with low-impact medium-intensity activities such as slow jogging, walking, cycling, swimming, hiking, or yoga, says Dr. Douillard.

Pitta. If you circled column two most often, you are the competitive pitta body type. You are medium-size with a muscular frame. You will excel at competitive sports that require strength, speed, and stamina such as tennis, track, skiing, weight lifting, and swimming. For balance, you should work into your routine activities that you find purely enjoyable and noncompetitive such as dancing, says Dr. Douillard.

Kapha. If you circled column three most often, you are the calm kapha body type. You excel in endurance and mind/body sports such as golf. But you have a natural tendency toward lethargy. You will be drawn to relaxing activities such as golf, cycling, hiking, and horseback riding. But you should sometimes challenge yourself with more vigorous exercise such as tennis, rowing, running, and swimming, says Dr. Douillard.

Advice for the Starting Line

Don't worry about false starts. Don't worry if you trip. Don't even worry if you're in the wrong race. "Just like smokers quit a number of times before they are successful, people who are trying to increase their physical activity may have to make several attempts before they succeed in making it a habit," says Dr. Howze. "Don't get discouraged."

Here's some advice to help you keep your perspective.

You don't have to be perfect. Consider the first weeks of exercise a trial run, a time to find out what you like and don't like, a time to identify your obstacles and adjust your plan, says Dr. Howze. Even the carefully planned program can lead you into unexpected difficulties. When you hit a problem, reassess your exercise decisions and, if you need to, make a change, she says.

Keep trying. Finding the right exercise program is a lot like finding the right outfit, says Butterfield. Sometimes you have to try on lots of different outfits before you find the one you like. Sometimes you have to try out lots of different activities before you discover what works best for you.

Set reachable goals. Your main goal may be to lose 20, 30, 40,

Discover Your Exercise Body Type

Circle all of the words that you feel describe you, even if you need to circle more than one in a category. Then add up the number of circled responses in each column. The column with the most responses is your body type, says John Douillard, D.C., a chiropractor and certified fitness trainer, who is president of the Life Spa Clinic in Boulder, Colorado, and author of *Body, Mind, and Sport.*

Characteristics	Vata	Pitta	Kapha
Mind	Quick	Aggressive	Calm
Mental activity	Restless	Sharp	Stable
Memory	Best short term	Good in general	Best long term
Sleep	Light, short	Sound, medium-length	Heavy, long
Talk	Fast	Sharp, clear-cut	Slow, sweet
Eating speed	Quickly	Medium pace	Slowly
Food	Prefer warm	Prefer cold	Prefer dry
Moods	Change quickly	Change slowly	Nonchanging
Weather	Dislike cold	Dislike hot	Dislike damp
Sex drive	Variable to low	Moderate	Strong
Hair type	Dry	Medium	Oily
Hair amount	Average	Thin	Thick
Skin temperature	Cold hands and feet	Warm	Cool, moist
Weight	Hard to gain	Medium	Hard to lose
Elimination	Dry, hard	Many, soft	Regular, thick
Reaction time	Quick	Average	Slow
Running speed	Very fast	Fast	Not so fast
Runs like a	Deer	Tiger	Bear
Muscle tone	Lean, thin	Defined	Fleshy, large
Totals	**Vata** ____	**Pitta** ____	**Kapha** ____

or 50 pounds—and you may not reach that goal for a while. So set small goals, says Butterfield: walking a mile, working out three times a week, or reducing body fat by 1 percent. It's important to have a goal, and it's important for it to be reachable. "When people don't set goals for themselves, they don't know when they are succeeding at their programs. They don't know they are making progress," he says.

Part 4

**Looking
Beautiful,
Feeling
Great**

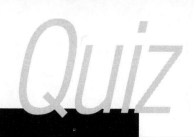

The Body Image Challenge

You can start feeling better about yourself and your body right now—no matter how much weight you want to lose. The following quiz was designed by James C. Rosen, Ph.D., professor of psychology at the University of Vermont in Burlington. It was created to help you find out what you like and what you don't like about yourself—and then to use that information to feel good about yourself today.

Use the following scoring system for questions 1 to 10. Rate yourself on a scale from 0 to 6, where:

0 = Not at all
2 = Slight
4 = Moderate
6 = Extreme

Rate yourself for the past *four weeks.*

_____ **1.** How dissatisfied are you with your overall appearance?

_____ **2.** How much have you worried or felt embarrassed about your appearance in social situations?

_____ **3.** How upset have you been when you felt someone noticed your appearance?

_____ **4.** How much has your appearance influenced how you evaluate yourself as a person? (For example, 2 = "It's one aspect of my self-evaluation"; 4 = "It's one of the main aspects"; 6 = "Nothing is more important.")

_____ **5.** How negatively have you thought of yourself as a person because of your appearance? (For instance, 6 = "I cannot find any positive qualities in myself because of my looks.")

_____ **6.** How much have you avoided public areas (such as restaurants and stores) or social situations (such as work, parties, family gatherings, and dates) because you felt uncomfortable about your appearance?

_____ **7.** How much have you avoided physical contact or intimacy (like lovemaking, hugging, kissing, dancing, touching, shaking hands) because of your appearance?

_____ **8.** How much have you avoided physical activities such as exercise or outdoor recreation because of your appearance?

_____ **9.** How much have you avoided other people seeing your body unclothed?

_____ **10.** How attractive physically have you felt that other people thought you were? (For example, 0 = Attractive or at least not unattractive; 2 = Slightly unattractive; 4 = Moderately unattractive; 6 = Extremely unattractive.)

Using the following scale, choose the best number, from 0 to 6, for questions 11 to 16. Rate yourself for the past *four weeks:* 0 = 0 days (not at all); 1 = 1 to 3 days; 2 = 4 to 7 days (once or twice a week); 3 = 8 to 11 days; 4 = 12 to 16 days (about half the days); 5 = 17 to 21 days; 6 = 22 to 28 days (almost every day).

_____ **11.** How often have you scrutinized your appearance?

_____ **12.** How often have you thought about your appearance *and* felt upset as a result?

_____ **13.** How often have you tried to cover up or camouflage your appearance with clothes or makeup?

_____ **14.** How often have you avoided looking at your body?

_____ **15.** How often have you compared your appearance with that of other people?

_____ **16.** How frequently have you tried to get reassurance from someone that your appearance is okay?

_____ **Total Score**

Scoring: After adding up your responses for questions 1 to 16 to get your total body-image score, read on to discover what your score means.

(continued) ▶

The Body Image Challenge—Continued

If you scored less than 30, congratulations! Out of a possible 96 points, the average score for working women is 23. Women who score less than 30 have a reasonably happy body image, with a minor amount of dissatisfaction.

If you scored 31 to 50, you have a normal score for a woman who is overweight. The average score for overweight women trying to lose weight is 41. So a score in this range means your self-image is holding up well, given the challenge of our weight-conscious world. Regardless of how much weight you lose, you can develop a more positive body image if you follow the tips in upcoming chapters.

If you scored above 50, you have some work ahead of you. It's not uncommon for women to worry too much about their looks or to feel that their body image interferes with the rest of their self-image. The average score for women seeking professional help for body-image concerns is 57. If you scored around this level or higher, you should allow time every day for about six weeks to work on your body image. Although becoming more physically fit will help you feel more confident, a score in this range says that you might need to deliberately practice new body-image attitudes and behaviors to make a lasting change in your self-image.

Here is some advice from Dr. Rosen on how to bring up your score.

Questions 1, 2, 3, and 12 deal with self-consciousness. If you checked a 3 or greater on those questions, do the "mirror exercise." First, make a list of your body parts. Start with the ones you like the most and progress to the ones you like the least. Now stand clothed in front of a mirror and stare at each part for at least a minute. Once you feel comfortable with a body part, move on to the next one on the list. Then do the same exercise naked. Pay attention to your thoughts while you do the exercise. Instead of calling your body disgusting, gross, or some other negative word, use neutral words to describe your body. For example, try words such as *smooth skin, muscular, strong,* and *feminine.* Once you've overcome your negative thoughts while in front of the mirror, try talking more positively about yourself when in public.

Questions 4 and 5 deal with the importance you place on physical imperfections. If the sum of those two questions is above 7, try keeping a body-image diary. Divide the diary into four sections: A, B, C, and D. Whenever a body-image situation arises, write it down, detailing the situation in part A, how you felt in part B, and what you did about it in part C. When you write about how you felt, write more than just negative comments. Ask yourself questions about the event such as "What did I imagine people were thinking when they saw me?" Now, for the D section, write down disputing thoughts that can correct the beliefs in the B section that you feel are self-defeating, erroneous, or unreasonable. For instance, write down comments people actually did make about your appearance instead of what you thought they were thinking.

Questions 6, 7, 8, 9, 13, and 14 deal with avoidance. If you consistently checked 3 or greater on these questions, you need to start facing your fears. Make a list of situations, activities, and even clothing styles (such as swimsuits) that you avoid. For each, plan how to gradually expose yourself to the situation. For instance, a woman concerned about chubby cheeks and fleshy underarms could take the following baby steps: Wear her hair pulled back instead of combed over her face; apply rouge to her cheeks; wear a blouse with a scooped collar instead of a turtleneck; and finally, with the lights on, let her husband give her a neck massage.

Questions 11, 15, and 16 deal with body preoccupation. If you score 4 or higher, you need to set some limits. For instance, if you are always mentally comparing yourself to other people, monitor your negative self-talk, change your position in aerobics class so that you are not facing "better-looking" classmates, and begin appreciating beauty in others instead of thinking jealous thoughts. Or, if you are an excessive clothes changer, allow yourself only two changes before leaving for work. Or, start to stop yourself when you're about to ask your spouse, "Do I look fat?" Or, cut back on the time you spend on the scale.

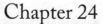

Chapter 24

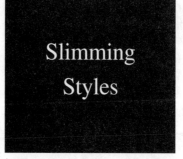

Slimming Styles

What's the easiest way to lose 5 to 10 pounds? Get dressed. (Use these wardrobe tricks.)

One day, while waiting for a bus, image consultant Lisa Cunningham saw the perfect example of how wearing certain styles can make a woman look slimmer.

She spotted a woman wearing a dress with one red diagonal line running from her right shoulder to her left hemline. "I thought, 'Wow, what a great dress. This woman is as thin as a rail,' " says Cunningham.

Then the woman turned sideways. And she realized just how slimming the dress was. "This woman was nine months pregnant," says Cunningham, who teaches at the Fashion Institute of Technology in New York City. "That long diagonal line took my attention straight down her body, and I never noticed her prominent tummy until the woman turned sideways."

As with this example of the pregnant woman, the right clothes can help you appear slimmer—5 to 10 pounds slimmer, says Cunningham. Certain styles can also hide body contours that you want to play down and accentuate others, or they can rebalance out-of-proportion hips or thighs. So in addition to showing you how to eat and exercise, the Fat-to-

Firm Program offers some clever tricks for dressing slim, right from the start.

The formula for dressing to look beautiful and feel great includes clothes that slim and elongate your body, flatter your individual body shape, and fit perfectly.

The Amazing Vertical Line

The basic principles of camouflage and diversion center on two simple principles: vertical and horizontal lines, says Cunningham. Horizontal lines tend to make you look wider. Vertical lines tend to make you look taller. The pregnant woman mentioned earlier had camouflaged her tummy by wearing a loose fitting dress. And she diverted attention away from it with a long diagonal line.

"When we look at people, we look top to bottom, right to left," says Cunningham. "Our eyes will always rest on a horizontal line. If we don't give the eyes a horizontal line to stop on, then the eyes go from top to bottom. So if your clothing and accessories create a vertical line, then you will appear taller and slimmer."

You can create vertical lines by wearing colored vertical stripes, having a row of buttons down the front of a dress, or opening your jacket. A long diagonal line that is more vertical than horizontal will make you look taller and slimmer. Diagonal lines that meet will make you look smaller where they come together and wider where they spread apart, says Jan Larkey, a fashion consultant in Pittsburgh and the author of *Flatter Your Figure*.

Other than lines, the color, shape, and fit of your garments also help subtract pounds instantly. For example...

Slim down with solid colors. When you wear a solid-colored outfit, whether it's red, black, or green, you minimize the number of noticeable horizontal lines that make your body look wider, says Cunningham.

Turn light and dark to your advantage. Portly opera divas sometimes wear dresses with lighter fronts and darker sides. For instance, a dress may have a bright red front panel with a darker cranberry color on the sides. "When the woman stands against the dark scenery, from a distance it is difficult to tell exactly where she ends and the scenery starts," says Jimmy Newcomer, professor of fashion at the Fashion Institute of Technology. To use the diva trick, look for solid-colored

► 353

Problem Solved

Financing Your Fat-to-Firm Wardrobe

Don't have the money to create a flattering wardrobe? Think again. Suzan G. Nanfeldt, an image consultant in New York City and author of *Plus Style: The Plus-Size Guide to Looking Great,* offers these money-saving strategies.

Take closet cues. One way to make sure that you invest in clothes that you will wear often is to take a look at your own closet. Without peeking, imagine the contents of your closet. The door is open. All of your clothes are there: clean, ironed, and ready to wear. (Remember, it's a fantasy.) Reach into that closet and pull out your two favorite outfits. Ask yourself, "Why do I like them so much?"

Pay attention to your answer. Those two favorite outfits are your closet "10s." They represent outfits where you got everything right.

"It looks terrific, it feels terrific, the color is good, the fabric is good, everything is good," says Nanfeldt. "Try to replicate those traits with future purchases. You might not find that same outfit again or the same color again, but you might find items that come close." And you'll minimize the number of times you spend money on clothes that you end up not wearing.

Calculate the long-term cost. Think of your clothes as an investment in your appearance. In investment dressing, you don't want to buy the cheapest clothes you can find. Instead, you want to buy the clothes with the most value. "If you have a blouse hanging in your closet that was the bargain of the century, but you've never worn it, it was not a steal," says Nanfeldt. Instead of focusing on the purchase price of the garment, focus on the cost per wear. In other words, if you pay $100 for a dress that you wear six times a year because you look great in it, the cost-per-wearing is lower than if you pay $100 for a dress that you only wear once because it is not flattering.

Factor in the cost of cleaning. If you have to pay to have a garment dry-cleaned every time you wear it, that adds to its real cost. To minimize costs, avoid high-maintenance fabrics like rayon and stick to easy-care fabrics such as washable silk and cotton knits, says Nanfeldt. Or go for wool or wool blends, which should be cleaned no more than once a year. (To keep wool fresh, hang garments on a hanger outside the closet for 12 hours after every wear to let the fiber breathe.)

clothing where the sides are slightly darker than the fronts, for instance, a green dress with darker green sides, he says.

Go princess. Dresses, swimsuits, or any other type of garment with a princess line—that is, cut in at the torso—make you look taller and create the illusion of a smaller waist, says Newcomer.

Expose your neck. When you wear V-neck and scoop-neck shirts, your neck will seem longer because your upper chest will look like an extension of your neck, says Newcomer. When you wear notched collars, you also look slimmer because they pull attention to your face and away from your body.

Loosen up. Stretch pants and other tight clothing may feel comfortable, but they will expose any rolls of fat on your legs, says Newcomer. "It's just doing the opposite of what you think it's doing," he says. "I know some women think that when they wear something that is tight it will make them look thin. But it just makes them look like they are stuffed into their clothes."

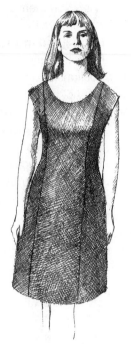

Dress with a Princess Line

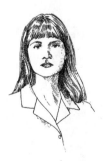

Notched Collar

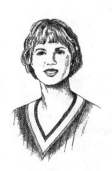

V-Neck Collar

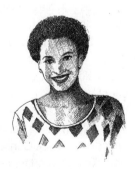

Round Scoop Neck

Dressing Slim from the Inside Out

What you wear underneath your clothes can further subtract pounds. Here are Fat-to-Firm foundation strategies from the experts.

Get a good bra that fits. When you wear worn, flimsy, or poorly fitted bras, they allow your breasts to sag, making your torso appear fatter, not firmer, says Cunningham. For the most slimming effect, look for a bra that holds your nipples no more than 2½ inches below an imaginary line connecting your underarms.

To determine your bra size, measure the circumference from your back, under your arms, and across your chest (above your breasts), says Leslie Rudisill, the women's sport shop department manager for Neiman Marcus in King of Prussia, Pennsylvania. If you measure an odd number such as 35, round up to the next even number. For your cup size, measure the circumference of your torso at fullest point of your bust. Then measure yourself under your breasts. Subtract the second measurement from the first. Use that number to determine your cup size.

Less than 5 = AA

5 = A

6 = B

7 = C

8 = D

More than 8 = DD

Finding a bra that creates the desired effect can take time, trying on bra after bra. So, once you find a bra that works for you, stick with the manufacturer, says Rudisill.

Wear camisoles. Camisoles—lightweight, silky, or satiny half-slips worn underneath blouses or dresses—have a slimming effect because they smooth over any bulges that may exist between your bra and your clothing, says Jennifer Maxwell Parkinson, president of Look Consulting International in New York City and founding president of the Association of Image Consultants International.

Try shapers. Body shapers and slimmers are a type of panty hose that hold in

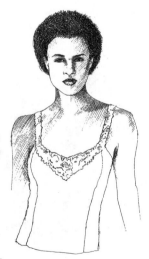

Camisole

your belly and buttocks while lifting and shaping your backside—even more so than control-top panty hose, says Rudisill.

"It's like having a girdle built into the hose, but it's not as constricting, says Rudisill. "I can tell you from personal experience that they really do work." Body shapers are sold in most department stores and cost about twice as much as other panty hose.

How to Match Your Clothes to Your Shape

Women who are proportioned like models—defined by the fashion industry as eight heads tall with hips and shoulders of equal width—can easily find clothes that fit and flatter. Problem is, very few women have

When clothing designers talk about the "proportional" woman, they're describing someone who is exactly eight heads tall, whose shoulders and hips measure the same width and whose waist is indented. A woman with such proportions can wear just about any outfit because her measurements fit the standard manufacturer's models.

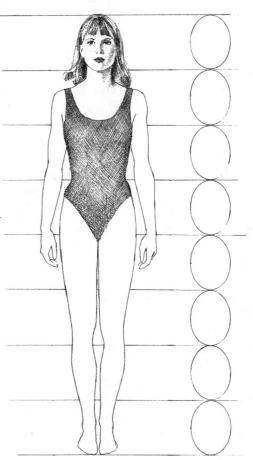

these proportions that match standard manufacturer's models. Most of us are a little too short for our width, or long-waisted, or have short legs, or some other deviation from an imaginary standard.

Not to worry. "Flattering styles exist for every body shape, says Carla Mason Mathis, founder of the ColorStyle Institute for Image Consultants in Menlo Park, California, and co-author of *Triumph of Individual Style*. The trick is knowing how to spot clothing colors, lines, styles, and features that enhance your unique body proportions.

"It's amazingly freeing when a woman realizes that her body is okay—it's her clothes that are all wrong," says Mathis. "If we choose clothes that are right for your body, you'll look beautiful no matter what your size or shape."

The Fat-to-Firm style guidelines take the guesswork out of finding what works best for you. For example, many of us inadvertently do the opposite of what fashion experts recommend. A pear-shaped woman, with slender shoulders and wide hips, might wear loose-fitting sweatpants or palazzo pants and loose, gathered skirts to hide her lower body and fitted tops to show off her slender upper body.

A pear-shaped woman should do the opposite, though. She should wear bulky clothing on her upper body to make her shoulders appear wider and wear more fitted (but not snug) clothing on her lower body to make her hips seem smaller, says Cunningham.

"Most often, when women think they are camouflaging something, they are actually accentuating it," says Cunningham. "They repeat their shape. What they really want to do is counteract their shape."

Though every woman is unique, most bodies are a variation of one of seven basic shapes: triangle, inverted triangle, rectangle, hourglass, diamond, rounded or oval, and tubular, says Judith Rasband, director of the Conselle Institute of Image Management in Provo, Utah, and author of *Fabulous Fit.*

Tubular women tend to be slim. Most women who want to lose weight tend to resemble one of the other six shapes. So the Fat-to-Firm strategies for dressing 5 pounds slimmer are based on these six shapes, and the guidelines that follow will help you find clothes and accessories that best flatter your figure and "erase" unwanted pounds.

Sources for the Fat-to-Firm dressing strategies include experts Jennifer Maxwell Parkinson, Carla Mason Mathis, Lisa Cunningham, Judith Rasband, Jan Larkey, and Jimmy Newcomer (all mentioned earlier), and Suzan G. Nanfeldt, an image consultant in New York City and author of *Plus Style: The Plus-Size Guide to Looking Great.*

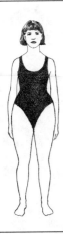

Triangle

✔ Body appears wider below the waist than above.

✔ Weight is centered on the buttocks, lower hips, and thighs.

✔ Shoulders are narrower than the hips.

✔ Bust is small to medium size.

✔ Waist is small to medium size.

✔ Hips measure at least 2 inches more in circumference than the bust.

Overall strategy: Fill out your shoulders and minimize your hips to create the illusion of a balanced figure.

Wear:

- Separates so that you can find clothes that fit both your upper and lower body equally well

- Straight skirts and pants with an even width up and down that don't balloon out on your lower body

- Shoulder pads, to make shoulders appear wider and steal the attention away from your hips

- Buttons, horizontal pins, scarves, and other details on your chest and shoulders, also to divert attention from your hips

- Shirts, dresses, blouses, or sweaters with a yoke (a horizontal, top section of fabric that makes the shoulders appear wider)

- Horizontal stripes along your shoulders

- Solid-colored outfits

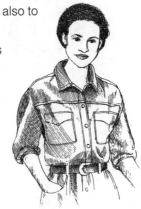

Yoke Collar

- V-shaped patterns, like chevrons, to make your hips seem slimmer and shoulders seem wider
- Earrings, to draw attention toward your face and away from your hips
- Stripes or prints on your upper body and solid colors on your lower body, also to draw attention from your hips

Avoid:

- Exercise tights and overly tight pants, which would tend to reveal any fatty lumps and bumps on your legs and rear end
- Bulky fabric such as denim and corduroy on your lower body
- A-line skirts, palazzo pants, pleated pants, and gathered skirts

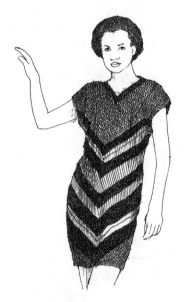

Chevron Pattern

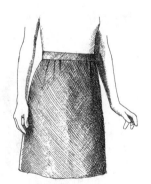

A-Line Skirt

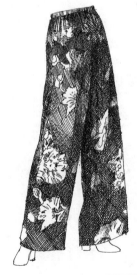

Palazzo Pants

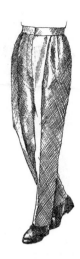
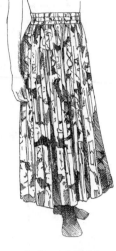

Pleated Pants **Gathered Skirt**

- Raglan, dolman, and other sleeves with sloping shoulders
- Contrasting belts, which create a reference point that make your hips seem larger (belts that match your pants, skirt or dress are fine)
- Jackets that flare out at the bottom
- "Big hair" that poofs more than halfway out to your shoulders
- Side pockets

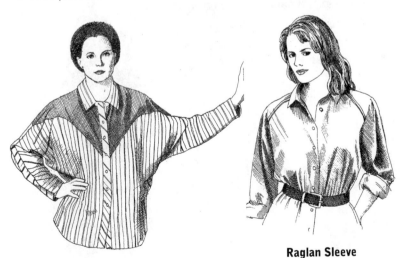

Dolman Sleeve **Raglan Sleeve**

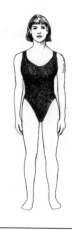

Inverted Triangle

✔ Body appears larger or wider above the waist than below.

✔ Weight is concentrated on the shoulders, upper back, and bust.

✔ The shoulders are wider than the hips.

✔ Bust is medium to large in size.

✔ Waist is medium to wide in size.

✔ Buttocks are often flat.

Overall strategy: Fill out your hips and lower body slightly and minimize your shoulders to create the illusion of a balanced figure.

Wear:

- Separates so that you can find clothes that fit both your upper and lower body equally well
- Raglan and dolman sleeves, to soften the line of your shoulder
- Vertical pins, to elongate and slim your upper body
- Fuller skirts and pants, such as palazzo pants
- Heavy fabric, such as denim and corduroy, on your lower body

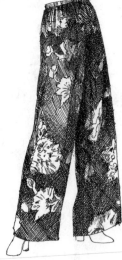

Palazzo Pants

- Open-necked collars, to lengthen the neck and focus the eye on the face and away from the bust and shoulders
- Bright colors, patterns, or horizontal stripes on your lower body, with solids on the upper body

Avoid:

- Shoulder pads, buttons, pins, and other accessories worn on or near your shoulders
- Fitted tank tops, which will overemphasize your bust

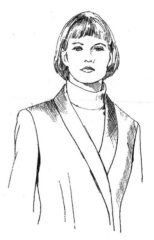

Open Tuxedo Collar

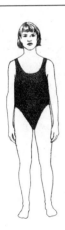

Rectangle

✔ Body appears to be nearly the same width at shoulders, waist, and hips.

✔ The waist is not noticeably indented. Appears wide in comparison with hips.

✔ Waist circumference is 7 inches or less than the bust or hip circumference.

✔ Thighs are the same width as hips.

✔ Bust is small to medium in size.

Overall strategy: Wear loose-fitting clothing that minimizes the waist and leads attention outward at the shoulders and hips, giving the illusion of more curves

Wear:

- Partially fitted clothing that flows over the waist and abdomen
- Belts with loose-fitting clothing above and below the waist

- Jackets, sweaters, and vests open in the front to draw attention to the middle of the body
- Tops that gather at the waist
- Complete elastic waist or elastic inserts at side or back

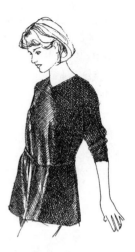

Belted Waist

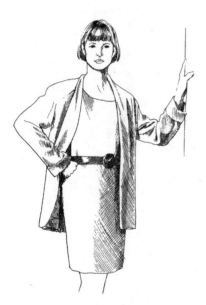

Open Jacket with Belt

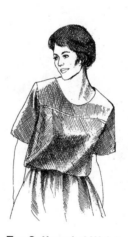

Top Gathered at Waist

Avoid:

- Long, straight hairstyles that have straight lines across the back, making the back appear wider
- Short jackets that stop at your waist

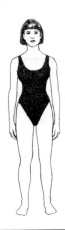

Hourglass

✔ Shoulders and hips are same width.

✔ Waist appears small in comparison to bust, shoulders, and hips. It measures at least 11 inches smaller than shoulders or hips in width. Makes bust and behind appear larger than they really are.

✔ Hips and buttocks are rounded.

Overall strategy: De-emphasizing the waist without overemphasizing the curves of the bust and hips

Wear:

- Clothes that fit loosely in the bust and hips, to minimize your curves (if you are extremely busty)
- Clothing with a princess line
- Lightweight, slimming fabrics with drape such as rayons and blends like combinations of rayon, silk, and synthetics
- Nonclingy, skirts with drape and flow, such as gently gathered skirts

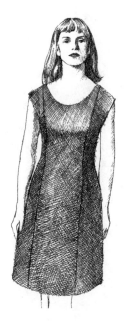

Dress with a Princess Line

- Pants and shorts that neither cling nor add bulk to your body, such as straight-legged jeans, culottes, Bermuda shorts, stirrups, and leggings

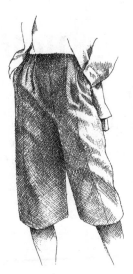

Culottes

Avoid:

- A belt worn at the waist, especially if you're extremely busty and round through the hips
- A seam line that circles your midsection, creating the effect of a belt

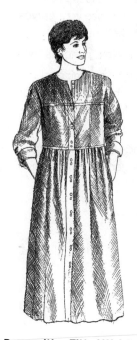

Dress with a Fitted Waist

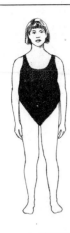

Diamond

✔ Shoulders and hips seem narrow compared to the waist and belly.

✔ Waist extends outward in front rather than inward.

✔ Bust is small.

✔ Buttocks are small, flat.

✔ Legs are thin.

Overall strategy: Create the illusion of wider shoulders and hips while simultaneously minimizing the waist and abdomen.

Wear:

- Shoulder pads

- Belts with noticeable buckles with an open jacket or tunic (the buckle will draw attention inward)

- Jackets, cardigans, and vests with hemlines that fall at least 7 inches below your waist (9 if you're very tall)

- Pleats that fall outward to the hips instead of inward toward belly

- Long tops such as tunics and overshirts that fall 7 to 9 inches below the waist

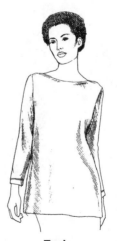

Tunic

- Flared tent, or float, dresses that flow easily over the figure (often have front tucks or empire waist but are very loose fitting)

Avoid:

- A long, straight hairstyle that stops at your waist, creating a horizontal line at your waist
- Wide, full, or gathered ankle-length skirts
- Jackets that stop at your waist

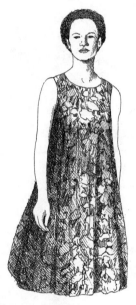

Tent Dress

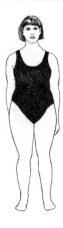

Round

✔ All body areas are rounded.

✔ Weight is above the average range.

✔ The bust, upper arms, upper back, midriff, waist, abdomen, buttocks, hips, and thighs are large and rounded.

✔ With weight loss, this type often changes into one of the other body shapes.

Overall strategy: Create straight lines, to counter roundness and draw attention into center front.

Wear:

- Loose-fitting belts with buckles to draw attention to the waist
- Loose-fitting, open jackets with a shirt or blouse in a contrasting color underneath, to create slimming vertical lines
- Shoulder pads to create an angle at your shoulder
- Light- to medium-weight fabric such as silk or cotton
- Cool, dark, muted slimming colors
- Notched collars to make your face and arms appear less round

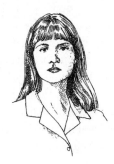

Notched Collar

Avoid:

- Round neck lines, which will make your face appear rounder
- Puffed sleeves, which will mimic the shape of your arms

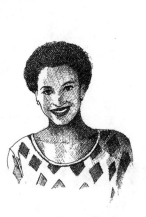

Round Scoop Neck

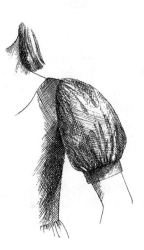

Puffed Sleeves

Problem Solved

You've Lost Weight—And Your Clothes Don't Fit

It's the classic dieter's dilemma: You start to lose weight, so your "fat clothes" hang on you. But few of us can afford to run out and buy a new wardrobe every time we drop a size.

"When you're losing weight, your clothes don't hang correctly on your body—you risk looking very unkempt, like you slept in your clothes," says Suzan G. Nanfeldt, an image consultant in New York City and author of *Plus Style: The Plus-Size Guide to Looking Great.*

Nanfeldt and other fashion experts offer the following strategies for adjusting your wardrobe as your weight changes.

Get a tailor. Figure that you'll drop a dress size for every 15 to 20 pounds you lose. "Make an investment with a good tailor who can tell you how and when to start taking in your clothes and how many times clothing can be altered before it's beyond redemption," says Nanfeldt.

Buy knits. Cotton, silk, or wool knits have more give, so they accommodate changes in body size more easily than nonstretch fabrics, giving you more leeway when your weight fluctuates, says Nanfeldt.

Make small additions. When you first begin to lose weight, pick a style and color scheme, then stick with it until you have reached your final goal, says Jennifer Maxwell Parkinson, president of Look Consulting International in New York City and founding president of the Association for Image Consultants International. For instance, you can get a navy blue suit with a few blouses and coordinating slacks. As you lose weight, you can gradually replace selected items in your new size, without replacing the whole outfit. For instance, after your lose the first 10 pounds, buy a new blouse. After the second 10 pounds, either buy another blouse or replace the jacket. That way, you will always have an outfit that fits.

Fat-to-Firm Fitting Tips

Once you find clothes that flatter your body type, you want those clothes to fit. "The difference between looking 'well-dressed' and 'well, dressed' is having something fit you correctly," says Nanfeldt.

Poorly fitted clothes wrinkle. They hug us in all the wrong places, drawing attention to the very features we don't want others to notice. They balloon out, making us actually appear larger than we are. And they are uncomfortable, making us feel unattractive, says Nanfeldt.

Unfortunately, finding clothes that fit can be as frustrating and confusing as it must have been for Prince Charming to find the right foot to wear the glass slipper.

Why is finding clothes that fit so difficult? Industry experts explain.

First, clothing sizes are not standardized. For instance, some sportswear manufacturers, such as American Eagle Outfitters, design their clothes to fit a younger, slimmer body. So in some lines of clothing, a "large" may fit an older woman's body snugly, even if she usually wears a medium, says Irene Mak, instructor of technical design at Parsons School of Design in New York City and technical designer at American Eagle Outfitters.

On the other hand, some manufacturers purposely design their clothes with extra fabric. So a woman who is usually a size 18 will put on a roomy size 16 garment and conclude that she lost weight, says Mak.

Second, designers often fit their outfits to the bodies of fashion models who are about as different from the average woman as bodies come. The average fashion model is 5 feet, 10 inches tall, wears a size 6, and is shaped like a rectangle—that is, her shoulders and hips are nearly as narrow as her waist. In contrast, 50 percent of American women wear size 14 or larger, the average height of the American woman is 5

The Truth about Turtlenecks and Double Chins

If you have a double chin, you should hide it with turtlenecks, jerseys, scarves, and high collars. Right?

Wrong.

"The higher the neckline and the rounder the neckline of the clothing, the less defined the woman's neck will appear," says Jennifer Maxwell Parkinson, president of Look Consulting International in New York City and founding president of the Association for Image Consultants International. In other words, a turtleneck isn't very slimming. Instead, a woman with a double chin should wear V-neck shirts or pointed collars to elongate her neck and make her chin appear more defined, she says.

Good Hair Days

As with clothing styles, the right hairstyle can make you appear slimmer, more proportioned and even more curvy.

Getting the right hairstyle is not difficult. Here is what you need to know.

Ask your stylist for advice. Often, finding a slimming hairstyle can be as simple as asking your stylist what she or he thinks would look best. "A good stylist should be able to give you ideas based on your face shape," says LeeAnn Nelbach, stylist and owner of the Kindest Cut Spa Salons in northern Virginia.

Consult your stylist before you're draped and shampooed. Your stylist will need to see what you look like with dry hair while you are wearing street clothes, so she can see your body and face shape as well, says Nelbach. That way, she will also be better able to suggest a flattering look by observing what sort of person you are.

In addition, Nelbach offers these general guidelines for choosing the most flattering style, based on body shapes and sizes.

Triangular bodies. Women with the classic pear shape—narrow shoulders, wide at the hips—should avoid short hair which will make the shoulders appear smaller. Long hair with a rounded V-cut in the back can be problematic for women with this body type because it directs the line of sight toward the rear end and hips.

Inverted triangular bodies. Women whose shoulders are broader than their hips should avoid angle-cut, wedge-shaped bobs or hairstyles that blend into the shoulders, which makes the shoulders appear wider. Instead, they should opt for a round cut that comes in toward the face.

---

feet, 4 inches tall, and they are just as likely to be triangular, diamond-shaped, or round.

Once a garment fits the model's proportions, the designer downsizes and enlarges it for various sizes. The more your size and shape differs from the size 6, rectangular fitting model, the more likely you will have fitting problems, says Nanfeldt.

Still, you should never settle for poorly fitted clothes. Here are some ways to help you find the right fit.

Research your choices. Find clothing by designers that cater to

Rectangular bodies. Women with straight bodies—their shoulders, hips, and waists are nearly the same width—should opt for shorter styles that fall above the collar line. Such a cut will break up the rectangular line of the body, creating a more attractive silhouette.

Hourglass bodies. For women whose shoulders and hips measure the same width and who have indented waists, any hairstyle suited to her hair type and lifestyle will also flatter her figure.

Diamond-shaped bodies. Women with thin arms and legs who carry most of their weight in their abdomens should avoid any hairstyle that contains a lot of volume at the shoulders because it will create a straight line from the waist up, making the entire body appear larger. Also, they should avoid a rounded cut in the back so that their hair won't point to the largest part of their bodies. Instead, they should opt for a rounded cut in the front that squares off in the back.

Round bodies. Women who carry their weight all over their bodies and are overweight should avoid a really short cut, which will make a large body appear larger. Instead, they should opt for a layered, flowing style, which is slimming.

Here are other features to take into consideration.

Round cheeks. Avoid a haircut that stops at the cheeks or chin. It will make the cheeks appear wider. Conversely, wearing the hair about an inch below the chin will flatter a round face.

Double chins. Wearing your hair pulled back, away from your chin and neck, will make a double chin look more pronounced. Opt for a cut that brings hair inward, cupping around the chin and neck. Also, avoid straight, angular cuts such as bobs that stop at the chin.

your body shape, then stick with them. For instance, Liz Claiborne designs a clothing line, Elisabeth, specifically designed for women size 14 and larger.

Many department stores train sales staff to know which designs work for which body shapes. So don't be afraid to ask for help, says Rudisill.

Ask questions. When catalog shopping, don't be afraid to call the customer service number and ask what types of clothes would fit your body shape. For instance, Lands' End has specialty shoppers trained to assist in choosing flattering clothes, particularly swimwear, for different figure types.

Call ahead. You can make your shopping experience somewhat easier by calling the department store ahead of time, telling a salesperson what you are looking for and having some things set aside for you when you arrive, says Rudisill. But you shouldn't skimp on your fitting-room time.

Spend time in the fitting room. A lot of time. No matter how much research you do, no matter how many questions you ask, no matter how much knowledge you have, you'll still have to give each outfit a test run. "Unless you like to return merchandise, try everything on," says Rudisill.

Put the clothes to this test. Nanfeldt recommends that in the dressing room, check the garments you're considering to be sure that they meet the following criteria.

- The garments are roomy enough for you to move comfortably.
- The fabric doesn't pull at the seams and create horizontal wrinkles.
- The fabric doesn't bunch up and create vertical wrinkles.
- Your blouse is not so small that the buttons, snaps, or other closures pull, even when you are sitting down.
- You can move your arms up and down, forward and backward, without the fabric of your blouse pulling against your body.
- When your arms hang at your sides, the sleeves don't fall below your wrists.
- Your blouse stays tucked into your skirt or pants when you move.
- The waistband of a skirt stays put when you walk. (If it gradually travels around your waist as you walk, it's too big.)
- When wearing pants, the crotch neither cuts into you, hugs your buttocks, or falls far below your body.
- Your pants fall in a straight line from the outermost curve of your buttocks to the floor. They should neither cup or bunch up under your buttocks.

Focus initially on how the clothes feel on the body instead of how they look. If clothes are not comfortable, you won't wear them.

Chapter 25

Overcome the Fitting-Room Jitters

Buying swimsuits, jeans, and workout clothes can intimidate any woman. Here's how to find styles that look great— no matter what your shape.

Image consultant Suzan G. Nanfeldt of New York City knows what happens when we step into the fitting room.

We take off our clothes and slip into new-smelling, stiff outfits with the tags and plastic alarm devices hanging off. We adjust our hair. Then two little voices start arguing in our heads.

VOICE #1: "You look fabulous."
VOICE #2: "Hey, this makes you look fat. Lady, whaddaya thinking?"
VOICE #1: "No, no. This is your color. You look radiant in green."
VOICE #2: "Did you check out the size? It's impossible—you don't wear that size."

And you go home empty-handed.

"When we're looking in the mirror, we're looking through the shade of what we want to see," says Nanfeldt, author of *Plus Style: The Plus-Size Guide to Looking Great.* "We're not getting a realistic picture of what is truly there."

Four Ways to Beat the Fitting-Room Blues

Fortunately, we can do some things to ban those bickering voices from the fitting room.

Go rested. Putting on and taking off clothes takes patience and energy. Avoid shopping on those days when your only true aspiration involves catching tonight's Movie of the Week. Otherwise, you'll step foot in the mall with imaginary voices already quibbling about how you look, says Nanfeldt.

Shop alone. You can catch negative moods from friends, says Nanfeldt.

Be prepared. You need to bring along or wear the right shoes and undergarments to make sure that what you are trying on fits and looks good. Shoes are most important because they help ensure that the pants length fits. When shopping, don't be afraid to bring along a bag of essentials: shoes, blouses, and tights, says Nanfeldt.

Talk to the sales help. In most upscale department stores, salespeople are trained to help you. You can even call ahead, let them know what you will be looking for, and have them set some outfits aside before you arrive, says Leslie Rudisill, the women's sport shop department manager for Neiman Marcus in King of Prussia, Pennsylvania.

Still, no matter how many precautions you take, some clothes will automatically set the critical voices astir.

Swimsuits, jeans, and workout clothes are the prime culprits. Buying these kinds of clothes need not, however, bring on that inner critic. Your main strategy for keeping such negative talk at bay during such trying times is education. What follows is all the information you need to pick out, try on, and purchase swimwear, jeans, and exercise clothes that flatter your body.

Swimsuits: Yes, You Can Wear One *Now*

Skin is skin. Fat rolls are fat rolls. And swimsuits show all. Or do they? Fashion designers and image consultants say that you have numerous strategies at your disposal for making that flimsy little piece of fabric flatter your body.

Create a diversion. If you don't want someone to look at your hips, thighs, belly, breasts, or behind, then give them a reason to look somewhere else, says Jan Larkey, a fashion consultant in Pittsburgh and author of *Flatter Your Figure.* "When I am at the beach, I wear the wildest pair of sunglasses or hat that I can," she says. "If you have good-looking legs, then wear something really crazy and colorful on your feet."

Hide a tummy with flowers. A swimsuit with an overall pattern of overlapping flowers will take the attention away from your abdomen, says Larkey.

Cover yourself. Beach cover-ups can get you to and from the water without revealing extra curves, says Larkey.

Check the arm and bra. A bad bra will push the breast tissue of large-breasted women to the sides, making the tops of your arms appear lumpy. The worst offender is the shelf bra, a piece of elastic that runs across the chest. "It's like putting your breast in a cone of soft, mushy fabric. It doesn't flatter," says Bill Indursky of New York City, formerly a designer for Anne Terry Designs, a manufacturer of plus-size swimwear.

Look for a suit with good support, enough room for your breasts, and small armholes. You want the armhole to be big enough to slide your arm through comfortably. But you also want to have fabric high enough under your armpit to help prevent your breasts from sliding to the side, he says.

Go for the V. A V-neck will elongate your upper body, bringing attention to your face, says Indursky.

Cover your rear. Don't settle for a suit that doesn't have enough fabric to contain your rump. For two-piece suits, you may be able to solve the problem by buying a larger bottom and a smaller-size top, says Indursky.

Go for elastic. Some suits contain an elastic meshing that creates more support around the tummy. While Indursky admits that the fabric probably does little to make your tummy actually appear smaller, it will soothe you psychologically, making you feel as if the suit is containing your bulge.

Do the stretch test. Suits are made of two different kinds of fabrics: one that stretches horizontally and one that stretches both horizontally and vertically. For a suit that holds you in, you want fabric that stretches only horizontally. You can tell which type of fabric the suit has by pinching the suit in two different places and gently pulling up and to the side to see which way it naturally stretches, says Indursky.

Stay away from a low-back. A suit that comes up to the mid-back is more flattering than a low-back suit because it covers up some bulges and bumps. Large-breasted women should, however, opt for a high-back or a racer-back swimsuit, which is shaped like a Y and covers most of the back, for more support. It will keep you from feeling as though you are going to fall out of your suit while you are swimming, says Indursky.

Get a transparent skirt. Skirts are one way to cover up your thighs. The problem is, the rest of the world will see the skirt and assume that you are wearing it because you have something to hide. If you want to hide your thighs, opt for a skirt made of a meshy material that is not opaque. "You'll have the feeling of hiding without being less sexy or frumpy," says Indursky.

Go gathered. To disguise a tummy bulge, get a suit that is gathered to one side and skirted just in the front. That will move the eye in an angular direction, away from your belly, says Indursky.

Accessorize. Suits with accessories such as rhinestone (or faux rhinestone) bobbles near the chest will bring the eye up and away from the lower body, says Indursky.

Find a vertical line. A suit with a princess line that runs from the shoulders down the sides creates the illusion of slimness. The closer those lines come to the front of the body, the greater the slimming effect, says Indursky.

Go high-cut. Moderately high cut swimsuits will create a slimming diagonal line across your thigh or hip, says Lisa Cunningham, an image consultant who teaches at the Fashion Institute of Technology in New York City. Of course, if you're modest or have an ample derriere, you'll probably want to steer clear of the super-high-cut, thong-type suits.

The Jeans Scene

Some women try on as many as 20 pairs of jeans before finding a pair that fits. Buying jeans should not be so trying.

In most cases, simply asking a salesperson for help can alleviate fitting frustrations, says Jill Lynch, brand communications manager for Levi Strauss and Co. in San Francisco. Most salespeople are trained to help you find the right jeans for your body shape.

You can also alleviate some of the frustration involved in finding the right jeans by following some advice from fashion experts and jeans manufacturers.

Know your options. Different styles of jeans suit different body shapes. For instance, Levi's 550 relaxed-fit jeans work well for the curvy woman with larger hips, while the classic Levi's 501 jeans for women work better for a woman with a straighter body. Generally, jeans are divided into three main categories: slim, relaxed, and loose. Slim usually fits a narrow, teenage body. Relaxed works more for a woman with a defined waist and round hips. Loose provides a comfortable fit that can be worn by all body shapes.

Unfortunately, no industry standard governs terminology for jeans styles. So one company's definition of *relaxed* might not be the same as another's. See the jeans cheat sheet in this chapter to get a better idea of how some of the styles of major jeans manufacturers will fit you.

Move over to the women's department. As teens, some of us got in the habit of shopping in the men's jeans department because our bodies were straighter, our hips were narrower, and well, we looked almost like a boy. If you are still buying men's jeans, you'll probably be plagued with fitting problems, the most common of which is a gap at the waistband along your back. Your adult body is now curvier than your teenage body. To get a better fit, try on the jeans in the women's department, says Lynch.

No side pockets. Jeans with pouch pockets on the side or in front bring attention to your hips, says Cunningham. If you have a triangular body—that is, if you are wider on the bottom half than the top—you should avoid pockets and other lines of accentuation. "Find jeans as plain as you can, without tucks, pleats, or extra bellowing pockets, especially on the sides," she says.

Get big back pockets. So many women agree that small back pockets make a rear end appear larger that Levi's has enlarged back pockets on its women's jeans in response to the demand, according to Lynch.

Get lighter fabric. Some denim is thicker than others. If you are heavier on the bottom half of your body, then you'll want to get the thinnest denim you can find, says Cunningham. For instance, Edwin has rayon jeans called Santa Cruz that fit more slimly than denim jeans.

Avoid tapered. A woman with wide hips or a large rear should avoid tapered jeans because the narrow fit at the ankle will actually make the hips and buttocks appear wider, says Cunningham.

Wear them the right way. Some jeans are designed to be worn on your hips. Others are made for your waist. Fortunately, some manufacturers provide an illustration attached to the jeans showing you how to wear the pants.

Get belly help. Women with belly bulges should opt for pleated jeans or jeans with elastic waistbands to offer more room in the abdomen,

(continued on page 382) ►

Picking the Right Pair of Jeans

The original blue jean was very basic and standard—heavy denim, five pockets, straight legs, and designed for guys. How things have changed. Here are how different jeans fit on different bodies.

Levi's

- Classic 501. A good place to start for all body types. These are the original jeans with the classic five-pocket, straight-leg fit.
- Relaxed 550. Made for the woman with larger thighs, these jeans fit looser through the seat and thigh.
- Loose 560. These provide even more room through the seat and thighs, all the way to the ankles.
- Slim 512. They work well for women with the Sharon Stone body: tall, thin, long-legged, and noncurvy.
- Guy's fit. Made to be worn low on the hips, these straight-leg jeans provide slightly more room in the seat and thighs (but not as much as relaxed jeans).
- Petite. These jeans are scaled for the woman under 5-foot-3.
- Plus-size. They are designed to fit the woman size 16 and up.
- Personal Pair. Available only at the Original Levi's Stores, these jeans are created to your individual body type.
- Wide-leg. Fitted at the waist with wide legs to the ankles, these are good for all body types except the very petite.

The Gap

- Classic. They provide some curve through the hips with narrow legs. Work well for women who are not excessively curvy and who do not have large thighs.
- Loose. The legs of these jeans offer more room through the hips and thighs.
- Slim. Narrow through the hips, thighs, and knees, they contain the smallest leg openings that the Gap makes. Work well for slim, noncurvy women who like tight-fitting jeans.

- Reverse. These sit high on the waist, covering the tummy. They also are roomy through the hips and thighs.
- Wide-leg. They provide more room through the hips and thighs, all the way to the ankles. The denim is lightweight, more slimming than other types of denim.

Lee

- Relaxed. These jeans have more room through the hips, thighs, and knees while tapering to the ankles.
- Easy. They provide some room through the hips and thighs (not as much as relaxed). Front waist dips.
- Classic. Front waist dips on these, with a slimmer fit through the hips and thighs and tapered legs.
- Big Easy. These jeans are loose-fitting through the thighs and hips with wide legs all the way to the ankles.

Guess

- The Melrose. Guess's traditional-fitting jeans with narrow legs. Because they provide some room in the hips, most body shapes can usually wear these jeans.
- The South Beach. Slim-fitting jeans with a low waist and narrow legs. Work well on straight bodies.
- The Westside. Relaxed jeans with tapered legs that fit pear-shaped and curvy women well.
- The Tomboy. Though slimmer women can wear them, these jeans provide a good fit for larger women. Work extremely well for women with wide hips and thighs.
- The Boyfriend. Designed to feel as though you are wearing your boyfriend's jeans. The waist is low and roomy. The legs are straight and loose. The jeans are comfortable and can provide a good fit for larger women.

recommends Lynch. Also, women who have belly bulges should look for high-waisted jeans (as opposed to hip huggers) to hold the belly in, she advises.

Get personal. If no matter what you do, if you still can't find jeans that match your body shape, then give customized jeans a try. For example, Levi's makes jeans called Personal Pair jeans, available at Original Levi's Stores.

Outfitting Your Exercising Body

Many women make the mistake of buying the least expensive exercise clothes that they can find. Why? Because they want to lose weight. They are exercising to lose weight. And why bother buying a nice outfit when they are only going to have to buy another one when they are thinner?

Buy something nice. You'll exercise more often.

"If you are going to be exercising, you want to buy quality clothing," says Carolyn Schmidt, who made exercise clothing for large women and taught an exercise class for large women in Chicago. "Buy a well-made outfit that has substantial, quality fabric, like Lycra. It feels better when it's on, it lasts longer, and it looks better."

Here are some ways to get exercise clothes that flatter you.

Go diagonal. If your body is triangular, try leotards with V-shaped patterns to accentuate your shoulders and bring attention away from your hips. The V shape can be made by the cut of the fabric or by color such as black and white diagonal lines, says Cunningham.

Go solid. If your weight and height are not evenly divided between your upper and lower body, then keep your outfit the same color from your top to your leotard to your leggings to create a slimming vertical line, says Cunningham.

Wear a loose top. If you have heavy legs and hips, wear a baggy top with leggings to accentuate your shoulders and bring attention away from your lower body, says Cunningham.

Hike up your leotard. High-cut leotards will create a slimming diagonal line across your thigh. If the leotard you wear is not high-cut, you can fake the effect by pulling the fabric of the leotard higher on your leg to your hipbone, suggests Cunningham. As with swimsuits, however, if you have a large derriere, you may look best in only moderately cut leg openings.

How to Pick the Perfect Exercise Bra

Exercise bras have been accused of lots of things. Women call them soggy, flimsy, abrasive, unflattering, uncomfortable—even stubborn (once you get some of them on, they are nearly impossible to remove).

Up until 1978, women who exercised didn't even have exercise bras. Some resorted to wearing regular bras and then wrapping elastic bandages around their breasts. Even after the invention of exercise bras, it wasn't until the 1990s that sports bras were made for large-breasted women. (Large-breasted women still have the most limited selection in exercise bras.) But today, a woman can find an exercise bra that fits, feels good, looks good, and controls bouncing—all she has to do is try it on and test the bra for comfort, support, and appearance, says Missy Park, founder of Title IX, a women's athletic supply company in Berkeley, California. Here are some things to look for when trying on exercise bras to help you avoid bouncing, chafing, wetness, and flattening. (We've also included a tip to save you money.)

These tips come from Park; Anne Kelly, president of Junonia, Ltd., a St. Paul, Minnesota, company that specializes in activewear for women size 14 and larger; and Deborah Compton, a sales representative and wear tester for Moving Comfort women's athletic wear in Chantilly, Virginia.

To Avoid Bouncing...

- If your breasts are a C-cup or larger, opt for bras with distinguishable cups rather than the type that push your breasts into a kind of uni-breast against the chest wall. Bras that hold each breast separately in a sturdy cup (called isolation bras) provide the most support for women with medium to large breasts. But they are hard to find in smaller cup sizes. Women with smaller breasts will find more support in compression bras, the type that smash the breasts as flat as a pancake against the chest wall.

- Look for exercise bras with two layers of fabric, one that forms around your breasts and another on top.

- Bras with straps that run toward the middle of the back in a T or X shape will pull the entire breast up, which controls bouncing better than straps that run straight over the shoulder. Large-breasted women, however, should make sure that such bras fit comfortably. Sometimes the T- and cross-backs can irritate muscles in the center of the back.

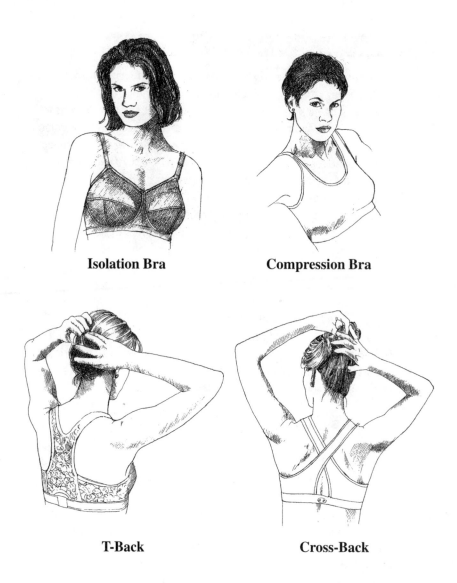

Isolation Bra **Compression Bra**

T-Back **Cross-Back**

- Look on the hang tag to see if the company performed wear-testing or breast-bounce studies. Buying a bra from a company that does wear-testing and bounce studies, such as Motion Control and Champion Jogbra, virtually guarantees the bra will have superior motion control.

- Some companies make bras designed for specific sports, usually based on wear-testing and breast-bounce studies. You won't need

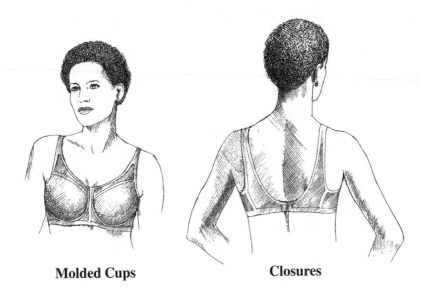

Molded Cups   **Closures**

as much support from a bra to play golf as you will to ride a horse. Look on the hang tag for such information.

- When trying on the bra, make sure your breasts don't spill out at the top or along the sides. You should not be able to see any part of your breasts.

- When in the fitting room, jump up and down while watching your breasts in the mirror. If your breasts bounce in the fitting room, they will also bounce while wearing the bra in an aerobics class.

To Avoid Chafing...

- When in the fitting room, move your arms forward and back. Bend. Twist. Do motions as if you were exercising. For instance, if you will wear the bra while playing golf, take several swings. If you feel any friction, don't buy it.

- Feel the seams with your fingers. They should feel soft and flat. If you feel bumps, the seams are likely to chafe your skin as you exercise.

- Look at where the seams are placed. No seams should run over a nipple.

- If the bra has underwires, make sure they are plush lined.

To Stay Dry...

- Look for bras made with moisture-wicking fabrics (made with spun polyester such as CoolMax or Supplex nylon) or fabrics treated with Intera, Polywick, or Quik-Wik. Such fabrics dry quickly as they pull the sweat away from your body.

- Avoid any bra that has cotton fabric next to your skin. Cotton gets soaked easily and dries slowly.

To Avoid the Flattening Effect...

- Look for bras that have molded cups. Such bras look like they already have breasts inside. They won't lie flat. Other than giving you a more curvy silhouette, such bras also feel more comfortable and control bouncing better in larger-breasted women.

For Easier Removal...

- Look for bras with closures in the front or the back rather than bras that you must pull over your head.

- If you buy bras made with moisture-wicking material, you'll have an easier time removing them because they won't get as wet. The wetter the bra, the more it glues itself to your skin.

- To get off the most stubborn, pull-over-your-head bra, make sure to remove it correctly. Cross your arms in front of your body, grab the bottom of the bra along the sides, and roll it off.

To Save Money...

- Along with your shoes, your exercise bra is your most important piece of equipment. You shouldn't skimp. Though quality exercise bras will cost you between $30 and $40, they will also last. Quality bras are made with elastics that are resistant to salt. Often they will last two years or longer.

Chapter 26

Feeling Good about Yourself

Don't wait until you reach your "ideal" weight. Self-esteem can start today.

If being one of the "beautiful people" meant a woman would love her looks, then Heather Locklear wouldn't have told *Cosmopolitan* magazine, "When I look in the mirror, I see the girl I was growing up: braces, crooked teeth, a baby face, and a skinny body. My legs are still too thin. And I'm knock-kneed. My knees can look at each other and have a conversation."

And Kirstie Alley wouldn't have revealed, "All I ever wanted to be was blonde, blue-eyed, short, and big-breasted. My prayers were obviously not answered."

And Dolly Parton wouldn't have said, "I know I'm not a natural beauty. I've got short legs, little hands, and a tiny frame. And, yes, I've had cosmetic surgery. I've had nips and tucks and trims and sucks, boobs and waist and butt and such, eyes and chin and back again."

From the famous to the unknown, from size 2 to size 32, from pear-shaped to hourglass—few woman can resist the urge to criticize their bodies, say experts. "You can't tell how a person feels about her body by how her body looks," says Cinder Ernst, a fitness consultant at World

Gym in San Francisco. "In my locker room, some of the most tortured people are the women whose bodies could go on the covers of magazines."

Learning to Hate Your Body

It's no wonder that women feel less than perfect. Ultra-thin fashion models—an impossible (and even unhealthy) ideal—mock us from every advertisement. Countless commercials coax us to change the color of our hair, the length of our nails, and the contour of our lips. The First Lady's haircut (what's wrong with it, that is) is national news. And the tabloids can't wait to tell us about Liz's and Roseanne's latest effort to lose weight.

Yes, the media can make us feel incredibly inadequate. In fact, research shows that the more time we spend reading women's magazines, the more dissatisfied we are with our bodies.

But the media only reflects an attitude found in society at large. And society reflects what's found in the media. From childhood on, women are praised for how they look rather than what they do, says psychologist Jan P. Ferris, Ph.D., who treats eating disorders in her private practice in North Hills, California.

And, with our girlfriends, we take up where our family and teachers left off. We teasingly (but seriously) attack body part after body part—from foreheads to thighs to ankles—turning the maligning of our bodies into a kind of perverse way of life.

Criticizing our bodies may be commonplace, but that doesn't mean it isn't damaging. In the most extreme cases, poor body image can lead to the three eating disorders: compulsive overeating, bulimia (in which women overeat and purge food from their bodies), or anorexia nervosa (in which they starve themselves in an attempt to get thinner and thinner). Such women have completely lost touch with what their bodies really look like, says Dr. Ferris.

But even much less severe body-image problems can turn women into "losers," according to Cheri K. Erdman, Ed.D., a counselor and professor at the College of DuPage in Glen Ellyn, Illinois, and author of *Nothing to Lose: A Guide to Sane Living in a Larger Body* and *Live Large! Ideas, Affirmations, and Actions for Sane Living in a Larger Body.* For example, we lose track of other positive traits, like our personalities, values, and actions. Some other losses we may experience include the following:

- Lost time. Because some of us spend so much time and energy thinking nasty thoughts about our bodies, we lose time that could be spent on other pursuits, such as furthering our careers or strengthening relationships.

- Lost dreams. Some of us avoid fun things like restaurants, swimming pools, and sporting events, putting our lives on hold until we lose weight.

- Lost enjoyment. Instead of enjoying life in the present, some of us fantasize about how happy we will eventually be in the future when we finally achieve the "perfect body."

Do You Need a New Body Image?

Even perfectly normal, attractive women can have poor body image. Because poor body image is so prevalent among women, just about all of us could use a boost in our self-esteem. Six clues, however, can let you know how urgently you should work on your body image. If any of the following are true for you, you should make improving your body image one of your top priorities, says Joni Johnston, Psy.D., a clinical psychologist in Del Mar, California, and author of *Appearance Obsession: Learning to Love the Way You Look.*

CLUE #1: How your thighs look or what you ate today can determine your mood.

CLUE #2: In your mind, you often hold beauty contests with other women where you are both judge and contestant. You still lose.

CLUE #3: You feel threatened by attractive women.

CLUE #4: You avoid social situations (such as going to the beach) because of your body.

CLUE #5: You often think negative thoughts about your body.

CLUE #6: You are in a relationship with a man you know is bad for you. You stay in it because either you feel that you don't deserve him because you think he is more attractive than you or you feel that you should be grateful to have any man at all.

Stand Up for Yourself

Even if you haven't come to terms with your body, even if you haven't gotten around to buying those flattering clothes, even if you haven't lost a pound—you can still appear thinner, more attractive, and more confident. How? By standing differently.

"If your self-confidence and self-esteem are low, go with the old acting line: Fake it until you make it," says Hilka Klinkenberg, managing director of Etiquette International in New York City and author of *At Ease...Professionally.*

Here are two ways to stand up for yourself.

Stop leaning. When you lean on the edge of a desk or against a wall, people think that you don't have the energy to stand up straight. "If you see a woman who looks tired and exhausted and she is also heavy, you automatically focus on her weight," says Klinkenberg. "If a woman is standing up straight with a presence, then the weight isn't an issue. She just seems to have a great deal of presence."

Work on your posture. Proper posture can make you feel better about yourself. It's also better for your spine and your balance. Rounding your shoulders can contribute to shoulder, neck, and lower back problems, according to Margot Putukian, M.D., assistant professor of orthopedic surgery and internal medicine at Hershey Medical Center in Pennsylvania. To correct your posture, keep your shoulders straight and your spine straight and neutral, not slouched. Hold your chin high. Tuck your buttocks under to help keep your pelvis in the correct position. Proper posture provides optimal positioning of the spine and surrounding structures.

Good posture is not only good for you, but also conveys your positive image of yourself to others, adds Dr. Putukian.

The Gradual Path to Loving Your Body

At World Gym in San Francisco, a woman in Ernst's exercise class grumbles about her thunder thighs. Ernst walks over and tells the woman that she just insulted her thighs. She asks the woman to apologize. The conversation evokes laughter. But it also makes a strong point. "If you could hate your body into changing, then we would all be on the covers of these magazines," says Ernst. "Hating your body is futile."

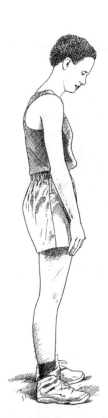 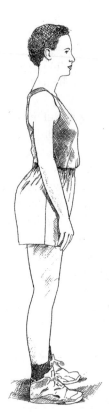 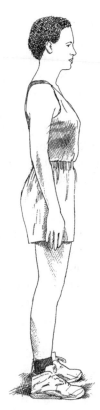

You look shorter and wider when you round your back, letting your shoulders sink down toward your knees.

You look shorter and wider when you allow your pelvis to fall forward, swaying your back.

You look taller and slimmer standing with your pelvis tucked under, shoulder blades down, and back straight.

Ernst speaks from experience. The size 12 fitness instructor did not always feel confident about how she looked.

"It has been a process of trying to go from not liking my body at all, to feeling neutral about my body, to liking my body sometimes, to liking my body more times than not, to liking my body mostly all the time," says Ernst. "Now, I can say that I like my feet, thighs, butt, hair, and cheeks. I'm working on accepting my varicose veins. I don't love them, but they can stay. I just won't look at them anymore."

(continued on page 394) ►

Don't Postpone Your Life

Carolyn Schmidt, 45, of Tinley Park, Illinois, put most of her life on hold while she tried to lose weight. She avoided sports. She wore the cheapest clothes she could find (which fit poorly and made her feel ugly). And she dreamed of the day when she would be thin enough to get her pilot's license.

Carolyn never lost the weight. But the Chicago woman eventually got on with her life. She hired a wardrobe consultant who helped her replace all of those cheap clothes with clothes that make her feel beautiful. She began exercising. And she took flying lessons.

"I look back and I realize there was no good reason preventing me from exercising, buying the clothes, and taking the flying lessons," says Carolyn. "The only thing that was holding me back was my own perception that fat people can't do wonderful things."

Like Carolyn, many women unnecessarily postpone things that they could be doing now, says James Rosen, Ph.D., professor of psychology at the University of Vermont in Burlington. "If you start avoiding every situation that makes you feel self-conscious, then you are never going to feel confident."

Here are some common things women postpone "until they lose weight" that they could be doing right now—as well as some ways to tackle them.

Wearing a Swimsuit

Why: We are ashamed of our bodies.

How to overcome it: At first, put on your swimsuit when at home, but don't go out. Just walk around in it. Look at yourself in the mirror. Eventually, just the act of wearing one in private will make you more comfortable with wearing on in public. For your first few forays to a public swimming pool or beach, go with a large-size friend or a group of large women. Or take a water aerobics class designed for large women. Read through the advice about finding a bathing suit that flatters your body in "Swimsuits: Yes, You Can Wear One *Now*" on page 376.

Going to the Doctor

Why: Fear of harassment or abuse. Fear that the doctor will make treatment contingent on weight loss. Fear that doctor will blame all health problems on our weight.

How to overcome it: Keep shopping around until you find a doctor with whom you are comfortable. Know your body well enough that you can stick up for yourself when your doctor blames a nonrelated health problem on your weight. Be assertive. Tell the nurse that you prefer not to be weighed. Write to the National Association to Advance Fat Acceptance at P.O. Box 188620, Sacramento, CA 95818-8620. Ask for a copy of the pamphlet entitled "Bill of Rights of Fat People in Health Care."

Asserting Ourselves at Work and in Relationships

Why: We feel we don't deserve to have an opinion. We feel that the sort of person who speaks up must be thin and beautiful, a category in which we feel we don't belong.

How to overcome it: Know that everyone's opinion is valuable. Stop focusing on your body and focus on internal strengths, such as your intellect or your kindness.

Going Back to School

Why: We don't feel we have enough time to focus on school until we are finished "fixing" our bodies. We feel that our weight is the big problem and our lack of education the small problem in life. Also, for some people, there's the fear of not being able to fit in the desk.

How to overcome it: You're wasting more time than necessary worrying about your appearance. Put some of that time into your education. Know that your lack of education is the big problem and your appearance the small problem. If you are worried about fitting into a desk, go to the school's office for people with disabilities. They are required by law to make sure the desks are roomy enough for your body.

Dating

Why: Low self-esteem. The thought, "Any man who would want me must have something wrong with him." The assumption that men won't find us attractive.

How to overcome it: Focus on aspects of yourself that are appealing other than the flaw you usually obsess about. Mentally rehearse all the reasons someone would find you desirable. Remember that you are more likely to worry about minor imperfections in your

(continued) ▶

Don't Postpone Your Life—Continued

appearance than others do. Know that men are not as critical of women's bodies as women are of their own bodies. In the long run, mates choose one another based on personalities, values, and morals. Appearance may rank high during first dates. But meaningful relationships are based on deeper factors.

Exercise

Why: Worried what other people in the gym will think about how our bodies look. Worried we will look silly as we try to figure out how to use equipment or follow an aerobics sequence. If we were chubby during childhood, we may have been ridiculed during gym class, which eventually made us hate exercise.

How to overcome it: Build up your courage by starting your program in the privacy of your home. Or take low-impact classes designed for large women. Go to gyms during less busy hours.

Buying New Clothes

Why: We feel that we don't deserve the clothes unless we've lost the weight. We feel buying new clothes is futile since we'll just have to buy more when we are a smaller size. Trying on clothes also gives us more feedback than we want about our true body size. We must look at ourselves in the mirror and we must confront our clothing size.

How to overcome it: You'll look and feel better in clothes that fit. Go through your closet and set aside for charity all the clothes that are uncomfortable or don't fit well. Then, read the advice about dressing for a changing body in chapter 24 on page 352. To overcome fitting-room jitters, see chapter 25 starting on page 375.

Looking for a New Job

Why: We feel that we'll have more time to job search once we lose the weight. We feel that our weight hampers any success we might have in finding a new, better job.

Ernst's strategy for improving her body image may sound comical, but it works, say psychologists. This strategy starts to scratch the surface, to start to deal with the low self-esteem. But there's a need to go deeper into the issues driving this behavior, adds Dr. Ferris.

Most women cannot progress straight from low to high self-esteem.

How to overcome it: Don't let your appearance undermine your competence as a worker. Pinpoint your internal strengths such as reliability, energy, and intelligence. Focus on them. Tell yourself that a woman with such strengths deserves more now. Stop procrastinating. Prepare yourself for job interviews by mentally rehearsing thoughts about your competence and abilities. Remember that a new body is not your key to happiness—your new job is.

Family Reunions or Visiting with Relatives

Why: Our families are often at the root of our poor self-image. Brothers teased us about our thighs. Gramps always noticed every pound we gained—and made sure we noticed, too. With so much time passing between visits, we feel like relatives will criticize every change in our bodies.

How to overcome it: Prepare yourself for the reunion by mentally complimenting yourself over and over. Focus on the social event, not on your appearance. Don't assume relatives only care about how you look. In reality, families get together to enjoy spending time with one another, not to bring one another down. While at the reunion, do not act guilty by saying things like, "I should not be eating this" or "Every time I look at cake, I gain weight." Such comments invite relatives to pick your body apart. If people make unsolicited remarks about your appearance, tell them such comments are hurtful.

Traveling by Air

Why: Seats may not be wide enough for our bodies. We feel cramped.

How to overcome it: Ask for an aisle seat. Pre-board so that you can get to your seat early to put up the arm rest. When ordering your ticket, ask to have the seat next to you blocked if the flight isn't booked.

We need smaller steps to get us there, says Dr. Erdman. In order, those small steps are as follows.

- Acceptance. When you accept your body, you understand that you can't hate it away. You agree to not call it nasty names anymore.

- Like. Rather than liking the way it looks, focus on liking how it works. For instance, Dr. Erdman focuses on the strength of her thighs rather than the size.

- Transcendence. Yes, like can lead to love. But not always. Transcendence offers a more realistic goal, says Dr. Erdman. In transcendence, instead of focusing on the outside of your body, you focus on the inside. You cherish traits such as your honesty, your brainpower, or your cooking ability instead of your appearance.

Your progression through those stages won't come easily, says Dr. Johnston. To help you along, however, experts have offered the following strategies.

Draw yourself. Women with poor body image often think they look much larger than they are, says Dr. Johnston. To get an accurate gauge of your body size, draw how large you think you look on a banner of paper. Then have a trusted friend trace the shape of your body onto another piece of paper and compare the two, she suggests.

Make a list. Write down the ways that you are being hurt by obsessing about your appearance. For instance, your "hurt list" may include trying on one outfit after another in the morning in an effort to find one that doesn't make you feel fat, or not being able to go swimming because you won't wear a swimsuit. Once you see the consequences of poor body image, you'll be more motivated to change, says Dr. Ferris.

Take back your life. Make a list of the situations you avoid because of your body shape or size. Then rate those situations on a fear scale from 1 to 10. Pick the least scary situation, set a deadline for accomplishing it, and go do it, says Dr. Johnston.

To help motivate yourself, give yourself an out that will decrease your fear, but still let you accomplish the goal. For instance, if your goal is to wear a swimsuit at the beach, tell yourself that if your still uncomfortable after 15 minutes , you'll leave and do something else instead. Getting there is the hard part. That way, the trip won't seem so intimidating, says Dr. Johnston.

Physical activity. Physical activity will help you feel more confident about how your body functions. You'll become comfortable with the sensations of lifting, bending, stretching, and reaching. As you integrate physical activity into your life, you'll gain strength and endurance, making you proud of what your body can accomplish, says Debby Burgard, Ph.D., a psychologist in the San Francisco Bay area and co-author of *Great Shape: The First Fitness Guide for Large Women*. And because you're moving rather than exercising, you can see that your body can be used for fun.

Banish the thought. Even Dr. Erdman has her days when she curses her belly. When she finds herself thinking such thoughts, she stops herself. "I don't allow myself to get stuck there," she says. "I don't judge the thought as good or bad. I recognize that I have it, then I decide to let it go."

Get support. Working on your body image can become a difficult task, especially when you are surrounded by women who consistently say nasty things about their own or other women's bodies. For support, find some women who accept their bodies and the bodies of others exactly the way they are, says Dr. Burgard. You can find such women by contacting body-acceptance groups such as the Body Positive, 4962 El Camino Real, Suite 225, Los Altos, CA 94022-1410, for the moderately overweight; National Association to Advance Fat Acceptance, P.O. Box 188620, Sacramento, CA 95818-8620, for the extremely overweight and their families; and Largesse, the Network for Size Esteem, P.O. Box 9404, New Haven, CT 06534-0404, for the moderately overweight.

Read up. If you need further reassurance that your identity and worth goes beyond body shape, Dr. Erdman suggests that reading publications and books that support size acceptance can help remind you that you are normal. Good magazines include *Radiance* and *Big Beautiful Woman*. Some books on size acceptance include Dr. Erdman's *Nothing to Lose and Live Large,* Dr. Johnston's *Appearance Obsession: Learning to Love the Way You Look,* and Carol Johnson's *Self-Esteem Comes in All Sizes.*

Stay off the scales. Remember that your weight fluctuates up and down 5 pounds throughout the month. "I don't know that there is any single instrument in home more destructive than the scale," says Dr. Johnston. "When you weigh yourself more than once a month, you put yourself on an emotional roller coaster."

Keep a body journal. For a few weeks, keep a journal of the thoughts you have about your body, suggests Dr. Johnston. The journal helps because many of our negative thoughts are so common that we don't even realize we have them.

Judge others, not yourself. When someone tells you that your thighs are getting big, the comment provides information about them, not you. "People who love and accept their own bodies are accepting of anybody's body," says Dr. Johnston.

Remember that you have a choice when confronted with someone else's ideas about your body. You don't have to internalize the comment and accept it as true. If it is true, it's not someone else's right to judge your body anyway. Instead, you take the comment as a sign of the insensitivity or ignorance of that person, not a negative reflection of your own worth, says Dr. Ferris.

Talk to yourself. Instead of heaping criticism on thighs or other body parts when you look in the mirror, tell yourself that you are okay. "You have to say it until you believe it," says Dr. Ferris.

Visualize a bodiless you. Imagine yourself as a spirit, not a physical being. You are now a formless orb. Ask yourself: What would people admire about me? Because you are bodiless, you are forced to focus on internal traits such as morality, character, and intellect, says Dr. Ferris.

Part 5

The Fat-to-Firm Recipe Collection

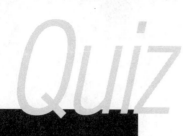

Is Your Kitchen Stocked for Healthy, Low-Fat Eating?

Cooking and eating the Fat-to-Firm way are easy when you have the right stuff on hand—from low-fat, high-flavor snacks to boneless chicken breasts, grains, and vegetables for fast, kind-to-your-waistline dinners.

Are you a savvy shopper? Are your pantry and refrigerator ready for action? Find out—and learn some new supermarket strategies that will help you stick with your new eating plan—with this quiz developed for the Fat-to-Firm Program by Cathy Kapica, R.D., Ph.D., associate professor of nutrition and clinical dietetics at Finch University of Health Sciences/Chicago Medical School in North Chicago. Read the following statements, then rate your habits by using this scoring system:

1 = Never;
2 = Rarely;
3 = Sometimes;
4 = Often;
5 = Always.

_____ **1.** I do the grocery shopping when I am not hungry.

_____ **2.** I make a list of the groceries I need, and I shop only from that list.

_____ **3.** When planning my shopping list, I assess my supply of kitchen basics—pasta, rice, cereal, tuna, beans, frozen vegetables, and fruit juice—and add them to my list.

_____ **4.** I keep my kitchen stocked with low-fat condiments like Worcestershire sauce, horseradish, Dijon mustard, teriyaki sauce, and pickle relish to add flavor to food.

_____ **5.** I keep a supply of cooking spray, broth, and canned tomatoes to use instead of butter and margarine when preparing food.

_____ **6.** I read the food labels for fat, calorie, and fiber content and check the packaging for food descriptions such as "reduced-fat," "low-fat," "less-saturated-fat."

_____ **7.** If a fresh fruit or vegetable is not in season, I choose frozen varieties without added sauces, sugar, or salt.

_____ **8.** I choose processed meats that are at least 90 percent fat-free.

_____ **9.** I look for whole-grain and whole-wheat bakery products, which list whole-wheat flour first on the ingredient list.

_____ **10.** If I buy candy or similar treats, I choose small, portion-controlled packages so that I'll be less likely to overindulge.

_____ **11.** I choose a breakfast cereal whose label says "high-fiber," "whole-grain," or "bran."

_____ **12.** When buying poultry, I choose low-fat, quick-cooking turkey or chicken pieces such as skinless, boneless breasts.

_____ **13.** I choose low- or nonfat dairy products.

_____ **14.** I keep shopping trips to a minimum—only once or twice a week.

_____ **15.** If at all possible, I do the grocery shopping alone, without children or spouse, to avoid impulse purchases.

_____ **Total Score**

Scoring: To determine your score, add up your points for all statements, then read on for the results.

If you scored 60 to 75, congratulations, you are supermarket-smart and on your way to fitness. To improve your health, try at least one new food per week to increase the variety and taste of your diet. (Have you had a papaya? Basmati rice? Endive? Goat cheese?)

If you scored 45 to 59, your shopping habits are on their way to improving your health. Just be more vigilant at the supermarket. Plan ahead, read package labels, and keep your cabinets stocked with low-fat, healthy choices.

If you scored 15 to 44, you need to work on your grocery-shopping habits. Begin by always planning your supermarket trips and reading food labels. Don't be rushed as you shop, but make conscious choices. After two weeks, retake this quiz to measure your improvement in shopping skills.

Chapter 27

Your Favorite "Fat" Foods— Made Thin

You can still eat the foods you love—now they're not only tasty but also slimming. Cook on.

Macaroni and cheese, onion rings and french fries, coleslaw and potato salad, pizza and cheeseburgers. Bet you think that those are the foods you'll have to give up on the Fat-to-Firm Program. After all, they're fattening. Not anymore. Our chefs at the Rodale Test Kitchen have worked overtime concocting delicious low-fat versions of your favorite dishes. They cut the fat calories way, way back but never sacrificed an iota of great taste. So remember: The Fat-to-Firm Program isn't a diet. You can (and should) eat plenty of delicious low-fat, high-fiber, nutrition-rich foods like the ones you're about to discover here. Keep in mind, too, that there's no hunger and no deprivation on the Fat-to-Firm Program. (And there's no out-of-control bingeing because you've gone for days on tuna fish, grapefruit, and melba toast.) Instead, you'll find yummy, low-fat foods of all kinds that tell your stomach that the good times are here and your extra fat that it can get out of town.

Nutritional analysis for all recipes is per serving.

Spicy Chicken Fingers

Standard Recipe	Fat-to-Firm Makeover
236 calories	*77 calories*
13 g. fat (50% of calories)	*1.6 g. fat (19% of calories)*

Traditional deep-fried chicken fingers are loaded with fat and calories. To slim down these appetizers, eliminate the breading, mix the spices right into the chicken, and quickly pan-sear the chicken instead of deep-frying it. They're irresistibly delicious.

  1 pound boneless, skinless chicken breasts, cut into 1" cubes
  3 cloves garlic, minced
  1 tablespoon chopped fresh chives
1½ teaspoons red-wine vinegar
 ¾ teaspoon chili powder
 ¼ teaspoon hot-pepper sauce
 ½ cup nonfat plain yogurt or sour cream
1½ teaspoons Dijon mustard

In a food processor, combine the chicken, garlic, chives, vinegar, chili powder, and hot-pepper sauce. Process for 12 to 15 seconds, or until finely chopped. Shape the mixture into 2"-long football-shaped logs or "fingers." Set aside.

Coat a no-stick skillet with no-stick spray and warm over medium-high heat. Add the chicken fingers and cook for 2 to 4 minutes per side, or until all sides are lightly browned and the meat is cooked through.

In a small bowl, combine the yogurt or sour cream and mustard. Serve as a dipping sauce with the chicken. For easier dipping, serve the chicken with short wooden skewers.

Makes 6 servings

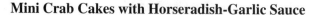

Mini Crab Cakes with Horseradish-Garlic Sauce

Standard Recipe	Fat-to-Firm Makeover
192 calories	*111 calories*
15.5 g. fat (73% of calories)	*2.5 g. fat (20% of calories)*

Crab cakes with tartar sauce can pack a hefty wallop of fat. But you can still enjoy them in this savory appetizer. The cakes are cooked in a small amount of oil rather than deep-fried. The zesty horseradish-garlic sauce easily replaces fatty tartar sauce for a total fat savings of 13 grams.

    1 tablespoon prepared horseradish
    1 tablespoon nonfat mayonnaise
    1 tablespoon chopped fresh dill
    2 cloves garlic, minced
    1 teaspoon lime juice
    ½ cup + 2 tablespoons nonfat plain yogurt
    ¼ cup fat-free egg substitute
    1 tablespoon Dijon mustard
    2 teaspoons low-sodium soy sauce
    ¼ teaspoon hot-pepper sauce
    8 ounces crabmeat, cartilage removed
    2 stalks celery, finely chopped
    ¼ cup finely chopped scallions
    1 teaspoon canola oil
       Paprika

In a small bowl, whisk together the horseradish, mayonnaise, dill, garlic, lime juice, and ½ cup of the yogurt. Set aside.

In a medium bowl, whisk together the egg substitute, mustard, soy sauce, hot-pepper sauce, and the remaining 2 tablespoons yogurt. Stir in the crabmeat, celery, and scallions. Mix well. Form the crab mixture into 16 small patties.

Warm the oil in a large no-stick skillet over medium heat. Add 8 of the patties and sprinkle each with paprika. Cook for 4 minutes. Turn the patties over, sprinkle with paprika, and cook for 4 minutes more, or until golden. Repeat with the remaining patties. Serve with the sauce.

Makes 4 servings

Onion Rings

Standard Recipe	Fat-to-Firm Makeover
225 calories	94 calories
11 g. fat (44% of calories)	2 g. fat (19% of calories)

Here's a snack-food success story. This one went out of the deep fryer and into the oven. The fat savings is 9 grams per serving. Now you can enjoy onion rings without worrying about your waistline. For best results, use large, sweet onions such as Vidalias.

2 egg whites
2 sweet onions, cut crosswise into ¼"-thick slices and
   separated into rings
2 cups crushed cornflakes
1 teaspoon chili powder

Preheat the oven to 375°F. Coat a baking sheet with no-stick spray and set aside.

In a large bowl, beat the egg whites until foamy. Add the onions and toss to coat.

In another large bowl, combine the cornflakes and chili powder. Dip the rings into the mixture until well-coated. Place the coated rings in a single layer on the prepared baking sheet. Bake for 15 minutes, or until the onions are tender and the coating is crisp.

Makes 8 servings (5 rings each)

Herbed Oven-Baked French Fries

Standard Recipe	Fat-to-Firm Makeover
352 calories	236 calories
18 g. fat (46% of calories)	2 g. fat (8% of calories)

Thought you would never eat french fries again? Try these. They're baked—not fried—and full of satisfying flavor.

   1½ teaspoons canola oil
   1 tablespoon finely chopped fresh thyme or 1 teaspoon
      dried
   ¼ teaspoon salt
   ¼ teaspoon ground black pepper
   4 baking potatoes, cut lengthwise into eighths

Preheat the oven to 400°F. Coat a large shallow baking pan with no-stick spray and set aside.

In a large bowl, combine the oil, thyme, salt, and pepper. Add the potatoes and toss to coat. Place the potatoes in a single layer in the prepared baking pan. Bake, turning occasionally, for 20 to 25 minutes, or until browned and crispy.

Makes 4 servings

Creamy Onion-Pepper Dip

Standard Recipe	Fat-to-Firm Makeover
156 calories	*100 calories*
10 g. fat (58% of calories)	*1.8 g. fat (16% of calories)*

The key to a delicious low-fat dip is switching from high-fat cream cheese and yogurt to nonfat versions. Try it with fresh-cut peppers, carrots, celery, and broccoli.

   1 red onion, chopped
   2 teaspoons olive oil
   ¾ cup drained water-packed chopped roasted red peppers
   3 ounces nonfat cream cheese
   6 tablespoons nonfat plain yogurt
   2 tablespoons fat-free Italian dressing

In a small no-stick skillet over medium-high heat, sauté the onions in the oil for 6 to 8 minutes, or until very tender.

Transfer to a food processor. Add the peppers, cream cheese, yogurt, and dressing. Process until smooth. Transfer to a serving bowl, cover, and refrigerate for at least 1 hour before serving.

Makes 8 servings

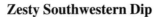

Zesty Southwestern Dip

Standard Recipe	Fat-to-Firm Makeover
137 calories	61 calories
10 g. fat (66% of calories)	0.5 g. fat (7% of calories)

You and your guests will love this traditional layered party dip. The recipe was slimmed down by replacing fatty refried beans and sour cream with black beans and nonfat yogurt cheese. Use baked tortilla chips to keep this snack at its healthiest.

1½ cups nonfat yogurt cheese (see hint)
2 tablespoons chopped fresh cilantro
1 teaspoon seeded, minced jalapeño peppers (wear plastic gloves when handling)
1 can (15 ounces) black beans, rinsed and drained
¼ cup chunky salsa
½ cup seeded, diced sweet red peppers
¼ cup sliced scallions

In a small bowl, stir together the yogurt cheese, cilantro, and jalapeño peppers. Spread in a circle on an 8" serving plate.

In another small bowl, mix the beans and salsa. Spoon over the yogurt mixture, leaving a 1" border all around.

Sprinkle with the red peppers, leaving a 1" border of the beans showing. Place the scallions in a circle in the center.

Makes 8 servings

Hint

■ *To make yogurt cheese, spoon 4 cups of nonfat plain yogurt into a colander lined with cheesecloth. Cover the colander with plastic wrap and place it over a large bowl. Refrigerate overnight to drain the liquid from the yogurt. Discard the liquid. You'll be left with about 2 cups of yogurt cheese in the colander.*

Classic Potato Salad

Standard Recipe	Fat-to-Firm Makeover
218 calories	*208 calories*
21 g. fat (87% of calories)	*2.4 g. fat (10% of calories)*

Summer wouldn't be summer without this picnic standard. While there are many international variations on potato salad, this low-fat version is distinctly American. A mixture of nonfat mayonnaise and sour cream replaces full-fat mayonnaise—and saves 18 grams of fat per serving.

2	pounds red potatoes, quartered
2	stalks celery, sliced
¾	cup nonfat sour cream
3	tablespoons nonfat mayonnaise
3	tablespoons chopped fresh parsley
1	tablespoon Dijon mustard
2	teaspoons chopped fresh dill
1	teaspoon minced garlic
¼	teaspoon ground black pepper
4	slices crisply cooked bacon, drained, patted dry, and crumbled
1	hard-boiled egg, sliced
3	tablespoons minced scallions

Place the potatoes in a large saucepan. Add cold water to cover. Bring to a boil over high heat. Reduce the heat to medium and cook for 15 minutes, or until the potatoes are easily pierced with a knife. Drain. If desired, set aside to cool.

In a large bowl, mix the celery, sour cream, mayonnaise, parsley, mustard, dill, garlic, and pepper. Add the potatoes and toss gently to coat. Top with the bacon, egg slices, and scallions. Cover and refrigerate for at least 30 minutes before serving.

Makes 8 servings

Creamy Coleslaw

Standard Recipe	Fat-to-Firm Makeover
102 calories	38 calories
8.7 g. fat (77% of calories)	0.4 g. fat (9% of calories)

For anyone who loves creamy coleslaw, this makeover is a god-send. A simple switch from regular mayo to nonfat saves more than 8 grams of fat per serving.

- ¼ cup nonfat mayonnaise
- 2 tablespoons white-wine vinegar
- 2 tablespoons water
- 1 tablespoon chopped fresh dill
- 1 teaspoon poppy seeds
- ¼ teaspoon ground black pepper
- 2 cups shredded green or red cabbage
- 1 cup diced celery
- 1 carrot, shredded

In a large bowl, whisk together the mayonnaise, vinegar, water, dill, poppy seeds, and pepper. Add the cabbage, celery, and carrots. Toss until well-combined. Cover and refrigerate for at least 1 hour before serving.

Makes 4 servings

Party Pizza

Standard Recipe	Fat-to-Firm Makeover
202 calories	149 calories
13 g. fat (58% of calories)	4 g. fat (24% of calories)

Pizza can be a healthy food if you avoid fatty toppings. Here, pizza gets a nutritious makeover with part-skim mozzarella and a topping of roasted peppers, olives, and fresh oregano.

Crust

1⅓	cups warm water (115°F)
1	package (¼ ounce) quick-rising active dry yeast
1	tablespoon olive oil
1	teaspoon salt
1	cup whole-wheat flour
2–3	cups unbleached flour
1–2	tablespoons cornmeal

Pepper Topping

1	clove garlic, minced
2	plum tomatoes, thinly sliced
1	tablespoon chopped fresh oregano
¾	cup shredded part-skim mozzarella cheese
2	sweet red, yellow, or green peppers, seeded, roasted, peeled, and cut into thin strips
¼	cup sliced black olives

To make the crust: Place the water in a large bowl. Sprinkle with the yeast and stir to combine. Set aside for 5 minutes, or until the yeast is foamy. Stir in the oil and salt. Add the whole-wheat flour. Stir in enough of the unbleached flour, ½ cup at a time, to make a soft dough.

Turn the dough out onto a lightly floured surface. Knead (adding unbleached flour as necessary) for 10 minutes, or until the dough is smooth and elastic. Cover with plastic wrap and let rest for 15 minutes.

Preheat the oven to 450°F. Coat a large baking sheet with no-stick spray, sprinkle lightly with the cornmeal, and set aside.

Using your hands, shape the dough into a 16"-round crust. Carefully transfer to the prepared baking sheet.

To make the pepper topping: Sprinkle the crust with the garlic, tomatoes, and oregano. Top with the mozzarella, peppers, and olives.

Bake on the bottom rack of the oven for 10 to 12 minutes, or until the crust is crisp and lightly browned.

Makes 8 servings

Speedy Sloppy Joes

Standard Recipe	Fat-to-Firm Makeover
484 calories	408 calories
20 g. fat (37% of calories)	8.5 g. fat (19% of calories)

Replacing some of the ground beef with ground turkey and adding lentils makes this homestyle sandwich healthy.

 1 onion, chopped
 1 green pepper, seeded and chopped
 1 clove garlic, minced
 8 ounces extra-lean ground round or sirloin
 4 ounces ground turkey breast
 1 cup low-sodium ketchup or barbecue sauce
 1 cup cooked lentils
 1 tomato, diced
 ¼ teaspoon black pepper
 8 whole-wheat kaiser rolls, split and warmed

Coat a large no-stick skillet with no-stick spray and warm over medium heat. Add the onions, green peppers, and garlic. Sauté for 5 to 10 minutes, or until the vegetables are tender.

Crumble the beef and turkey into the skillet. Cook, breaking up the meat with a wooden spoon, until browned. Drain off any juices and fat. Return the mixture to the skillet. Add the ketchup or barbecue sauce, lentils, tomatoes, and black pepper. Simmer for 15 to 20 minutes.

Serve on the rolls.

Makes 8 servings

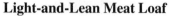

Light-and-Lean Meat Loaf

Standard Recipe	Fat-to-Firm Makeover
445 calories	*399 calories*
26 g. fat (53% of calories)	*9.4 g. (21% of calories)*

You can still enjoy meat loaf and stay thin. This version cuts the fat by replacing some of the ground beef with ground turkey. It also adds some vegetables and grains to boost the flavor and give your body the nutrients it needs.

1½	cups diced carrots
1½	cups diced onions
1	cup seeded, diced sweet red or green peppers
1	pound ground turkey
12	ounces extra-lean ground round or sirloin
1½	cups rolled oats
2	cups cooked rice
1½	cups tomato juice
½	cup fat-free egg substitute
1	teaspoon dried oregano
1	teaspoon dried thyme
½	teaspoon hot-pepper sauce
½	teaspoon ground black pepper
¼	cup ketchup
¼	cup water

Preheat the oven to 450°F. Coat two 8" × 4" loaf pans with no-stick spray and set aside.

Coat a large no-stick skillet with no-stick spray and warm over medium heat. Add the carrots, onions, and red or green peppers. Sauté for 5 to 10 minutes, or until the vegetables are tender. Transfer to a large bowl.

Crumble the turkey and beef into the bowl. Add oats and rice. Toss to mix.

In a small bowl, combine the tomato juice, egg substitute, oregano, thyme, hot-pepper sauce, and black pepper. Add to the meat mixture and mix well. Divide the mixture between the pans and pat it into place.

In a small bowl, combine the ketchup and water. Brush some over the top of each loaf.

Place the pans in the oven. Reduce the oven temperature to 350°F. Bake for 45 to 50 minutes, or until the meat is no longer pink in the center when tested with a sharp knife. (If the tops begin to brown too much, cover them with foil.)

Makes 8 servings

Italian Cheeseburgers

Standard Recipe	Fat-to-Firm Makeover
359 calories	*290 calories*
19.8 g. fat (50% of calories)	*6.4 g. fat (20% of calories)*

All you need for a healthy cheeseburger is some part-skim mozzarella cheese and extra-lean ground beef. This version gives you the taste you crave without all the fat and calories.

    1   pound extra-lean ground round or sirloin
    ¼   cup finely chopped onions
    ¼   cup seeded, finely chopped sweet red or green peppers
    ½   teaspoon dried basil
    ½   teaspoon dried oregano
    1   clove garlic, minced
    ¼   teaspoon ground black pepper
    1   can (14½ ounces) low-sodium stewed tomatoes
    8   thick slices Italian bread, toasted
    ¼   cup shredded part-skim mozzarella cheese

In a medium bowl, mix together the beef, onions, red or green peppers, basil, oregano, garlic, and black pepper. Shape into 4 burgers.

Coat a no-stick skillet with no-stick spray and warm over medium-high heat. Add the burgers and cook for 2 to 4 minutes per side, or until browned on both sides. Reduce the heat to medium, add the tomatoes, and cook for 10 minutes.

Place each burger on a toast slice and top with 1 tablespoon mozzarella, an equal amount of tomatoes, and another toast slice.

Makes 4 servings

Creamy Macaroni and Cheese

Standard Recipe	Fat-to-Firm Makeover
813 calories	*485 calories*
47.7 g. fat (53% of calories)	*9.1 g. fat (17% of calories)*

Here is the quintessential comfort food. It has a reputation as a high-fat food, but low-fat dairy products put it back on the healthy menu. This creamy and delicious version has 38 grams less fat than the original.

- 2 cups elbow macaroni
- 1 cup nonfat cottage cheese
- ¾ cup nonfat sour cream
- ⅓ cup skim milk
- 1 egg white, lightly beaten
- 4 ounces shredded reduced-fat Cheddar cheese
- 4 ounces shredded reduced-fat Monterey Jack cheese
- ¼ cup chopped onions
- 1 tablespoon light margarine or butter, melted
- 1 tablespoon cheese-flavored sprinkles
- 1 teaspoon dry mustard
- ¼ teaspoon ground black pepper
  Pinch of ground red pepper
- 2 tablespoons reduced-fat butter-flavored crackers, crumbled
- ½ teaspoon paprika

Preheat the oven 350°F. Coat a 2-quart casserole with no-stick spray and set aside.

In a large pot of boiling water, cook the macaroni according to the package directions. Drain, reserving 2 tablespoons of the cooking water. Return the macaroni to the pot.

In a large bowl, whisk together the cottage cheese, sour cream, milk, and egg white until well-blended. Stir in the Cheddar, Monterey Jack, onions, margarine or butter, cheese-flavored sprinkles, mustard, black pepper, red pepper, and the reserved cooking water.

Pour mixture over the macaroni and stir well. Spoon into the prepared casserole and sprinkle with the cracker crumbs and paprika.

Cover and bake for 25 minutes. Uncover and bake for 5 minutes, or until golden brown and bubbly.

Makes 4 servings

Quick Turkey and Stuffing

Standard Recipe	Fat-to-Firm Makeover
549 calories	*338 calories*
28.3 g. fat (46% of calories)	*6.1 g. fat (16% of calories)*

Bet you never guessed turkey was high in fat. Well, it isn't—until you pair it with the typical stuffing, which adds 26 grams of fat per serving. This unique twist on turkey and stuffing cuts the fat down to just 6 grams per serving. Plus, it cooks quickly on the stovetop instead of slowly in the oven.

    2 teaspoons margarine or butter
    1 pound turkey tenderloin
 1¾ cups water
    1 package (6 ounces) cornbread stuffing with seasoning
          mix
  ½ cup whole cranberry sauce

In a large no-stick skillet, melt the margarine or butter over medium heat. Add the turkey and brown on all sides. Transfer to a plate.

Add the water and seasoning mix from the stuffing to the skillet. Bring to a boil. Return the turkey to the skillet. Cover and cook over medium-low heat for 20 minutes, or until the turkey is no longer pink in the center when tested with a sharp knife.

Sprinkle the stuffing crumbs into the liquid around the turkey. Reduce the heat to low, cover, and cook for 5 minutes, or until the liquid is absorbed. Slice the turkey and serve with the stuffing and the cranberry sauce.

Makes 4 servings

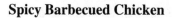

Spicy Barbecued Chicken

Standard Recipe	Fat-to-Firm Makeover
536 calories	*174 calories*
29 g. fat (49% of calories)	*1.6 g. fat (8% of calories)*

Barbecued chicken is as American as apple pie. And you don't have to give it up to stay trim. Boneless, skinless chicken breasts and a fat-free barbecue sauce update this American classic for today's healthy lifestyles. Because the barbecue sauce doesn't come into contact with uncooked chicken, you can use it as a sauce at the table.

¼ cup chili sauce
2 tablespoons low-sodium ketchup
1 tablespoon honey
1 tablespoon red-wine vinegar
1 teaspoon ground ginger
1 teaspoon Dijon mustard
¾ teaspoon ground black pepper
1 clove garlic, minced
¼ teaspoon ground red pepper
1 pound boneless, skinless chicken breasts

Coat a grill rack with no-stick spray. Light the grill according to the manufacturer's instructions. Place the rack on the grill.

Meanwhile, in a small saucepan, combine the chili sauce, ketchup, honey, vinegar, ginger, mustard, black pepper, garlic, and red pepper. Bring the mixture to a boil. Remove from the heat and set aside.

Place the chicken on the preheated grill rack. Grill, uncovered, for 10 minutes. Turn the chicken over and brush the cooked side with the sauce. Grill for 5 to 10 minutes, or until the chicken is no longer pink in the center when tested with a sharp knife. Brush generously with the remaining sauce before serving.

Makes 4 servings

Chicken Parmesan

Standard Recipe	Fat-to-Firm Makeover
529 calories	149 calories
23 g. fat (39% of calories)	2.8 g. fat (17% of calories)

A thick, gooey layer of melted mozzarella cheese is the hallmark of most Parmesan dishes. Here, a slightly thinner layer of reduced-fat mozzarella tops pan-seared herb-crusted chicken. Fat savings for you? A cool 20 grams.

> 2 tablespoons unbleached flour
> 2 tablespoons cornmeal
> 1 tablespoon chopped fresh parsley
> ½ teaspoon dried oregano
> ½ teaspoon dried basil
> ¼ teaspoon ground black pepper
> 4 boneless, skinless chicken breast halves (4 ounces each)
> 2 cans (8 ounces each) no-salt-added tomato sauce
> ¾ cup shredded reduced-fat mozzarella cheese
> 2 tablespoons grated Parmesan cheese

Preheat oven to 350°F. In a shallow bowl, combine the flour, cornmeal, parsley, oregano, basil, and pepper. Dip the chicken into the mixture to coat. Shake off any excess.

Coat a no-stick skillet with no-stick spray and warm over medium-high heat. Add the chicken and brown for 3 minutes per side.

Spread ½ cup of the tomato sauce across the bottom of an 11" x 7" baking dish. Top with the chicken and pour the remaining tomato sauce over the chicken. Sprinkle with mozzarella and Parmesan. Bake for 20 minutes, or until the cheese is melted and the chicken is cooked through when tested with a sharp knife.

Makes 4 servings

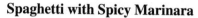

Spaghetti with Spicy Marinara

Standard Recipe	Fat-to-Firm Makeover
365 calories	*308 calories*
11 g. fat (27% of calories)	*3.7 g. fat (11% of calories)*

This pasta dish gets its rich, intense flavor from sun-dried tomatoes and garlic. A reduced amount of olive oil cuts the fat way down.

- 2 teaspoons olive oil
- 1 onion, chopped
- 3 cloves garlic, minced
- 1 jalapeño pepper, seeded and chopped (wear plastic gloves when handling)
- ½ teaspoon dried basil
- ½ teaspoon crushed red-pepper flakes
- ¼ teaspoon dried thyme
- ¼ teaspoon ground black pepper
- 1 bay leaf
- ¾ ounce dry-pack sun-dried tomatoes, finely chopped
- 1 can (28 ounces) crushed tomatoes
- 1½ tablespoons no-salt-added tomato paste
- 8 ounces spaghetti

Warm the oil in a large no-stick skillet over medium-high heat. Add the onions, garlic, jalapeño peppers, basil, red-pepper flakes, thyme, black pepper, and bay leaf. Sauté for 2 minutes. Reduce the heat to medium low, cover, and cook, stirring often, for 10 minutes, or until the onions are very tender.

Stir in the sun-dried tomatoes, crushed tomatoes, and tomato paste. Bring to a boil over high heat. Reduce the heat to medium low, cover, and simmer, stirring occasionally, for 15 minutes. Uncover and simmer for 10 minutes, or until the sauce is slightly thickened.

Meanwhile, in a large pot of boiling water, cook the spaghetti according to the package directions. Drain and return to the pot. Remove the bay leaf from the sauce and discard it, then add the sauce to the spaghetti and toss to coat.

Makes 4 servings

Fettuccine Alfredo

Standard Recipe	Fat-to-Firm Makeover
644 calories	398 calories
44 g. fat (62% of calories)	4.7 g. fat (11% of calories)

Trimmed of fat and brimming with flavor, this classic creamy dish is ready to eat in less than 20 minutes. Evaporated skim milk and nonfat sour cream replace the heavy cream in the original recipe—with a total fat savings of 39 grams. For best results, stir the sauce constantly as it cooks.

    1   pound fettuccine
    2   teaspoons olive oil
    1   can (12 ounces) evaporated skim milk
    ½   cup nonfat sour cream
    6   tablespoons grated Parmesan cheese
    2   tablespoons chopped fresh parsley
    ½   teaspoon dried basil
        Pinch of crushed red-pepper flakes
        Pinch of ground black pepper
    2   cloves garlic, minced

In a large pot of boiling water, cook the fettuccine according to the package directions. Drain and return to the pot. Add the oil and toss to coat.

In a medium bowl, whisk together the milk and sour cream until smooth. Add the Parmesan, parsley, basil, red-pepper flakes, black pepper, and garlic. Mix well. Pour over the fettuccine in the large pot.

Cook over low heat, stirring constantly, just until thick and bubbling.

Makes 6 servings

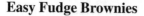

Easy Fudge Brownies

Standard Recipe	Fat-to-Firm Makeover
135 calories	*92 calories*
8 g. fat (53% of calories)	*2.1 g. fat (21% of calories)*

The calories and fat in these rich, chocolaty brownies come down with small adjustments to the eggs, sugar, and butter.

1½ cups sugar
⅓ cup margarine or butter
¼ cup buttermilk
¾ cup Dutch-process cocoa
1¼ cups unbleached flour
¼ teaspoon baking soda
2 eggs
2 teaspoons vanilla

Preheat the oven to 350°F. Coat a 13" × 9" baking dish with no-stick spray and set aside.

In a medium saucepan, combine the sugar, margarine or butter, and buttermilk. Stir over medium heat until the sugar is dissolved. Remove from the heat. Stir in the cocoa. Set aside for 10 minutes to cool.

In a small bowl, whisk together the flour and baking soda.

Add the eggs, one at a time, to the cooled cocoa mixture, stirring well after each addition. Stir in the vanilla, then stir in the flour mixture. Pour the batter into the prepared baking dish.

Bake for 18 to 20 minutes, or until a toothpick inserted in the center comes out almost clean. (Do not over bake.) Cool in the pan on a wire rack.

Makes 24

Hint

■ *For a low-fat cream cheese frosting, beat together until smooth: 3 ounces softened low-fat cream cheese, 3 ounces softened nonfat cream cheese, 1 cup confectioners' sugar, and 2 tablespoons skim milk. Spread over the cooled brownies.*

Apple Crisp à la Mode

Standard Recipe	Fat-to-Firm Makeover
443 calories	*262 calories*
11 g. fat (22% of calories)	*0.5 g. fat (2% of calories)*

Tender cooked apples and a sweet, crisp topping make an unbeatable warm dessert. Plus, this version of the all-American favorite has less than 1 gram of fat per serving (including the frozen yogurt or ice cream).

    4 cups peeled and thinly sliced Granny Smith apples
    3 tablespoons packed light brown sugar
    ¼ teaspoon ground nutmeg
    ½ cup unbleached flour
    ⅓ cup sugar
    ½ teaspoon baking powder
    ¼ teaspoon ground cinnamon
    2 tablespoons fat-free egg substitute
    1 cup nonfat vanilla frozen yogurt or ice cream

Preheat the oven to 400°F. Coat an 8" × 8" baking dish with no-stick spray.

Place the apples in the baking dish. Sprinkle with the brown sugar and nutmeg, and toss lightly. Spread the apples evenly over the bottom of the baking dish.

In a small bowl, whisk together the flour, sugar, baking powder, and cinnamon. Add the egg substitute and mix with a fork until crumbly. Sprinkle the crumb mixture evenly over the apples.

Bake for 30 minutes, or until the apples are tender and the topping is browned. Serve warm with the frozen yogurt or ice cream.

Makes 4 servings

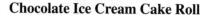

Chocolate Ice Cream Cake Roll

Standard Recipe	Fat-to-Firm Makeover
281 calories	*213 calories*
10 g. fat (32% of calories)	*0.3 g. fat (1% of calories)*

This dessert is perfect for birthday parties, holidays, or other special occasions and ultra-simple to prepare.

 1 tablespoon + ¼ cup cocoa
 1 package (1 pound) angel food cake mix (see hint)
 2 tablespoons water
 1 quart nonfat chocolate, vanilla, strawberry, or raspberry
 ice cream, softened

Preheat the oven to 350°F. Coat a 15" × 10" jelly-roll pan with no-stick spray. Line it with a large piece of wax paper, pressing the paper into the corners.

Sprinkle a tea towel with 1 tablespoon of the cocoa. Set aside.

Empty the cake mix into a large bowl. Stir in the remaining ¼ cup cocoa and mix well. Prepare the cake according to the package directions, adding an additional 2 tablespoons water. Spread the batter evenly in the prepared pan. Bake for 15 to 20 minutes, or until the top springs back when lightly touched.

Immediately loosen the edges of the cake and turn it out onto the prepared towel. Carefully remove the wax paper. Starting from one long side, roll up the cake with the towel. Cool on a wire rack.

Unroll the cake. Spread with the ice cream to within ½" of the edges. Reroll the cake without the towel. Wrap in plastic and freeze for at least 4 hours, or until ready to serve.

Makes 12 slices

Hint

■ *For this recipe, buy "just add water" angel food cake mix. We've added an additional 2 tablespoons water to help absorb the cocoa that's stirred into the mix.*

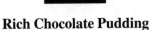

Rich Chocolate Pudding

Standard Recipe	Fat-to-Firm Makeover
192 calories	129 calories
6.2 g. fat (29% of calories)	3.7 g. fat (26% of calories)

Here's a creamy dessert that tastes decadent on the lips but won't cling to your hips. For an even slimmer pudding, replace the low-fat milk with skim milk.

2 cups 1% low-fat milk
2 tablespoons sugar
1 tablespoon cornstarch
1 tablespoon cocoa
1 square (1 ounce) semisweet chocolate, finely chopped
1 teaspoon vanilla
1 banana (optional)
6 strawberries (optional)
1 cup nonfat whipped topping (optional)

In a medium saucepan, whisk together the milk, sugar, cornstarch, and cocoa until well-blended. Whisk over medium heat until the mixture just comes to a boil.

Remove the saucepan from the heat; stir in the chocolate. Over low heat, slowly bring the mixture to a boil, stirring constantly. Boil for 2 minutes. Stir in the vanilla.

Spoon the pudding into four 6-ounce dessert glasses or custard cups. Cover with plastic wrap (be sure the plastic touches the surface of the pudding to prevent a skin from forming). Refrigerate for at least 3 hours, or until well-chilled.

If desired, serve garnished with sliced bananas and strawberries and whipped topping.

Makes 4 servings

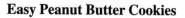

Easy Peanut Butter Cookies

Standard Recipe	Fat-to-Firm Makeover
245 calories	*45 calories*
14 g. fat (51% of calories)	*1.5 g. fat (30% of calories)*

These cookies are so easy to make, it's kids' stuff. And they have only a fraction of the fat that the original ones had. Keep the cookies on hand for a quick low-fat snack.

  1 can (14 ounces) low-fat sweetened condensed milk
¾ cup reduced-fat peanut butter
¼ cup fat-free egg substitute
  1 teaspoon vanilla
2¼ cups reduced-fat biscuit mix
¼ cup sugar

In a large bowl, combine the milk, peanut butter, egg substitute, and vanilla. Using a mixer at low speed, beat the mixture until smooth. Add the biscuit mix and mix well. Cover and chill for at least 3 hours.

Preheat the oven to 350°F. Coat two large baking sheets with no-stick spray. Drop teaspoonfuls of the dough onto the baking sheets, leaving 1" between mounds. Sprinkle the cookies evenly with the sugar. Bake for 6 to 8 minutes, or until lightly browned. Remove from the baking sheets and cool on wire racks.

Makes about 60

Hint

■ *To make the classic look of peanut butter cookies, slightly flatten each cookie with a fork before baking.*

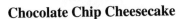

Chocolate Chip Cheesecake

Standard Recipe	Fat-to-Firm Makeover
427 calories	*179 calories*
30 g. fat (63% of calories)	*6.9 g. fat (35% of calories)*

Chocolate-lovers can replace the graham crackers with re-duced-fat chocolate wafer cookies or chocolate graham crackers.

2 cups graham cracker crumbs
¼ cup seedless raspberry jam, melted
3 tablespoons sugar
1 package (8 ounces) nonfat cream cheese, softened
1 package (8 ounces) low-fat cream cheese, softened
1 can (14 ounces) low-fat sweetened condensed milk
4 egg whites
1 egg
2 teaspoons vanilla
¾ cup mini semisweet chocolate chips
1 teaspoon unbleached flour

Preheat the oven to 325°F. Coat a 9" springform pan with no-stick spray. Set the pan on a large square of aluminum foil and wrap the foil securely around the bottom and up the sides of the pan.

In a small bowl, mix the crumbs, jam, and sugar. Press the mixture evenly in the bottom of the prepared pan.

In a medium bowl, using a mixer at medium speed, beat the nonfat cream cheese and low-fat cream cheese until light and fluffy. Add the milk, egg whites, egg, and vanilla. Beat until smooth.

In a small bowl, toss ½ cup of the chocolate chips with the flour. Fold into the batter. Pour the batter over the crust in the pan. Sprinkle with the remaining ¼ cup chocolate chips.

Place the springform pan in a large baking pan on the middle oven rack. Pour 1" of hot water into the larger pan. Bake for 50 to 55 minutes, or until the edges of the cake are lightly golden and a knife inserted into the center comes out clean. Remove the pan from the hot water. Cool in the pan on a wire rack for 30 minutes. Refrigerate overnight before slicing.

Makes 16 servings

Chapter 28

Free Yourself from the Salad Trap

A few dollops of fatty salad dressing can derail weight loss. Try these low-fat (and high-yum) versions—they're a salad-lover's best friend.

Salad—one of the best slimming foods around. Brimming with low-fat, high-fiber vegetables, plus lean protein and other goodies, it's one bowlful of goodness that's guaranteed to take you from fat to firm. Until you pour on a salad dressing loaded with cheese, oil, mayonnaise, or sour cream. The way you dress your salad can bring the calorie and fat count to that of a bowl of premium ice cream.

If you've fallen into the salad-dressing snare, you're not alone. Researchers have revealed that innocent-looking salad dressing is the biggest source of fat in many women's diets—ranking ahead of fat-laden red-alert foods like meat and cheese.

Nutrition experts say that by switching to low-fat dressings, your weight-loss efforts are far more likely to succeed. So the Fat-to-Firm Program devotes an entire recipe section to low-fat salad dressings because just using these recipes on your salads could make all the difference in shedding pounds. Don't be surprised if you love your salads even more with these super-tasty concoctions. Nutrition experts consulted for the Fat-to-Firm Program replaced all the fatty ingredients with other savory flavors: delicious flavored vinegars; reduced-fat mayonnaise; wonderful, zero-calorie herbs; nonfat yogurt; Dijon mustard; buttermilk. And the calorie savings are as fantastic as the taste. The Russian dressing, for example, has no calories from fat. So enjoy—and don't worry about an extra tablespoon or two.

Nutritional analysis for all recipes is per tablespoon.

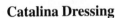

Catalina Dressing

Standard Recipe	Fat-to-Firm Makeover
67 calories	14 calories
6.4 g. fat (86% of calories)	0 g. fat (0% of calories)

This zesty dressing makes low-fat living easy. Cider vinegar, ketchup, sweeteners, and spices are quickly thickened with unflavored gelatin. It's perfect for almost any salad.

½ cup water
½ teaspoon unflavored gelatin
3 tablespoons apple cider vinegar
2 tablespoons ketchup
2 tablespoons corn syrup
1 tablespoon honey
⅛ teaspoon garlic powder
   Pinch of onion powder
   Pinch of ground red pepper
   Pinch of paprika

Place the water in a small saucepan. Sprinkle with the gelatin and allow to stand for 3 minutes to soften the gelatin. Stir over medium heat until the gelatin dissolves. Remove from the heat. Whisk in the vinegar, ketchup, corn syrup, honey, garlic powder, onion powder, red pepper, and paprika. Pour into a jar with a tight-fitting lid. Cover and refrigerate until serving time, or up to one week. Shake well before serving.

Makes 1 cup

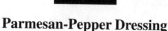

Parmesan-Pepper Dressing

Standard Recipe	Fat-to-Firm Makeover
38 calories	13 calories
3.5 g. fat (83% of calories)	0.4 g. fat (28% of calories)

Cottage cheese and buttermilk replace the fatty sour cream in this popular dressing. White-wine vinegar lends extra zip and flavor.

- ⅔ cup dry-curd or 1% low-fat cottage cheese
- ⅓ cup buttermilk
- 1 tablespoon white-wine vinegar
- 2 tablespoons grated Parmesan cheese
- 1 teaspoon ground black pepper

In a food processor or blender, puree the cottage cheese until smooth. With the machine running, pour in the buttermilk and vinegar. Process until smooth. Add the Parmesan and pepper. Process using on/off turns until just combined. Transfer to a small bowl. Cover and refrigerate until serving time, or up to three days.

Makes 1 cup

Creamy Buttermilk Dressing

Standard Recipe	Fat-to-Firm Makeover
58 calories	11 calories
5 g. fat (78% of calories)	0.5 g. fat (41% of calories)

This delicious dressing adds flavor to any salad without blowing your fat budget. Buttermilk and nonfat mayonnaise replace the full-fat mayonnaise in the original.

- ¾ cup buttermilk
- ¼ cup nonfat mayonnaise
- 2 tablespoons lemon juice
- 1 tablespoon olive oil

  2 tablespoons minced scallion tops or chopped chives
  1 tablespoon minced fresh tarragon
  ½ teaspoon ground black pepper

In a small bowl, whisk together the buttermilk, mayonnaise, lemon juice, and oil. Stir in the scallions or chives, tarragon, and pepper. Cover and refrigerate until serving time, or up to three days.

Makes 1 ¼ cups

Ranch Dressing

Standard Recipe	Fat-to-Firm Makeover
55 calories	*15 calories*
5.5 g. fat (90% of calories)	*0.4 g. fat (24% of calories)*

Most ranch dressings get their richness from fatty mayonnaise. This trimmed-down version gets full-bodied flavor from a combination of nonfat plain yogurt, low-fat mayonnaise, and tarragon vinegar.

  ¾ cup nonfat plain yogurt
  ½ cup low-fat mayonnaise
  2 tablespoons tarragon vinegar
  1 tablespoon minced onions
  2 teaspoons minced fresh parsley
  ¼ teaspoon celery seeds
  ¼ teaspoon Dijon mustard
  ⅛ teaspoon garlic powder

In a small bowl, whisk together the yogurt, mayonnaise, vinegar, onions, parsley, celery seeds, mustard, and garlic powder. Cover and refrigerate until serving time, or up to three days.

Makes 1 ¼ cups

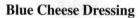

Blue Cheese Dressing

Standard Recipe	Fat-to-Firm Makeover
78 calories	*9 calories*
8 g. fat (92% of calories)	*0.3 g. fat (30% of calories)*

A little real blue cheese goes a long way in this high-flavor dressing. In fact, the blue cheese flavor is more pronounced than in most commercial dressings. Nonfat cottage cheese replaces regular mayonnaise for a fat savings of more than 7 grams per tablespoon.

 1 cup nonfat cottage cheese
 2 tablespoons crumbled blue cheese
 2 tablespoons skim milk
 1 clove garlic, minced

In a food processor or blender, process the cottage cheese, blue cheese, milk, and garlic using on/off turns until the mixture is slightly chunky. Transfer to a small bowl. Cover and refrigerate until serving time, or up to three days.

Makes 1 cup

Russian Dressing

Standard Recipe	Fat-to-Firm Makeover
76 calories	*9 calories*
8 g. fat (95% of calories)	*0 g. fat (0% of calories)*

Nonfat ingredients make this dressing a fat-fighter's dream. And the taste? It's great! The additional horseradish adds just the right zip.

 1 cup nonfat mayonnaise
 ½ cup nonfat plain yogurt
 ½ cup ketchup
 2 tablespoons prepared horseradish, drained

In a small bowl, whisk together the mayonnaise, yogurt, ketchup, and horseradish. Cover and refrigerate until serving time, or up to three days.

Makes 2 cups

Tomato Vinaigrette

Standard Recipe	Fat-to-Firm Makeover
70 calories	5 calories
7.8 g. fat (100% of calories)	0.2 g. fat (36% of calories)

Here's a tantalizing oil-free tomato vinaigrette flavored with white-wine vinegar, basil, thyme, and Dijon mustard. Eliminating the oil saves more than 7 grams of fat per tablespoon of dressing.

    1   cup peeled and chopped tomatoes
    ¼   cup white-wine vinegar
    1   teaspoon dried basil
    1   teaspoon dried thyme
    1   teaspoon Dijon mustard

In a food processor or blender, process the tomatoes, vinegar, basil, thyme, and mustard until well-combined. Transfer to a jar with a tight-fitting lid. Cover and refrigerate until serving time, or up to two days. Shake well before serving.

Makes ⅔ cup

Balsamic Vinaigrette

Standard Recipe	Fat-to-Firm Makeover
70 calories	*9 calories*
7.8 g. fat (100% of calories)	*0.1 g. fat (10% of calories)*

Balsamic vinegar is now readily available in most supermarkets. Here, it's mixed with defatted chicken broth, ketchup, and seasonings for an irresistibly rich dressing. These ingredients re-place the olive oil found in the original recipe.

½ cup defatted chicken broth
¼ cup balsamic vinegar
2 tablespoons ketchup
2 tablespoons Dijon mustard
½ teaspoon dried savory
½ teaspoon dried thyme
¼ teaspoon ground red pepper

In a small jar with a tight-fitting lid, combine the broth, vinegar, ketchup, mustard, savory, thyme, and pepper. Cover and shake until well-combined. Refrigerate until serving time, or up to one week. Shake well before serving.

Makes 1 cup

Lemon Vinaigrette

Standard Recipe	Fat-to-Firm Makeover
70 calories	*8 calories*
7.8 g. fat (100% of calories)	*0.5 g. fat (56% of calories)*

Here's a light and tangy dressing tailor-made for a quick salad. Defatted chicken broth replaces most of the oil. Shallots, parsley, thyme, and garlic give the dressing its savory flavor.

¼ cup lemon juice
¼ cup defatted chicken broth
2 tablespoons minced shallots
1¼ teaspoons olive oil
1 tablespoon minced fresh parsley
1 teaspoon minced fresh thyme
1 clove garlic, minced

In a jar with a tight-fitting lid, combine the lemon juice, broth, shallots, oil, parsley, thyme, and garlic. Cover and shake until well-combined. Refrigerate until serving time, or up to one week. Shake well before serving.

Makes ¾ cup

Orange Vinaigrette

Standard Recipe	Fat-to-Firm Makeover
70 calories	14 calories
7.8 g. fat (100% of calories)	0.1 g. fat (6% of calories)

You'll love this vinaigrette on spinach salad. Or try it on fruit salads. Orange juice and balsamic vinegar replace the olive oil found in the original.

½ cup orange juice
¼ cup balsamic vinegar
2 tablespoons Dijon mustard
4 teaspoons honey
¼ teaspoon cracked black pepper

In a jar with a tight-fitting lid, combine the orange juice, vinegar, mustard, honey, and pepper. Cover and shake until well-combined. Refrigerate until serving time, or up to one week. Shake well before serving.

Makes 1 cup

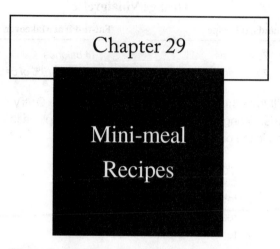

Chapter 29

Mini-meal Recipes

There's nothing "mini" about the taste, nutrition, and stomach-satisfying gusto of these low-fat treats.

Mini-meals—eating four to eight smaller meals every day rather than the typical three squares—is one of the best eating styles offered by the Fat-to-Firm Program. You're never hungry. And because you don't go hours without eating, your body switches to a higher metabolic rate. This means that you're eating the same amount of food as before but burning *more* calories. (There's nothing "mini" about that.) But the key to this style of eating is to make your mini-meals tasty, fun, varied, and low-fat. And that's what these recipes are all about. You'll find bagels, pizza, potato skins, chicken salad—all super-filling but still super-low in calories and fat. So go ahead, eat six times a day. You have nothing to lose but your weight.

For all recipes, nutritional analysis is per serving. Most recipes serve two people. So make sure to share them with your family to keep your portion mini. Or split the dish in half, eating part of it for your meal and part of it another time. Though we have given you serving sizes, use your stomach as a guide: Always stop when you're full.

Morning Recipes

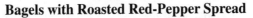

Bagels with Roasted Red-Pepper Spread

Standard Recipe	Fat-to-Firm Makeover
359 calories	*276 calories*
21 g. fat (53% of calories)	*4 g. fat (13% of calories)*

Bagels are healthy, right? They are until you spread the typical 2 tablespoons cream cheese on each bagel half. Then this innocent breakfast packs more than 350 calories and 21 grams of fat. Here's a better alternative, packed with the rich flavor of roasted red peppers. Grab one of these sandwiches on your way to work for a filling and nutritious breakfast.

    ½ cup water-packed roasted red peppers, well-drained
    ¼ cup nonfat cream cheese, softened
    ¼ cup low-fat cream cheese, softened
    ¼ teaspoon dried oregano
    ⅛ teaspoon garlic powder
    2 whole-grain bagels, split and toasted
    2 tablespoons alfalfa sprouts (optional)

In a mini food processor, puree the peppers, nonfat cream cheese, low-fat cream cheese, oregano, and garlic powder until smooth.

Spread the bottom half of each bagel with 2 tablespoons of the mixture. Add the sprouts (if using) and bagel tops.

Makes 2 servings

Hints

▪ *The spread can be made ahead and refrigerated in an airtight container for up to four days.*

▪ *To take it along, pack the spread in an airtight container. Pack the sprouts and untoasted bagels in separate resealable plastic bags. Refrigerate the spread and sprouts. At mealtime, toast the bagels and spread with the cream cheese mixture; add the sprouts.*

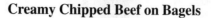

Creamy Chipped Beef on Bagels

Standard Recipe	Fat-to-Firm Makeover
352 calories	*321 calories*
14 g. fat (36% of calories)	*8.3 g. fat (23% of calories)*

Creamed chipped beef is a down-home classic. A combination of light cream cheese and nonfat sour cream brings down the fat so that you can enjoy it once again.

- 3 ounces low-fat cream cheese
- 1 tablespoon nonfat sour cream
- ¼ cup chipped dried beef
- 2 plain bagels, split and toasted

Place the cream cheese and sour cream in a medium bowl. Using a mixer on medium speed, beat until fluffy. Stir in the beef.

Spread the bottom half of each bagel with 2 tablespoons of the mixture. Add the bagel tops.

Makes 2 servings

Hints

- *The spread can be made ahead and refrigerated in an airtight container for up to one week.*
- *For breakfast on the run, grab one of these bagel sandwiches and a napkin as you head out the door.*
- *To eat these bagel sandwiches later in the day, pack the spread in an airtight container. Pack untoasted bagels in a resealable plastic bag. Refrigerate the spread. At mealtime, toast the bagels and spread them with the cream cheese mixture.*

Easy Fruit Salad

Standard Recipe	Fat-to-Firm Makeover
246 calories	*119 calories*
11.9 g. fat (44% of calories)	*0.7 g. fat (5% of calories)*

Fruit salad is one of the healthiest snacks. To keep it low in fat, just avoid things like shredded coconut and nuts. Here, assorted fruits and citrus juice deliver a bowlful of flavor—without the fat. Feel free to vary the fruit according to your taste and what's in season.

$\frac{1}{2}$ cup sliced bananas
2 teaspoons orange juice
1 tangerine, sectioned
$\frac{1}{2}$ cup chopped Golden or Red Delicious apples
$\frac{1}{2}$ cup seedless red or green grapes
$\frac{1}{4}$ teaspoon grated lemon rind
Pinch of grated nutmeg

In a medium bowl, combine the bananas and orange juice. Toss to coat the bananas. Add the tangerines, apples, grapes, lemon rind, and nutmeg. Toss gently.

Cover and refrigerate for at least 20 minutes, to allow the flavors to blend.

Makes 2 servings

Hint
▪ *This fruit salad makes a great midmorning pick-me-up. To take it along, assemble the salad in the morning and pack it in an airtight container. Refrigerate until needed.*

Afternoon Recipes

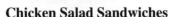

Chicken Salad Sandwiches

Standard Recipe	Fat-to-Firm Makeover
506 calories	*352 calories*
24 g. fat (43% of calories)	*6.9 g. fat (18% of calories)*

Mayonnaise is the fat culprit in most chicken salads. Switching to low-fat mayonnaise saves 17 grams of fat per serving. Grapes, raisins, and toasted walnuts give the sandwich delightful crunch and bright flavor.

      1 cup cubed cooked chicken
    ¼ cup low-fat mayonnaise
      2 tablespoons chopped toasted walnuts
      1 tablespoon raisins
      1 tablespoon small seedless grapes
      1 teaspoon warmed honey
      2 pita breads, split
    ½ cup shredded lettuce

In a medium bowl, combine the chicken, mayonnaise, walnuts, raisins, grapes, and honey. Stir well.

Line each pita with equal amounts of the lettuce. Top with the chicken salad.

Makes 2

Hint
■ *To take it along, pack the chicken salad in an airtight container. Pack the pita breads and lettuce in separate resealable plastic bags. Refrigerate the salad and lettuce until mealtime, then assemble the sandwiches.*

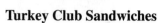

Turkey Club Sandwiches

Standard Recipe	Fat-to-Firm Makeover
310 calories	*251 calories*
13.4 g. fat (39% of calories)	*5.5 g. fat (20% of calories)*

Does bacon belong on a healthy menu? It does if it's Canadian bacon. Canadian bacon has only 2 grams of total fat per ounce, while regular bacon has 14 grams. These turkey club sandwiches contain nearly 8 grams less fat than traditional turkey clubs. Dig in!

4 slices whole-wheat bread, toasted
2 tablespoons nonfat mayonnaise
2 slices Canadian bacon
2 ounces cooked turkey breast, thinly sliced
4 tomato slices
4 lettuce leaves, torn

Spread the mayonnaise on the bread. Divide the Canadian bacon, turkey, tomatoes, and lettuce between two of the slices. Top with the remaining bread slices.

Makes 2

Hint

■ *These sandwiches can be made in the morning and packed in a resealable plastic bag. Refrigerate until mealtime.*

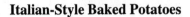

Italian-Style Baked Potatoes

Standard Recipe	Fat-to-Firm Makeover
294 calories	*273 calories*
6.3 g. fat (19% of calories)	*0.9 g. fat (3% of calories)*

Here's a baked potato topper that won't leave you missing the sour cream. Low-fat cottage cheese provides the same tangy flavor with much less fat. If you want the smooth texture of sour cream, puree the cottage cheese in a food processor for a couple of minutes.

> 2 hot baked potatoes
> ½ cup 1% low-fat cottage cheese
> ½ cup chopped tomatoes
> 2 tablespoons chopped fresh basil
> ¼ teaspoon ground black pepper

Using a kitchen towel to protect your hands from the heat, gently roll the potatoes on a countertop to crumble the flesh inside. Cut a long slit in the top of each potato and push the sides to open the center. Divide the cottage cheese, tomatoes, and basil between the potatoes. Sprinkle with the pepper.

Makes 2

Hints

■ *To bake the potatoes, place in a 400°F oven for about 1 hour or microwave for about 7 minutes.*

■ *To take it along, cool the potatoes to room temperature and pack in a resealable plastic bag. Pack the tomatoes and basil together in another bag. Pack the cottage cheese in an airtight container. Refrigerate all until mealtime. Microwave each potato on high for 2 minutes, or until heated through. Add the toppings.*

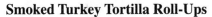

Smoked Turkey Tortilla Roll-Ups

Standard Recipe	Fat-to-Firm Makeover
289 calories	*232 calories*
11.2 g. fat (35% of calories)	*6.3 g. fat (24% of calories)*

These quick roll-ups make a great alternative to the traditional turkey sandwich. Just roll them and go. Low-fat cream cheese replaces mayonnaise for substantial fat savings.

2 flour tortillas (8" diameter)
2 tablespoons low-fat cream cheese
½ teaspoon dried dill
4 ounces smoked turkey breast, sliced
¼ cup alfalfa sprouts or shredded lettuce

Lay the tortillas flat on a work surface. Spread with the cream cheese and sprinkle with the dill. Add the turkey and top with the sprouts or lettuce. Roll up each tortilla.

Makes 2

Hint
- *To eat later, wrap the rolls in plastic and refrigerate for up to two days.*

Greek Salad

Standard Recipe	Fat-to-Firm Makeover
272 calories	*218 calories*
12.6 g. fat (42% of calories)	*7 g. fat (29% of calories)*

Low-fat Greek salad is easy to achieve. Reduce the oil in the dressing, omit the olives, and use diced toast instead of butter-drenched croutons.

        1 tomato, quartered
        1 small cucumber, halved lengthwise and sliced $\frac{1}{4}$" thick
        1 small sweet red pepper, seeded and diced
      $\frac{1}{2}$ small onion, sliced crosswise and separated into rings
        1 tablespoon crumbled feta cheese
    $2\frac{1}{2}$ tablespoons lemon juice
    $1\frac{1}{2}$ teaspoons olive oil
      $\frac{1}{2}$ teaspoon dried oregano
        1 small clove garlic, minced
        2 slices Italian bread, toasted and diced

In a medium bowl, combine the tomatoes, cucumbers, peppers, onions, and feta. Toss to mix.

In a small bowl, whisk together the lemon juice, oil, oregano, and garlic. Pour over the vegetables and toss gently.

Serve the bread with the salad.

Makes 2 servings

Hint

▪ *To take the salad with you, toss the vegetables and feta, then pack them in an airtight container. Pack the dressing in a separate container. Pack the untoasted bread in a resealable plastic bag. At mealtime, toast and dice the bread and pour the dressing over the salad.*

Southwest Corn Salad

Standard Recipe	Fat-to-Firm Makeover
236 calories	*196 calories*
11.8 g. fat (45% of calories)	*2.8 g. fat (13% of calories)*

Corn salad is a great alternative to a tossed salad as long as you go easy on the corn oil. This version uses just a teaspoon. Two kinds of peppers, scallions, and cilantro jazz up the corn's mild flavor.

    2 cups frozen corn
    1 small sweet red pepper, seeded and finely chopped
    1 scallion, thinly sliced
    2 teaspoons chopped canned green chili peppers (wear
         plastic gloves when handling)
    2 teaspoons lemon juice
    1 teaspoon olive oil or corn oil
    ½ teaspoon chopped fresh cilantro
    ¼ teaspoon chili powder

In a medium saucepan over high heat, bring about 1 quart water to a boil. Add the corn and red peppers. Cook for 45 to 60 seconds, or until just crisp-tender. Drain and transfer to a medium bowl.

Stir in the scallions, chili peppers, lemon juice, oil, cilantro, and chili powder. Toss to mix. Cover and refrigerate for 30 minutes, or up to two days.

Makes 2 servings

Hint
■ *To take it along, pack the entire salad in an airtight container. Refrigerate until mealtime.*

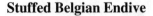

Stuffed Belgian Endive

Standard Recipe	Fat-to-Firm Makeover
149 calories	*68 calories*
14.5 g. fat (88% of calories)	*4.5 g. fat (60% of calories)*

Why turn to celery stuffed with cream cheese for a snack? These endive leaves are filled with tasty nonfat yogurt cheese. A small amount of toasted nuts adds crunch and flavor without contributing too much fat.

1 head Belgian endive
1 cup nonfat yogurt cheese (see hint)
2 tablespoons chopped, toasted walnuts or pecans

Separate the endive into individual leaves. Spread each leaf with yogurt cheese. Sprinkle with the walnuts or pecans.

Makes 2 servings

Hints

▪ *To make 1 cup yogurt cheese, spoon 2 cups nonfat plain yogurt into a colander lined with cheesecloth. Cover the colander with plastic wrap and place it over a large bowl. Refrigerate overnight. Discard the liquid in the bowl.*

▪ *To take it along, pack the endive and walnuts or pecans in separate resealable plastic bags. Pack the yogurt cheese in an airtight container. Refrigerate until mealtime.*

Evening Recipes

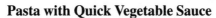

Pasta with Quick Vegetable Sauce

Standard Recipe	Fat-to-Firm Makeover
493 calories	*473 calories*
16.5 g. fat (30% of calories)	*6.2 g. fat (12% of calories)*

This tomato sauce comes together quickly and beats bottled sauce by a mile—with less fat, less sodium, and more flavor.

    3 canned peeled plum tomatoes
    1 tablespoon lemon juice
    1 teaspoon olive oil
    2 teaspoons chopped fresh basil or parsley
    1 clove garlic, minced
    6 ounces medium-shell pasta
    ½ cup frozen cut green beans
    ⅔ cup frozen corn
    ¼ cup seeded, chopped sweet red peppers
    1 tablespoon crumbled feta cheese

In a food processor or blender, combine the tomatoes, lemon juice, and oil. Process until smooth. Add the basil or parsley and garlic. Process using on/off turns just until combined. Set aside.

In a large pot of boiling water, cook the pasta for 5 minutes. Add the beans. Return to a boil and cook for 2 minutes. Add the corn and peppers. Return to a boil and cook for 1 to 2 minutes, or until the pasta is tender and the vegetables are crisp-tender. Drain well.

Transfer to a large bowl. Add tomato mixture and feta. Toss to combine.

Makes 2 servings

Hint
■ *This pasta dish can be packed in an airtight container and served cold as a pasta salad. Melba toast or garlic breadsticks make a nice accompaniment.*

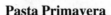

Pasta Primavera

Standard Recipe	Fat-to-Firm Makeover
508 calories	*451 calories*
28 g. fat (50% of calories)	*10.2 g. fat (20% of calories)*

This version of pasta primavera doesn't need a high-fat cream sauce for flavor. Mixed vegetables, sweet basil, and a bit of Parmesan contribute plenty. Serve this pasta dish with Italian bread to complete the meal.

6 ounces rotini or penne
8 ounces frozen mixed vegetables (see hint)
1 tablespoon olive oil
2 cloves garlic, minced
2 tablespoons chopped fresh sweet basil
2 tablespoons grated Parmesan cheese
¼ teaspoon salt
¼ teaspoon ground black pepper

In a large pot of boiling water, cook the rotini or penne for 5 minutes. Add the vegetables. Return to a boil and cook for 2 to 4 minutes, or until the pasta is tender and the vegetables are crisp-tender. Drain and set aside.

Warm the oil in the same pot over medium-low heat. Add the garlic and cook for 5 minutes, or until fragrant. Return the pasta and vegetables to the pot. Toss to coat with the oil and rewarm.

Add the basil and toss to mix. Sprinkle with the Parmesan, salt, and pepper.

Makes 2 servings

Hints

▪ *For the vegetables, use half of a 16-ounce bag of frozen mixed vegetables, such as carrots, broccoli, and cauliflower. This combination is often referred to as California mix.*

▪ *For a thinner sauce, reserve some of the pasta cooking water. Add it along with the basil.*

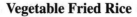

Vegetable Fried Rice

Standard Recipe	Fat-to-Firm Makeover
279 calories	184 calories
10 g. fat (32% of calories)	2.8 g. fat (14% of calories)

Eliminating the eggs and reducing the amount of oil saved 7 grams of fat in this popular take-out dish. Broccoli and sweet red peppers add crunch, flavor, and vitamin C.

- ¾ cup chopped broccoli
- 2 teaspoons water
- ½ cup seeded, chopped sweet red peppers
- 1 tablespoon chopped scallions
- 1 teaspoon sesame oil
- ½ teaspoon grated fresh gingerroot
- 1¼ cups cold cooked rice
- 4 teaspoons low-sodium soy sauce
- ¼ teaspoon ground black pepper

Place a wok or large no-stick skillet over medium-high heat until hot. Add the broccoli and water. Cover and cook, stirring occasionally, for 3 to 4 minutes, or until the broccoli is crisp-tender.

Add the red peppers, scallions, oil, and gingerroot. Cook, stirring periodically, for 2 to 3 minutes, or until the peppers are crisp-tender. Add the rice. Cook, stirring often, for 3 to 4 minutes, or until the rice is heated through. Add the soy sauce and black pepper. Stir well.

Makes 2 servings

Hint

■ *To take it along, pack in an airtight container. Refrigerate until mealtime. Microwave on high for 2 minutes, or until heated through.*

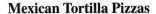

Mexican Tortilla Pizzas

Standard Recipe	Fat-to-Firm Makeover
280 calories	*205 calories*
6.4 g. fat (21% of calories)	*5.3 g. fat (23% of calories)*

This multinational twist on an American favorite saves you calories and fat. But the big news is the boost in both fiber and flavor.

  2 flour tortillas (8" diameter)
$\frac{1}{2}$ cup salsa, drained
$\frac{1}{4}$ cup canned black beans, rinsed and drained
$\frac{1}{4}$ cup canned red kidney beans, rinsed and drained
$\frac{1}{3}$ cup shredded reduced-fat hot-pepper Monterey Jack cheese
  1 tablespoon chopped fresh cilantro

Preheat the oven to 375°F. Coat a baking sheet with no-stick spray.

Place the tortillas on the baking sheet. Coat each tortilla with no-stick spray. Divide the salsa between them. Sprinkle with the black beans, kidney beans, Monterey Jack, and cilantro. Bake for 10 to 15 minutes, or until the cheese melts.

Makes 2

Hint

■ *These pizzas can be made anywhere you have access to a toaster oven. To take it along, wrap the tortillas in plastic. Mix the salsa and beans, then place them in an airtight container. Combine the cheese and cilantro in a resealable plastic bag. At mealtime, assemble the pizzas and bake (if necessary to fit the toaster oven, cut the tortillas in half).*

Cheese Quesadillas

Standard Recipe	Fat-to-Firm Makeover
414 calories	*134 calories*
27 g. fat (59% of calories)	*3.9 g. fat (26% of calories)*

A good ol' grilled cheese sandwich can sure hit the spot. Unfortunately, the spot it hits is your waist. Two slices of American cheese, two slices of white bread and 2 teaspoons of butter add up to a hefty 27 grams of fat. These Southwestern-style quesadillas are a healthier alternative. Plus, they're packed with the bright flavors of salsa, olives, and two cheeses.

     2 fat-free flour tortillas (8" diameter)
     2 tablespoons shredded reduced-fat Cheddar cheese
     2 tablespoons shredded reduced-fat hot-pepper Monterey
          Jack cheese
     1 tablespoon chopped canned green chili peppers (wear
          plastic gloves when handling)
     1 tablespoon chopped or sliced black olives
     1 tablespoon thinly sliced scallions
     ¼ teaspoon chili powder
     ½ cup warmed salsa

Warm a medium no-stick skillet over medium-low heat. Place a tortilla in the skillet. Quickly sprinkle with the Cheddar, Monterey Jack, peppers, olives, scallions, and chili powder. Top with the second tortilla. Using a spatula, gently press to combine the layers.

Cook for 3 to 4 minutes per side, or until lightly browned and the cheese is melted. Cool slightly and cut into wedges. Serve warm with the salsa.

Makes 2 servings

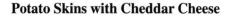

Potato Skins with Cheddar Cheese

Standard Recipe	Fat-to-Firm Makeover
311 calories	*187 calories*
18 g. fat (52% of calories)	*4.1 g. fat (20% of calories)*

Potato skins are often deep-fried just like french fries. Or they are slathered with butter and baked. Add the Cheddar cheese, and these snacks pack more fat than you can imagine. Here, the skins are baked and topped with reduced-fat Cheddar that delivers melt-in-your-mouth texture.

> 2 large baked potatoes, quartered lengthwise
> $\frac{1}{2}$ cup shredded reduced-fat Cheddar cheese
> 2 tablespoons chopped scallions or chives
> Paprika (optional)

Preheat the oven to 425°F. Coat a baking sheet with no-stick spray.

Scoop out the potato flesh, leaving a $\frac{1}{4}$" to $\frac{1}{2}$" shell. Reserve the flesh for another use (see hint).

Coat the insides of the potato skins with no-stick spray. Place, cut side up, on the baking sheet and bake for 10 to 15 minutes, or until crisp. Sprinkle with the Cheddar and scallions or chives. Bake for 2 minutes, or until the cheese is melted. Sprinkle with the paprika (if using).

Makes 2 servings

Hint

■ *The reserved potato flesh can be used to make home fries for breakfast. Coat a large no-stick skillet with no-stick spray. Add chopped onions and green peppers. Sauté over medium heat for 4 minutes, or until soft. Add the potato flesh, paprika, salt, and black pepper. Gently flatten the mixture with a spatula. Cook for 3 to 4 minutes, or until browned on the bottom. Flip the mixture and cook for 3 to 4 minutes more.*

Index

Boldface references indicate primary discussions. Underscored page references indicate boxed text. *Italic* references indicate illustrations.

H

I

M

T

U

Y